Clinical ECGs in Paramedic Practice

Charles L. Till

Disclaimer

Printing history

This edition first published 2021

The authors and publisher welcome feedback from the users of this book. Please contact the publisher:

Class Professional Publishing,
The Exchange, Express Park, Bristol Road, Bridgwater TA6 4RR
Telephone: 01278 427 800
Email: post@class.co.uk
www.classprofessional.co.uk

Class Professional Publishing is an imprint of Class Publishing Ltd

A CIP catalogue record for this book is available from the British Library

Paperback ISBN: 9781859598696
eBook ISBN: 9781859598702

Cover design by Hybert Design Limited, UK
Designed and typeset by S4Carlisle Publishing Services

This book is dedicated to my parents, Ann and Richard.

Your unwavering support and enthusiastic encouragement throughout my career have helped me to become the professional I am today. Thank you.

Contents

About the Author

Charles L. Till

Charles is the Head of Clinical Improvement and Development within the Medical Directorate at East Midlands Ambulance Service NHS Trust. His previous professional experience includes the education of student paramedics as a Senior Lecturer and as a Paramedic Education Specialist within higher education institutions and the NHS. He also has experience as a Paramedic Practitioner and Practice Educator. He continues to work clinically within the medical directorate and has gained experience in several NHS ambulance services across the UK, including London Ambulance Service NHS Trust, the Scottish Ambulance Service, and South Central Ambulance Service NHS Foundation Trust.

Charles entered the profession as a graduate paramedic with a FdSc in Paramedic Science from the University of Northampton. He holds a BSc in Healthcare Practice and a PgC in Learning and Teaching in Higher Education. He is currently reading for an MSc in Internal Medicine with Edinburgh University (2019–2022).

Acknowledgements

I would like to thank everyone that has been involved in this project, including the contributors and reviewers, Lianne, Katherine and the rest of the team at Class Professional Publishing and Professor Douglas Chamberlain for his foreword and involvement.

Contributors:

Douglas Chamberlain

Gary Rutherford

Reviewers:

Steven Carter

Rhiannon Davies

Scott Diamond

Celia Exon

James Gardner

Rebecca Spence

Owen Williams

Mark Whitbread

I would also like to thank the hundreds of student paramedics who have attended my ECG lectures over the last few years. Your enthusiasm and questions have helped my vision for this book take shape and maintained my motivation whilst writing it. I would especially like to thank students of the September 2019 DipHE Cohort, Coventry University, for your thoughts and opinions in the later stages of this project.

Charles L. Till, 2021

*　　*　　*　　*

The publishers would like to thank Keith Cameron and Richard Pilbery for kindly supplying ECG scans as examples for the book, as well as the anonymous reviewers of the text. The following ECGs have been drawn by Charles L. Till for the purposes of the book:

- ECG 1.3 - Asystole
- Test ECG 1.1 - Sinus Rhythm
- Test ECG 1.5 - Asystole
- ECG 2.2 - Absolute Bradycardia
- ECG 2.15 - 1st Degree AV Block
- ECG 2.16 - 2nd Degree AV Block
- ECG 2.17 - 2nd degree AV Block
- ECG 2.18 - 2nd Degree AV Block 2
- ECG 2.19 - 3rd Degree AV Block

- ECG 2.21 - Ventricular Escape Rhythm
- ECG 2.24 - Premature Junctional Contractions
- ECG 2.26 - Multifocal Premature Ventricular Contractions
- ECG 2.29 - Couplets
- Test ECG 2.1 - Sinus Bradycardia
- Test ECG 2.9 - 2nd Degree AV Block
- ECG 3.1 - ST Depressions
- ECG 3.2 - De Winter's Sign
- ECG 3.3 - Inverted T Waves
- ECG 3.4a (left) and ECG 3.4b (right) - Wellen's Syndrome
- ECG 3.23 - Hypokalaemia
- Practice ECG 1.1 - Couplets (Chapter 4)
- Practice ECG 1.2 - Idioventricular Rhythm (Chapter 4)
- Practice ECG 1.3 - 2nd Degree AV Block 2 (Chapter 4)
- Practice ECG 1.4 - PAC (Chapter 4)
- Practice ECG 1.5 - Multi PVC (Chapter 4)
- Practice ECG 1.6 - PJC (Chapter 4)
- Practice ECG 1.7 - Junctional (Chapter 4)
- Practice ECG 1.8 - 2nd degree block (Chapter 4)
- Practice ECG 1.9 - Sinus (Chapter 4)
- Practice ECG 1.10 - MAT(Chapter 4).

Remaining artwork has been supplied by S4 Carlisle © Class Professional Publishing.

Foreword

Ideally, and for many reasons, everyone should have at least some knowledge of the heart and its function, but those with any involvement in patient care need to have more. This includes knowledge of the heart's electrical activity as shown on the electrocardiogram (ECG), as well as an appreciation that a normal tracing does not preclude serious heart disease. An abnormal tracing is, however, a matter for possible concern that may be trivial or serious. This is also true of effort tests in which an apparently abnormal tracing may have no functional significance and should not be regarded alone as evidence of heart disease.

Most physicians are in the challenging specialty of general practice and should know something of ECGs, however many do not. Cardiologists also have an extensive remit and must learn as much as possible from their own sub-specialty which usually involves interventional procedures. They may find little of interest in the basic pattern of the ECG, but therefore miss important evidence of true abnormalities which deserve consideration for further investigation, notably, but not exclusively, echocardiography.

Paramedics were introduced to Britain a little over 50 years ago and to part of the United States a short while earlier. These days, they are usually the first to see individuals who have developed evidence of ischaemia or arrhythmias out-of-hospital and they have become experts at providing appropriate medical care.

This excellent book will be of interest, and indeed of much value, to all of these groups. It is one that I can enthusiastically recommend.

Douglas Chamberlain CBE MD FRCP EFACC

Introduction

Reading and interpreting electrocardiograms (ECGs) is a fundamental skillset for paramedics. We come across ECGs on almost every shift and make treatment decisions based on our interpretation. But how many paramedics can confidently say that they are 'good' at ECGs?

The subject of cardiac electrophysiology is a medical specialty in itself. There is no expectation for all paramedics to know everything about ECGs. That would be an unrealistic goal. As with any topic, some people seem to just 'get' ECGs from the first lesson. They immediately take it all in and feel comfortable with interpreting them. This is not the case for all students. In the course of the many ECG lectures I have delivered over the years, I have found countless students who seem to almost fear reading an ECG. At the same time, I have come to believe that every person who is capable of becoming a paramedic is also capable of reading and interpreting an ECG to a sufficient standard for paramedic practice. The challenge lies in helping each student and paramedic to understand ECGs, but also to believing that they, in themselves, are capable. In a classroom where often a handful of students' voices may dominate, perhaps also asking complex questions, it can be easy to feel left behind. Whereas the reality is that usually a large proportion of the class are in the same boat, trying to grasp and consolidate the basics.

I have aimed this book from first-year student all the way through to experienced paramedic. If you are already the ECG wizard of your cohort or station, you will find it a useful resource for confirmation and reference. But if you feel a bit daunted by ECGs, or you are never sure where to start or what you *need* to know, then this book will help you, not only to increase your ECG knowledge, but also to feel more comfortable and in control when faced with an ECG in your clinical practice as a paramedic.

I find that all registered paramedics tend to fall into the same broad groups as the students: those who 'get' ECGs and those who always feel they *should* know more about ECGs. This text will be particularly useful to those in the latter group. The format and layout lets you dip in and out of the book to target the subjects you feel you need to cover, whilst also building on your existing knowledge and experience.

When approaching the topic of ECG interpretation in the out-of-hospital setting, it is vital that consideration is given to the overall clinical presentation of the patient and how their signs and symptoms relate to their ECG. Throughout the book, the ECG and the heart are considered from a holistic perspective. There is discussion throughout on how ECG changes and their underlying causes affect the differential diagnoses, our clinical decisions and patient management in the out-of-hospital setting.

Many ECG changes have primary causes originating outside of the heart, just as many cardiac conditions may present with symptoms which initially lead the clinician towards a different body system when seeking a diagnosis. Making a correct diagnosis on a difficult ECG can be professionally satisfying, but it is important to consider that it is not always necessary to definitively diagnose an obscure ECG abnormality. Recognising that an abnormal arrhythmia is present and understanding how it may affect your patient is key. Spending too much time analysing the ECG may be detrimental to patient care if it delays vital treatment or a time-critical transfer. Never let personal pride harm your patient.

It is important to remember that interpreting an ECG rhythm and formulating a working diagnosis for the clinical management of the patient are, while linked, often different. However, a correct ECG diagnosis will certainly offer useful information which may help with formulating the clinical working diagnosis. An example of this would be a patient with an ECG showing sinus tachycardia, a heart rate above 100 beats per minute. This could be caused by a multitude of pathologies or physiological changes. Consideration needs to be given to all of the information obtained through your history taking and physical examination, alongside the ECG findings, to formulate a clinical working diagnosis for the patient.

In this book, we will look at both the common and the important ECG changes and arrhythmias which paramedics may encounter. The in-depth study of cardiology and electrophysiology and discussion of every potential ECG arrhythmia are left in the realm of other textbooks. By stripping away vast amounts of information which may be of little relevance in the out-of-hospital setting, readers can focus on understanding and putting into practice the core ECG knowledge which is essential to our clinical paramedic practice.

Equipped with the knowledge within this book, you can feel confident in identifying key ECG abnormalities. If you are unable to identify a particular ECG change in clinical practice, you will be equipped, nonetheless, with the skills to manage the patient and transport them safely and appropriately.

The patient care discussed in this book is in-line with, and informed by, the Joint Royal College Ambulance Liaison Committee and Association of Ambulance Chief Executives and the Resuscitation Council (UK) guidelines. As with all clinical care episodes, sound and reasonable clinical judgement should be used in combination with relevant guidelines to inform patient care on a case specific basis.

How to Use this Book

This book has been written as both a study resource and a reference guide. If you are revising for an exam or taking the first steps to learning about ECGs then you can work through this book from beginning to end, increasing your knowledge with each section which builds up on your learning from the last. Each entry is also designed to be accessible independently, as a quick reference or recap.

As well as discussing the identification of abnormalities on the ECG, this book will also consider the potential clinical presentations, causes, and out-of-hospital management of patients presenting with each abnormality.

You can practice ECG interpretation and test your knowledge with the practice ECGs and case scenario questions throughout the book. There is also a whole section at the back of the book dedicated to practice ECGs and case scenarios for revision and assistance in consolidating your learning.

The physical skill of obtaining an ECG is separate from reading and interpreting an ECG. Appendix 1 on page XXX covers the process of obtaining an ECG.

This book also uses boxes and symbols to help you easily find information:

Green boxes are used in Section 1 to highlight fundamental core components of ECG understanding. They are also used throughout the book to highlight key points after certain sub-sections.

Beige boxes contain useful additional information or further discussions on a topic. If you are new to ECGs, you might decide to come back to these later in your studies, or if you are already experienced in ECG interpretation, the beige boxes have a higher potential for you to find something new to learn.

Alert boxes draw your attention to important information you need to be aware of. They may highlight information which you need to ensure your patient does not come to harm. !

The following four boxes and symbols are used with most ECG rhythms in the book:

ECG identification boxes tell you the criteria related to specific ECG abnormalities and how to identify them.

Clinical presentation boxes tell you about the potential signs and symptoms a patient may present with that are associated with the underlying illness causing the ECG abnormality, or the abnormality itself.

Causes boxes tell you about the different causes of an ECG abnormality, to help with formulating a working diagnosis.

Management boxes tell you about potential interventions and treatments for the ECG abnormality or the underlying illness.

The Golden Rule

A 12-lead ECG is a fantastic diagnostic tool; it tells you about the electrical activity occurring within the heart. However, it does not tell you if the patient has a pulse and it does not provide comprehensive information about the patient or their haemodynamic state. We must remember that the printed ECG is only a snapshot of the heart's electrical activity. It becomes historic the moment it has finished printing. Do not let yourself become so distracted and task-focused while analysing a printed ECG that you miss a change or deterioration in your patient's clinical condition.

'Always look at the patient'

When used appropriately alongside the rest of the clinical observations and findings from the physical exam, and most importantly the clinical history that has been obtained, the ECG provides information to allow the formation of a working diagnosis which otherwise may not be possible. It is all too common for a paramedic to become fixated on a single clinical finding, observation or ECG print-out and let this wrongly influence the rest of their assessment and the formation of a working diagnosis. Endeavour to never let confirmation bias influence your decision making.

Human Factors and ECG Interpretation

It is important to be aware of how human factors affect us and our decision making, see Appendix 3 on page 268 for more information on human factors in the context of ECG interpretation.

Fundamentals of Cardiac Function and ECG Interpretation

In this section we will discuss the essential information necessary to understand the human heart and the ECG. We will explore the physical and electrical functions of the heart and how it operates to maintain cardiac output and keep the body supplied with oxygen. We will then go on to learn the basics of the ECG and the fundamental skills needed when analysing an ECG in a clinical context.

Physical Heart Function, Electrical Heart Function and the Cardiac Cycle

The physical and electrical functions of the heart are directly related and work together to produce a heartbeat.

The cardiac muscle acts as a pump, pushing blood around the body and maintaining blood pressure. The pump is controlled by the electrical functions of the heart by way of electrical impulses. It is these electrical impulses that are detected by our monitor's electrodes and that are represented as a printed graph, what we know as an ECG tracing.

Key Concepts: Physical Heart Function[1, 2, 3]

- The heart is located in the **mediastinum** within the thoracic cavity and sits inside the pericardium.
- The heart is a muscle which works as a pump, creating the pressure needed to move blood through the body and maintain blood pressure.
- The **pericardium**, also known as the pericardial sac, is a double-layered membrane which envelops and protects the heart and the roots of the great vessels as they emerge from the heart.
- The **great vessels** are the large blood vessels that transport blood directly to and from the heart. They consist of two arteries which transport blood out of the heart, the **aorta** and **pulmonary artery**, and three veins which deliver blood to the heart, the **superior vena cava**, **inferior vena cava** and the **pulmonary vein** (Figure 1.1).
- The heart has four chambers, the **right atria**, **right ventricle**, **left atria** and **left ventricle** (Figure 1.1).
- The right and left sides of the heart pump at the same time, but function as **two separate pumps** creating a **dual circulation**.
  - The right side of the heart takes **deoxygenated blood** from the body into the right atrium and pumps it to the lungs via the right ventricle.
  - The left side of the heart takes **oxygenated blood** from the lungs into the left atrium and pumps it through the body via the left ventricle.

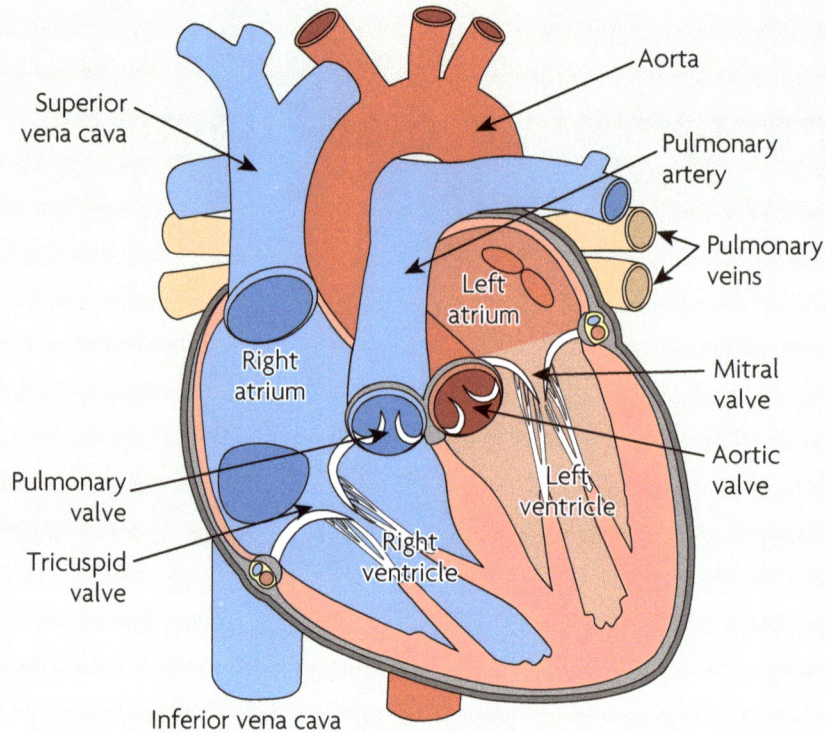

Figure 1.1 Cross-sectional view of the heart.

- The heart has four valves to prevent blood from flowing in the wrong direction (Figure 1.1):
  - The **tricuspid valve** sits between the right atrium and right ventricle.
  - The **pulmonary valve** sits between the right ventricle and the pulmonary artery.
  - The **mitral valve** sits between the left atrium and the left ventricle.
  - The **aortic valve** sits between the left ventricle and the aorta.
- Heart valves, when functioning correctly, predominantly only allow blood to flow in **one direction**. This creates a one-way system, helping to maintain blood pressure by preventing blood from flowing backwards.
- When a heart chamber is contracting, the phase is termed **systole**.
- When a heart chamber is in a relaxed phase, it is termed **diastole**.
- To pump blood during a heartbeat, the myocardial (cardiac muscle) cells that form the walls of the heart's chambers contract. This reduces the volume within the chambers, increasing pressure and forcing blood out through the heart valves.
  - When the atria contract (atrial systole), they push blood into the ventricles (Figure 1.2).
    - The right atrium pushes blood through the tricuspid valve into the right ventricle.
    - The left atrium pushes blood through the mitral valve into the left ventricle.
  - When the ventricles contract (ventricular systole), they push blood out of the heart into the great vessels (Figure 1.2). The tricuspid and mitral valves prevent the blood from being pushed back into the atria during ventricular contraction.
    - The right ventricle pushes blood through the pulmonary valve into the pulmonary artery to the lungs.
    - The left ventricle pushes blood through the aortic valve into the aorta to the rest of the body.

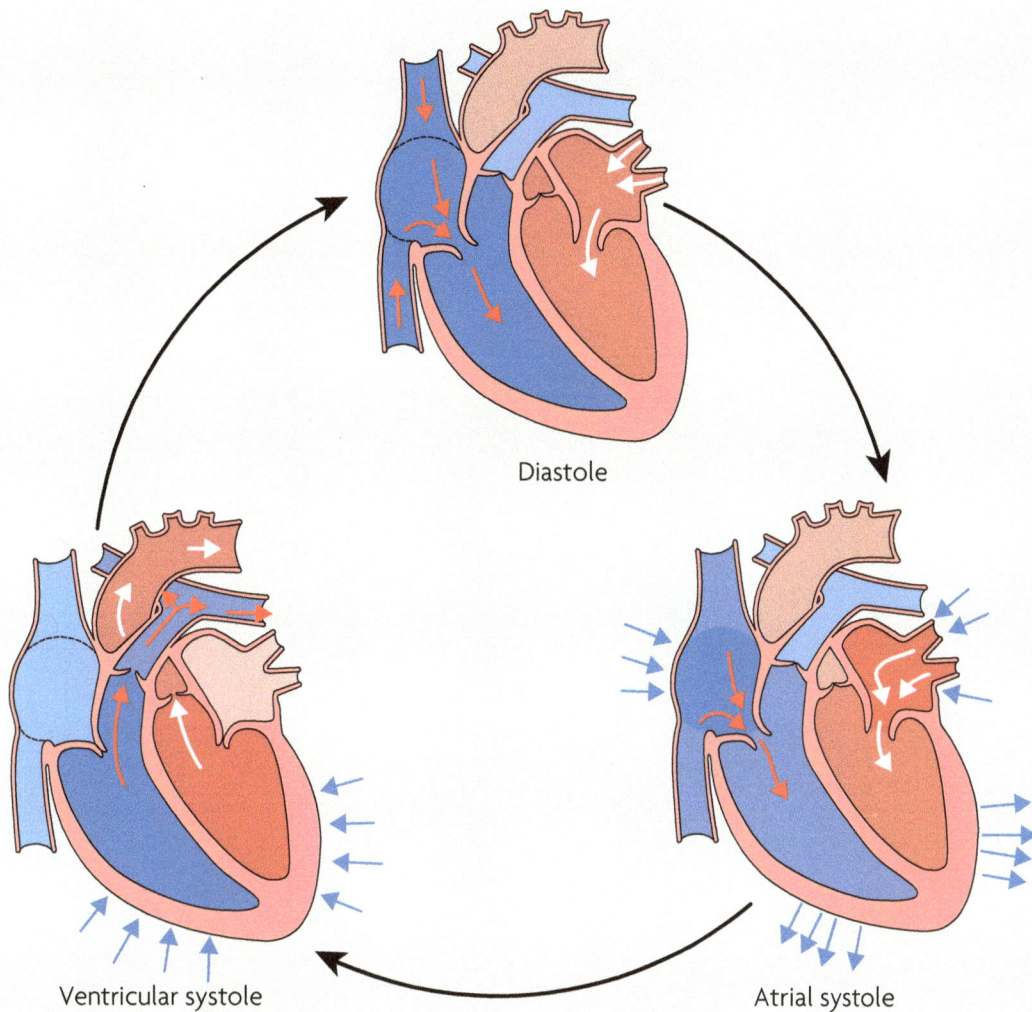

Figure 1.2 Physical cardiac cycle.

- The heart wall is made up of three layers:
  - ▶ The **epicardium** forms the outer layer, consisting of mesothelial cells and connective tissue. Its primary function is to reduce friction of movement between the heart and the inside of the pericardial sac as the heart pumps. The epicardium forms the innermost layer of the pericardium.
  - ▶ The **myocardium** forms the middle, and thickest, layer and consists of cardiac muscle tissue. Its primary function is to allow the heart to operate as a pump.
  - ▶ The **endocardium** forms the innermost layer of the heart, lining the inside of the heart chambers, valves and large blood vessels.

Key Concepts: Circulation[3, 4]

- Blood is the medium by which **oxygen** and **carbon dioxide** are transported around the body. Oxygen enters the blood and carbon dioxide leaves the blood in the lungs during gas exchange.
- All the cells in the body require oxygen to produce energy via **aerobic respiration**; this process produces carbon dioxide as a waste product. Cells can produce energy without oxygen via **anaerobic respiration**, but this produces lactic acid and other harmful metabolites and is therefore not sustainable.

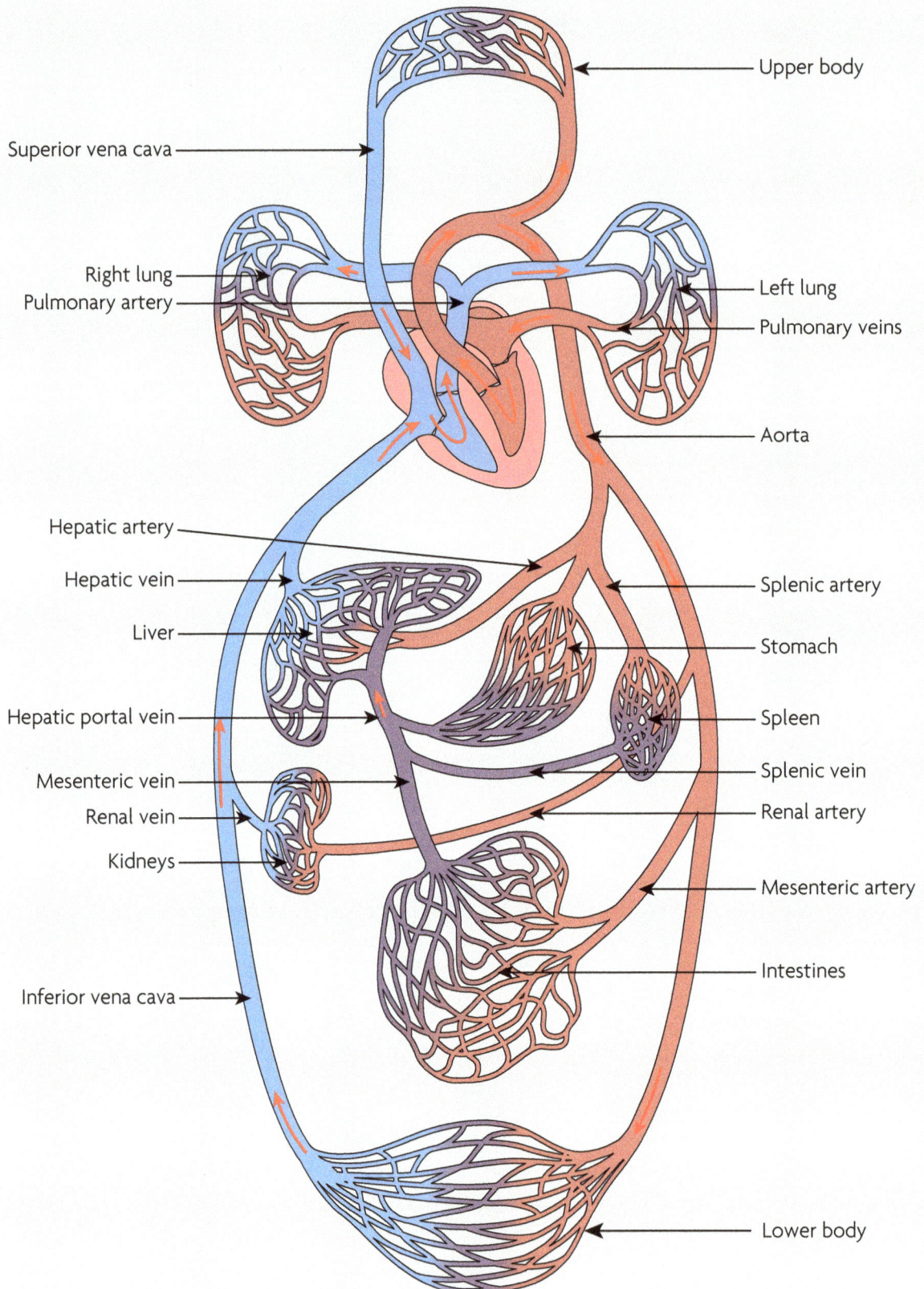

Figure 1.3 The circulatory system.

Upper body

Superior vena cava

Right lung
Pulmonary artery

Left lung
Pulmonary veins

Aorta

Hepatic artery

Hepatic vein

Splenic artery

Liver

Stomach

Hepatic portal vein

Spleen

Mesenteric vein

Splenic vein

Renal vein

Renal artery

Kidneys

Mesenteric artery

Intestines

Inferior vena cava

Lower body

- The **circulatory system** (Figure 1.3) transports blood between the body and the lungs, via the two sides of the heart, delivering oxygen and removing carbon dioxide. The heart produces and maintains blood pressure and facilitates a constant flow of blood through continuous pumping, normally at a rate of between 60 and 80 pumps, or beats, per minute. There are two main parts of the circulatory system, **systemic circulation** and **pulmonary circulation**.
  - Systemic circulation is responsible for transporting blood between the heart and the body:
    - Oxygenated blood is pumped from the left ventricle, through the aorta, into the systemic arterial circulation, to the rest of the body where it delivers oxygen to cells and becomes deoxygenated. The blood also collects carbon dioxide from the cells. Deoxygenated blood still contains some oxygen within the red blood cells; it can be thought of as 'less oxygenated'.
    - Deoxygenated blood returns from the body via the systemic venous circulation, into the superior and inferior vena cava and then to the right side of the heart. First into the right atrium, then the right ventricle.
  - Pulmonary circulation transports blood between the heart and the lungs:
    - Deoxygenated blood is pumped from the right ventricle, through the pulmonary artery, into the lungs where it takes on oxygen, becoming oxygenated again and offloading carbon dioxide.
    - Oxygenated blood travels from the lungs through the pulmonary vein and into the left side of the heart. First into the left atrium, then the left ventricle.

Key Concepts: Electrical Heart Function[1, 4, 5]

- The heart contains two main types of **myocardial cell**:
  - **Cardiomyocytes** (cardiac muscle cells) form the muscular walls of the heart and make up around 99% of the bulk of cells in the heart. They possess these key properties:
    - **Contractility**: The cell can shorten and lengthen its fibres.
    - **Extensibility**: The cell can stretch.
    - **Conductivity**: The cell responds to electrical impulses and transmits them from cell to cell, though not as rapidly as cardiac pacemaker cells.
  - **Cardiac pacemaker cells** are modified cardiomyocytes that do not have the ability to contract and instead have an improved ability to generate and conduct electrical impulses rapidly. They form the cardiac conduction system and account for around 1% of the bulk of cells in the heart. They often present in groups or 'clusters' in the sinoatrial and atrioventricular nodes and in conducting pathways such as the bundle of His and the bundle branches. They possess these key properties:
    - **Conductivity** and **excitability**: The ability to respond to electrical impulses and rapidly transmit them from cell to cell.
    - **Automaticity**: The ability to spontaneously self-generate an electrical impulse in the heart. This is an important distinction from cardiomyocyte cells which cannot normally spontaneously generate their own electrical impulses.
- An electrical impulse is generated at a group of cardiac pacemaker cells. In sinus rhythm the impulse is generated at the **sinoatrial node** (SA node) at a rate faster than that of any other cardiac pacemaker cells, typically 60–100 times a minute.
- Cardiac cells at rest, with no electrical activity taking place, are termed to be **polarised**.
- An electrical impulse, known as an **action potential**, causes cardiomyocyte cells to **depolarise**. Every cardiac cell that depolarises causes a chain reaction in adjacent cardiac cells also depolarising, allowing the electrical impulse, the action potential, to move through the heart.

- Cardiomyocytes contract and shorten as they depolarise, causing the walls of their heart chamber to contract (systole), reducing the volume of the chamber. A reduction in volume causes an increase in pressure and thus blood is pushed out.
- **Repolarisation** is the recovery of cardiac cells to a polarised state, becoming ready to depolarise again. A cardiac cell cannot depolarise again until it is repolarised; this is known as the **refractory period**.
- The refractory period is important as it creates a maximum contraction rate for the heart; it cannot beat faster than it can recover.

The Cardiac Conduction Pathway[1, 4, 5]

The cardiac conduction pathway (Figure 1.4) is made up of conductive cardiac pacemaker cells and forms a 'motorway' through the heart. This conductive pathway allows electrical impulses, called action potentials, to travel rapidly across the heart. Cardiomyocytes do not have the ability to transmit electrical impulses rapidly enough through the heart, so the cardiac conduction pathway is needed to facilitate the delivery of these impulses throughout the cardiac muscle in a rapid and timely manner, so that the cells can all function synchronously to form each heartbeat. Each stage of the cardiac conduction pathway is reflected on the ECG tracing (Figure 1.5).

- The **SA node** is located in the right atrium and is the **primary pacemaker** within the heart which means that it sets the heart rate. It does this by spontaneously generating an electrical impulse.
- The impulse passes across the right, then the left atria causing the atrial cardiac muscle cells to depolarise and contract. On the ECG this is seen as the **P wave**.
- The impulse reaches the atrioventricular node (AV node) where it is delayed for a few milliseconds before being allowed to continue. This short delay, seen as the PR interval on the ECG, allows the ventricles sufficient time to fill from the contracting atria before they themselves contract.

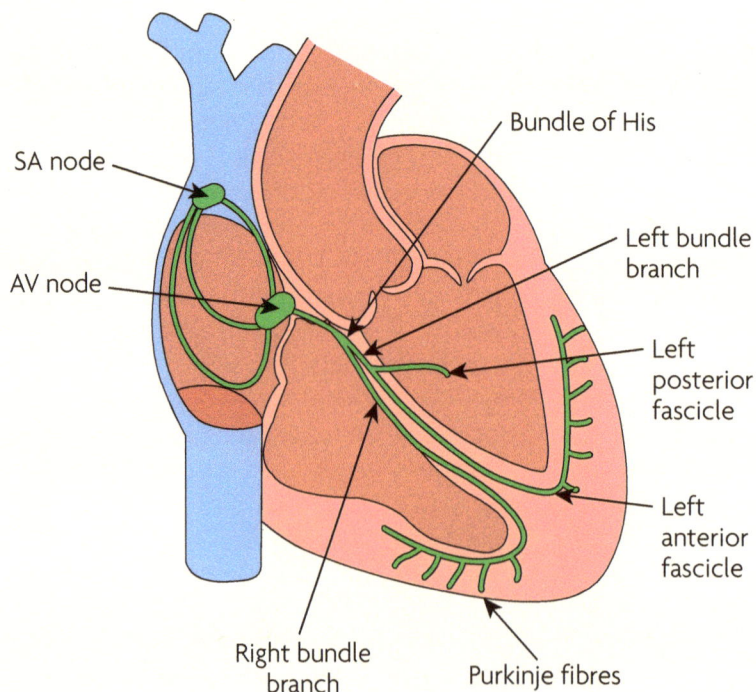

Figure 1.4 The electrical conduction system of the heart.

- The impulse moves down from the AV node, passing through the **bundle of His** before dividing into the **left and right bundle branches**. The left bundle branch subdivides into the Left Anterior Fascicle (LAF) and the Left Posterior Fascicle (LPF). The right bundle branch does not subdivide.
- The impulse spreads across and depolarises the ventricular walls through the many **Purkinje fibres** which spread out from the bundle branches, causing the ventricles to contract. The depolarisation of the ventricles is seen as the **QRS complex** on the ECG.
- Ventricular repolarisation occurs as the ventricles get ready to receive another impulse; this period is seen as the **T wave** on the ECG.
- Atrial repolarisation occurs at the same time as the QRS complex and is not normally visible on the ECG.

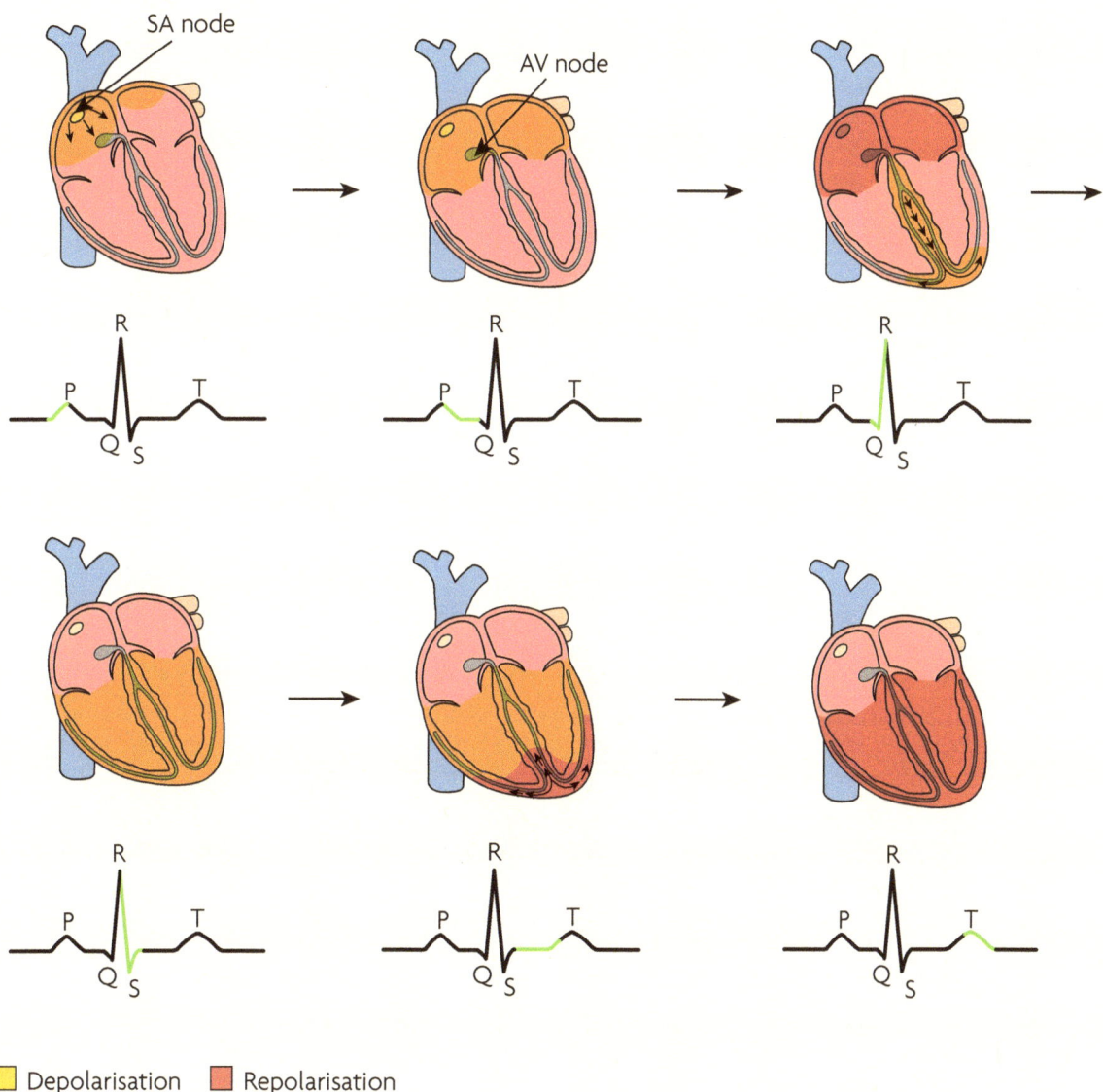

Depolarisation   Repolarisation

Figure 1.5 The electrical conduction system of the heart in relation to the ECG.

Example

Imagine a polarised cardiac cell as an upright domino ready to be knocked down. When the domino is knocked over it has depolarised. In falling, it also knocks over (depolarises) the dominoes that are standing up (polarised) around it. Now imagine a table covered in dominoes all standing up (polarised). When one domino falls over it creates a wave of falling (depolarising) dominoes from that point and moving across the table. In this analogy, repolarisation is the domino returning to a standing position and becoming ready to fall again.

Escape Rhythms

Each electrical cell possesses automaticity; it can spontaneously generate an electrical impulse. In sinus rhythm the SA node is in control of the heart as the primary pacemaker and initiates each heartbeat. It also controls the heart rate (page 11). Throughout the cardiac conduction pathway there are groups of pacemaker cells which act as back-up should the SA node fail. These pacemaker cells will start to produce their own impulses and take on the role of an ectopic pacemaker for the heart if they stop detecting electrical impulses from further along the cardiac conduction pathway. Escape rhythms are discussed in more detail on page 65.

U Waves

The U wave is a small deflection that occurs immediately after the T wave and can also merge with the end of the T wave. The U wave is not always present on an ECG. The U wave becomes more visible in slower heart rates. It is usually concordant with the T wave (in the same direction). An abnormal U wave can occur in several arrhythmias discussed throughout this book.

Key Concepts: Cellular Electrophysiology of the Heart[4, 6, 7]

At a cellular level, the polarity of a cell and its depolarisation and repolarisation relate to the movement of sodium, potassium and calcium ions across the cell membrane. It is important to understand that an increased or decreased amount of any one of these ions in the interstitial fluid surrounding the cardiac cells can cause serious cardiac arrhythmias (page 143).

- The contraction of cardiomyocyte cells is triggered by an electrical impulse, called an action potential, which spreads through the heart from cell to cell. An action potential, which is the movement of an electrical impulse, is a momentary reversal of the polarity of a cell. The action potential is facilitated by voltage-gated ion channels, which are channels responsible for moving ions from one side of the cell membrane to the other and are activated and deactivated based on the voltage inside the cell.
- Cardiomyocytes are connected to neighbouring cells by gap junctions, which are channels that allow ions to pass freely between cells. The movement of these ions is the trigger for an action potential in each cell.
- This membrane potential exists due to the concentration gradients of several types of ions across the cell membrane (inside compared to outside of the cell).

- In its resting, polarised state, there is a higher concentration of potassium ions (K^+) inside the cell and a higher concentration of sodium ions (Na^+) and calcium ions (Ca^{2+}) outside the cell. Ion pumps on the cell membrane maintain this gradient by moving K^+ into the cell and shifting Na^+ and Ca^{2+} out of the cell.
- An electrical voltage exists across the cell membrane.
  - ▸ The resting membrane potential is the voltage that exists in a cell when it is at rest. This potential is negative, meaning that the inside of the cell is more negative than the outside. This is known as being polarised. The cell membrane is more permeable to potassium, allowing it to diffuse freely out of the cell, which contributes to a negative resting potential inside the cell.
  - ▸ When membrane voltage increases and becomes less negative it is said to be depolarised.
- Cardiomyocytes have a stable resting potential of –90 millivolts (mV); depolarisation is triggered when they are stimulated by neighbouring cells. A depolarised cell has a higher concentration of Na^+ and Ca^{2+} within the cell than its resting, polarised neighbours; this causes Na^+ and Ca^{2+} to travel to adjacent cells via the gap junctions. This movement of Na^+ and Ca^{2+} triggers depolarisation in those cells by increasing the membrane voltage of the cell from –90mV to a threshold potential of around –70mV, triggering phase 0.
- Phases of cardiac action potential (Figure 1.6):

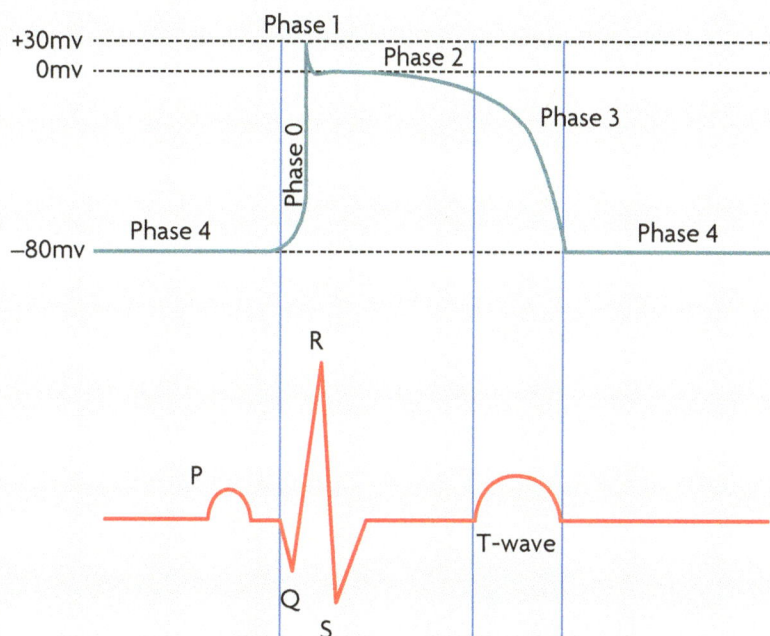

Figure 1.6 Action potential graph in relation to the ECG.

- ▸ **Phase 0: Rapid depolarisation**
  - ▸ With the movement of Na^+ and Ca^{2+} ions from neighbouring cells, membrane potential increases, reaching the threshold potential of around –70mV. This triggers voltage-gated fast Na^+ channels to open, causing a rapid influx of Na^+ from outside to inside the cell. This causes a rapid increase in membrane potential to +20mV.
  - ▸ During this rapid depolarisation, at –40mV, voltage-gated slow Ca^{2+} channels open, causing a slow and constant influx of Ca^{2+} into the cell.
  - ▸ It is during this increase of Na^+ and Ca^{2+} within the cell that some of these ions travel through the gap junctions and trigger the same depolarisation (Phase 0) in neighbouring cells.

> **Phase 1: Early repolarisation**
>> When the membrane potential reaches around +20mV, the voltage-gated fast Na$^+$ channels close and voltage-gated K$^+$ channels open, moving K$^+$ from inside to outside the cell.
>> This causes a rapid but small decrease in membrane potential.

> **Phase 2: Plateau**
>> The slow-working Ca^{2+} channels move Ca^{2+} into the cell together with the K$^+$ channels, moving K$^+$ out of the cell balance while maintaining the membrane potential in a stable state for around 200 milliseconds.
>> The influx of Ca^{2+} into the cell triggers the release of Ca^{2+} from the sarcoplasmic reticulum within the cell. This large increase in Ca^{2+} from the sarcoplasmic reticulum triggers the muscle contraction of the cardiomyocytes via the sliding filament mechanism of the cell; muscle contraction starts around halfway through the plateau phase and takes place in the second half of this phase.
>> Towards the end of the plateau phase, the sodium calcium exchanging ion pump allows Na$^+$ to slowly enter the cell, helping to prolong the phase.

> **Phase 3: Final repolarisation**
>> Ca^{2+} channels close and K$^+$ channels remain open. The continued efflux of K$^+$ from inside to outside the cell causes the membrane potential to decrease and return to its resting potential of –90mV.
>> Ca^{2+} is transported via active transport both out of the cell and back into the sarcoplasmic reticulum.

> **Phase 4: Resting membrane potential**
>> The Na$^+$ and K$^+$ pump restores and maintains the ion balance and resting membrane potential until the next depolarisation is triggered by Na$^+$ and Ca^{2+} ions from neighbouring cells, repeating phase 0.

Key Concepts: Putting It All Together, the Cardiac Cycle and the ECG[2, 3, 4, 8, 9]

- The cardiac cycle is shown in Figure 1.7:
  - **Atrial systole**: The SA node generates an electrical impulse which depolarises the atria as it travels towards the AV node. This atrial depolarisation is seen as the P wave on the ECG. The atria contract and pump the remaining blood into the ventricles. Only around 30% of blood in the ventricles comes from atrial contraction; the other 70% comes from passive ventricular filling.
  - **Ventricular systole**: The electrical impulse leaves the AV node after a brief delay and travels down into the ventricles via the bundle of His before splitting into the left and right bundle branches. The ventricles depolarise and contract, pumping blood out of the heart. The right ventricle pumps blood through the pulmonary valve into the pulmonary artery towards the lungs. The left ventricle pumps blood through the aortic valve into the aorta towards the rest of the body. This ventricular depolarisation is seen as the QRS complex on the ECG. The tricuspid and mitral valves close and prevent blood from flowing back into the atria.
  - **Ventricular diastole**: The aortic and pulmonary valves close and prevent blood from backflowing into the ventricles. The ventricular myocardial cells begin to repolarise ready to contract again, seen as the T wave on the ECG. The atria and the ventricles are in diastole (relaxed), and passive filling begins. Blood flows through the atria and the open mitral and tricuspid valves, passively filling the ventricles in preparation for the next heartbeat. The cycle continues.

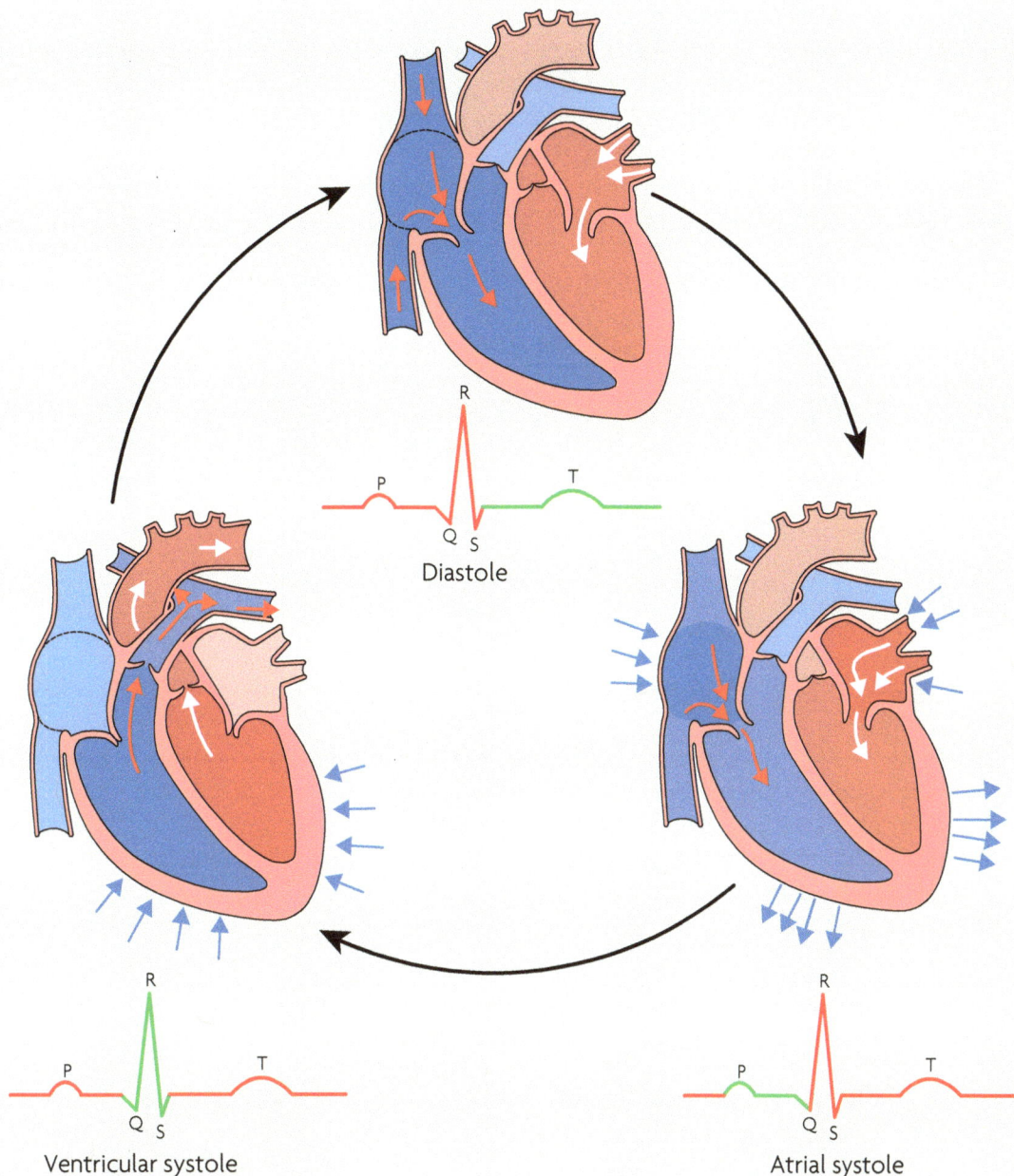

Figure 1.7 Cardiac cycle with ECG.

Heart Rate Control[3, 4]

The rate and contractility of the heart are controlled by the autonomic nervous system, changing in response to the needs and demands of the body (see cardiac output, page 13). The autonomic nervous system uses both neurological and chemical pathways to communicate with the heart. Messages to the heart via nerve pathways have a more rapid but short-lived influence over the heart than chemical pathways; this is important for understanding the regulation of blood pressure. Chemical messengers have a slower but more sustainable influence. These pathways primarily influence the SA node but also have effects on the AV node and both atria. The ventricles are not usually directly influenced by the autonomic nervous system, except for chemical messengers to increase or decrease their contractility.

The autonomic nervous system is divided into the sympathetic nervous system and the parasympathetic nervous system. Both systems have a constant effect on the heart and the two opposing effects compete to gain influence over control of the heart. Imagine a car being driven with both accelerator and brake pedals being pressed: when one is pressed a little more, and the other is pressed a little less, the car will change speed.

- **The sympathetic nervous system** acts to speed things up; it is the 'accelerator pedal' of the heart. It increases heart rate, increases contractility of cardiac muscle and accelerates conduction through the AV node. The primary sympathetic nerve pathway travels along the spinal column before reaching the heart. The main sympathetic chemical messenger is noradrenaline.
- **The parasympathetic nervous system** acts to slow things down; it is the 'brake pedal' of the heart. It decreases heart rate, decreases contractility and slows conduction through the AV node. The right and left vagus nerves (the 10th cranial nerve) act as the primary parasympathetic nerve pathway to the heart and travel directly from the brain, bypassing the spinal column. The main parasympathetic chemical messenger is acetylcholine.

Cardiac Circulation[3, 5, 10]

Like all other cells in the body, cardiac muscle cells need their own blood supply to provide them with oxygen and nutrients, as well as to remove toxins, carbon dioxide and other by-products of cellular respiration.

- The heart is continually working and requires a continuous and reliable blood supply; this is provided by the coronary arteries (Figure 1.8).
- If a coronary artery becomes blocked, the area of cardiac muscle tissue it supplies blood to will start to become ischaemic and damaged due to lack of oxygen and the build-up of toxins (see myocardial infarction, page 93).

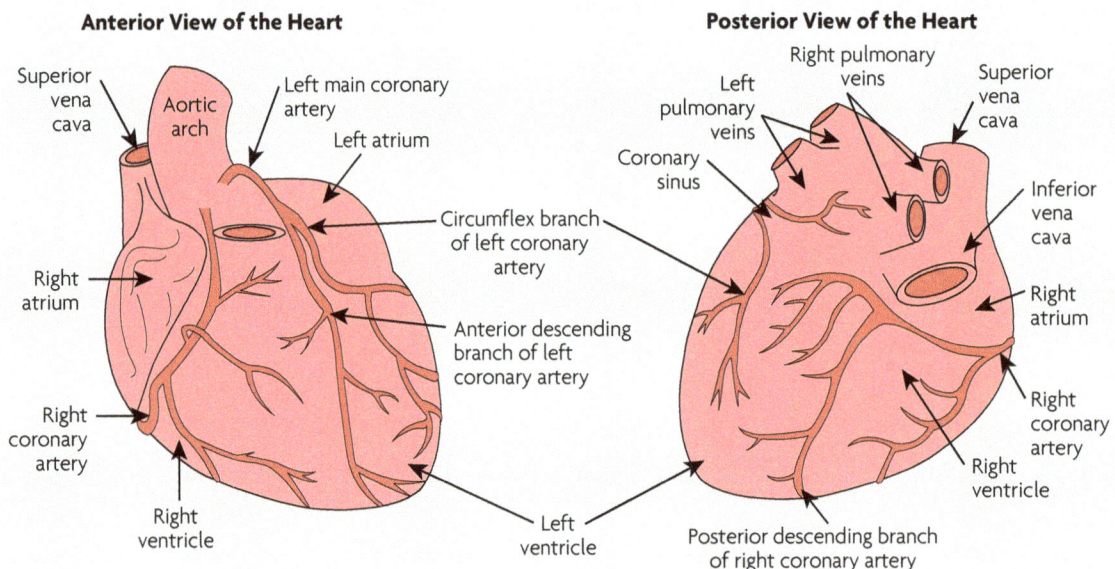

Figure 1.8 Coronary artery blood supply.

- Some parts of the heart are supplied by two coronary arteries. This is known as dual circulation, meaning that if one artery becomes blocked the cardiac muscle will continue to receive at least some blood flow from the other coronary artery source, minimising the area of ischaemia.
- The Left Main Coronary Artery (LMCA) and the Right Coronary Artery (RCA) both originate from the base of the ascending aorta and are the first arteries to leave the aorta. Blood pressure is highest here and thereby ensures a reliable supply of blood to meet the variable demands of the cardiac muscle.
- The LMCA supplies blood to the left ventricle, left atria and the interventricular septum. In a small number of people, it also supplies the posterior side of the heart.
  - The LMCA splits into two branches, the Left Circumflex artery (LCx) and the Left Anterior Descending (LAD) artery.
  - The LAD artery sits in the anterior interventricular sulcus and supplies blood to the anterior wall of the left ventricle and anterior septum.
  - The LCx supplies the lateral left ventricular wall. The posterior descending artery originates from the left circumflex artery in around 8% of people (5–10%); this is known as left dominant circulation.
- The RCA supplies blood to the right atrium and parts of both ventricles. In the majority of people, around 80%, the RCA also supplies the posterior side of the heart; this is known as right dominant circulation. The RCA sits in the coronary sulcus between the right atrium and right ventricle.
  - The RCA divides into two branches, the marginal branch and the posterior interventricular descending branch.
- In around 12% of people (10–20%), the posterior descending artery is supplied by both the LMCA and the RCA; this is referred to as codominance.

Cardiac Output and Circulatory Shock[2, 3, 11, 12, 13, 14]

As we know, the heart's primary function is to pump blood around the body to maintain sufficient blood pressure and maintain end-organ perfusion. Cardiac output is the term used to describe the volume of blood pumped from the heart each minute.

A significant and sustained drop in blood pressure can lead to impaired end-organ perfusion, causing irreversible injury and failure of the vital organs unless corrected rapidly. Many of the life-threatening arrhythmias that can occur in the heart are harmful primarily because they reduce cardiac output, leading to impaired end-organ perfusion and eventual failure of vital organs.

Cardiac output is calculated by multiplying the number of times the heart beats per minute (the heart rate) and the stroke volume (the volume of blood ejected from the left ventricle with each heartbeat).

- Heart Rate (bpm) [**HR**] × Stroke Volume (ml) [**SV**] = Cardiac Output (ml) [**CO**]
- **HR × SV = CO**
- Example: If HR is 80 beats per minute and SV is 65 ml, then: 80 × 65 = 5,200
  The cardiac output is 5,200 ml, or 5.2 litres, per minute.

In the out-of-hospital environment, we can measure heart rate, but we cannot measure stroke volume, meaning we are not able to calculate cardiac output. However, it is essential for us to understand how the heart can alter cardiac output and how problems with the heart can cause it to drop. (Understanding of cardiac output is also a popular pathophysiology exam question, so make sure you understand and are able to calculate it!).

The body uses arterial and cardiopulmonary baroreceptors (pressure sensors) to immediately detect any changes in blood pressure. If a reduction in blood pressure is detected, the sympathetic nervous system (page 12) communicates with the heart and utilises several mechanisms to increase cardiac output as it attempts to maintain sufficient blood pressure, such as:

- Increasing the heart rate.
- Increasing the force of ventricular contraction, which increases stroke volume.
- Increasing systemic vascular resistance by constricting blood vessels throughout the body, particularly the blood supply to the skeletal muscles and the renal and gastrointestinal systems.

Circulatory Shock

Circulatory shock is the state of insufficient blood flow to the tissues of the body, meaning that the perfusion of vital organs with oxygen is insufficient and they are at risk of permanent damage. There are multiple subtypes of circulatory shock. We will focus on those that relate directly to the heart.

Cardiogenic Shock

Also known as pump failure, cardiogenic shock is caused by the failure of the heart muscle, heart valves or the cardiac conduction system, resulting in the failure of the heart to function effectively as a pump. Damage to the heart muscle reduces its ability to function and this reduces stroke volume which in turn leads to decreased cardiac output.

As we know from page 2, the primary function of the heart valves is to prevent blood from flowing backwards during a heartbeat. Heart valve failure allows blood to backflow into the heart chambers; this reduces the amount of forward pressure created, again lowering cardiac output.

A problem with the cardiac conduction system causing the heart to beat either too fast or too slow can lead to rate-related cardiogenic shock. If the heart rate is bradycardic (page 35), the slow heart rate will proportionately reduce the cardiac output; as we understand from the equation $[\textbf{HR} \times \textbf{SV} = \textbf{CO}]$, if the value of **HR** is reduced, then so too is the resulting value of **CO**.

When the heart becomes extremely tachycardic (page 39), the speed of ventricular contractions can lead to reduced ventricular filling during diastole as the extreme heart rate does not allow adequate time between each contraction; therefore, stroke volume is decreased, which in turn decreases cardiac output.

Causes of cardiogenic shock are numerous and widely discussed in later chapters, including:

- Myocardial infarction (page 93).
- Heart failure (page 122).
- Bradycardia (page 35).
- 2nd or 3rd degree heart blocks (pages 62 and 64).
- Idioventricular rhythms (page 68).
- Narrow complex tachycardia (page 39) and ventricular tachycardia (page 49).
- Heart valve failure.

Hypovolaemic Shock

When blood is lost from the body, the overall circulating volume of blood within the circulatory system is reduced. Fluid loss through means other than blood loss, such as diarrhoea and vomiting, also reduces circulating volume. In extreme cases this can also lead to hypovolemic shock.

Stroke volume is reduced due to a lack of available blood for supplying the ventricles, leading to a decrease in cardiac output.

Causes of hypovolemic shock include:

- Haemorrhagic blood loss, internal or external, which can be traumatic or medical in origin.
- Severe dehydration, which can be due to severe vomiting and diarrhoea, profuse sweating, environmental illness (heat stroke / exhaustion), reduced oral intake of fluids.
- Transdermal fluid loss in severe burns.

Obstructive Shock

Obstructive shock occurs when blood flow is obstructed in the circulatory system or heart, usually by a blockage in a blood vessel. If a large blood vessel becomes obstructed, the blockage can lead to a reduction in cardiac output through an insufficient supply of blood returning to the heart.

Causes of obstructive shock include:

- Pulmonary Embolism (PE): A PE occurring in a large enough respiratory blood vessel will impair blood return to the left side of the heart, reducing cardiac output.
- Cardiac tamponade: Stroke volume is reduced due to constriction of the heart within the pericardial sac, preventing it from fully expanding and filling.

Other Types of Shock

Distributive shock: is an impaired and abnormal distribution of blood flow to body tissues. Distributive shock is further divided into three types:

- Septic shock: Vasodilation due to sepsis causes a reduction in blood pressure and cardiac pre-load.
- Anaphylactic shock: The extensive and excessive release of histamine causes widespread vasodilation, reducing blood pressure and cardiac pre-load.
- Neurogenic shock: Occurs in spinal cord injury when the sympathetic nervous system cannot communicate with the heart because of damage to the pathways within the spinal column. Separately, the vagus nerve is a cranial nerve and does not travel down the spinal column, so the parasympathetic nervous system still acts to slow down the heart and reduce contractility. This causes bradycardia and hypotension, resulting in neurogenic shock.

Clinical Signs and Symptoms of Shock

- Pallor and diaphoresis (pale and clammy skin).
- Cold peripheries and delayed capillary refill time.
- Tachycardia and tachypnoea.
- Hypotension and weak or absent peripheral pulses.
- Dizziness or near loss of consciousness.
- Loss of consciousness or reduced level of consciousness.
- Anxiety and confusion.

Cardiac Pre-load and Afterload

Pre-load is the volume of blood within the ventricles and the degree to which they are stretched prior to contraction. A reduction in pre-load leads to a reduction in cardiac output. An increase in pre-load will increase cardiac output. A significant decrease in pre-load can lead to cardiac arrest, especially if the heart muscle is weak and relies on pre-load to maintain cardiac output. This is of particular importance in right coronary artery myocardial infarction (page 114).

Afterload is the force which the heart has to overcome to eject blood through the aortic valve and into systemic circulation. The higher the afterload, the harder the heart has to pump to maintain cardiac output. If the heart cannot match the force required to exceed the afterload, then cardiac output will decrease.

ECG Interpretation

Now that we understand how the heart functions physically and electrically and how its operation relates to the rest of the body, we can begin to consider how we approach examining, analysing and assessing an ECG.

The 9-step ECG Interpretation Tool

By using a structured and systematic approach to assessing an ECG we can reduce the chances of missing potentially significant findings. Only by using this systematic approach consistently with every ECG we perform can we confidently apply it when we are under extreme stress. Think of this ECG interpretation tool as the 'ABC' or Primary Survey of ECG interpretation.

A structured aide-memoire may not be needed to discover abnormal changes on an ECG when you are rested and fresh, but during a busy night shift, in the early hours of the morning and faced with a complex ECG, you will be glad that you have the practised 'muscle memory' of this structured approach to rely on.

With the five-step approach to ECG interpretation we follow a pattern where we first assess ECG lead II and consider the rate and rhythm of the heartbeat. We then assess each stage of the heartbeat by systematically analysing the P waves, the QRS complexes and the T waves. We then consider a more global approach and look for any location-based abnormalities by analysing every ECG lead using the first five steps of the ECG interpretation tool.

There are an additional four steps which have been created specifically to prompt paramedics in the out-of-hospital setting, taking the tool beyond problem-finding to include prompts around circulatory management, diagnosis formation and paramedic clinical interventions.

We will be using this interpretation tool throughout this book to evaluate and discuss ECG rhythms and to complete the practice case scenarios.

The 9-Step ECG Interpretation Tool	
ECG Steps	**Remember to look at every ECG lead view, not just lead II**
1	What is the rate and rhythm?
2	Are there any P waves and what is their relationship with the QRS complex?
3	What is the duration and morphology of the QRS complex?
4	Is the ST segment isoelectric, depressed or elevated?
5	Are the QT intervals and T waves normal?
Clinical Steps	
6	Is the heart generating a palpable pulse of appropriate rate and providing adequate perfusion?
7	Is the rhythm unstable and at risk of deterioration?
8	Does the presenting rhythm support or change your working diagnosis?
9	Are any clinical interventions required?

Rate Calculation[1]

We need to be able to calculate the heart rate from an ECG. On a normally calibrated ECG printer, we know the speed is 25 mm per second and we know that 1 small square = 1 mm, meaning 1 small square = 0.04 seconds. Five small squares make up a larger one. One large square = 0.2 seconds and 5 large squares make up one second. There are multiple methods that may be used to estimate or calculate the heart rate.

- **Estimating methods:**
  - ▸ Both of the following estimation methods are only suitable for estimating the heart rate in regular rhythms. If used on irregular rhythms the estimation is likely to be considerably inaccurate. For irregular rhythms, a calculating method should be used.
- **Countdown method** (Figure 1.9):
  - ▸ By memorising the following number sequence, you can obtain a quick, rough estimation of heart rate.
  - ▸ Find an R wave sitting close to the thick line between two large boxes. Then count the number of full large boxes between that R wave and the next R wave.
  - ▸ The number sequence below relates to the number of large boxes between the R waves: **300, 150, 100, 75, 60, 50, 43, 37**.
  - ▸ So, if there were four complete large boxes between the R waves, we would know that the rate was below 75, but above 60.
  - ▸ Understanding the maths: Because each large square on the ECG represents 0.2 seconds, there are 300 large squares in one minute. To calculate the 'beats per minute', we need to divide 300 by the number of large squares between each QRS complex. For example, if there are 2 large squares between each QRS complex, this would be 300/2 = 150 beats per minute.
- **R-R interval method:**
  - ▸ This simple method often requires a calculator.
  - ▸ Equation: **Rate = 60/X**. Where X is the distance in seconds between two R waves.
  - ▸ Example: If the R-R interval comprises 16 small squares, then 0.04 seconds multiplied by 16 equals 0.64 seconds. Meaning, **Rate = 60/0.64. 60/0.64 = 94** beats per minute (or rather, 93.75, but we round up or down to the nearest whole number).
  - ▸ This method can also be used for the number of small squares without translating it into seconds. We know there are 1,500 small squares in one minute. To calculate the beats per minute we would then count the number of small squares between each R-R interval and use this to divide 1,500. Using the same example: 1,500/16 = 94, this gives the same results as above.
- **Calculating method:**
  - ▸ If the heart rate is irregular or you need a more accurate heart rate, then the calculating method can be used.
  - ▸ Count the number of R waves in 30 large boxes (six seconds). Then multiply this number by 10 to calculate the heart rate in 60 seconds.
  - ▸ **Y × 10 = Rate** where Y is the number of R waves in 30 large boxes.
  - ▸ Example: If there were 9 R waves in the 30 large boxes (six seconds), then **9 × 10 = 90** beats per minute.
  - ▸ The standard 12-lead ECG is 10 seconds long, meaning that you could also count the number of QRS complexes in those 10 seconds and multiply by six to estimate the irregular rate.
- All of the above three methods can also be used to calculate the atrial rate by counting P waves instead of R waves.

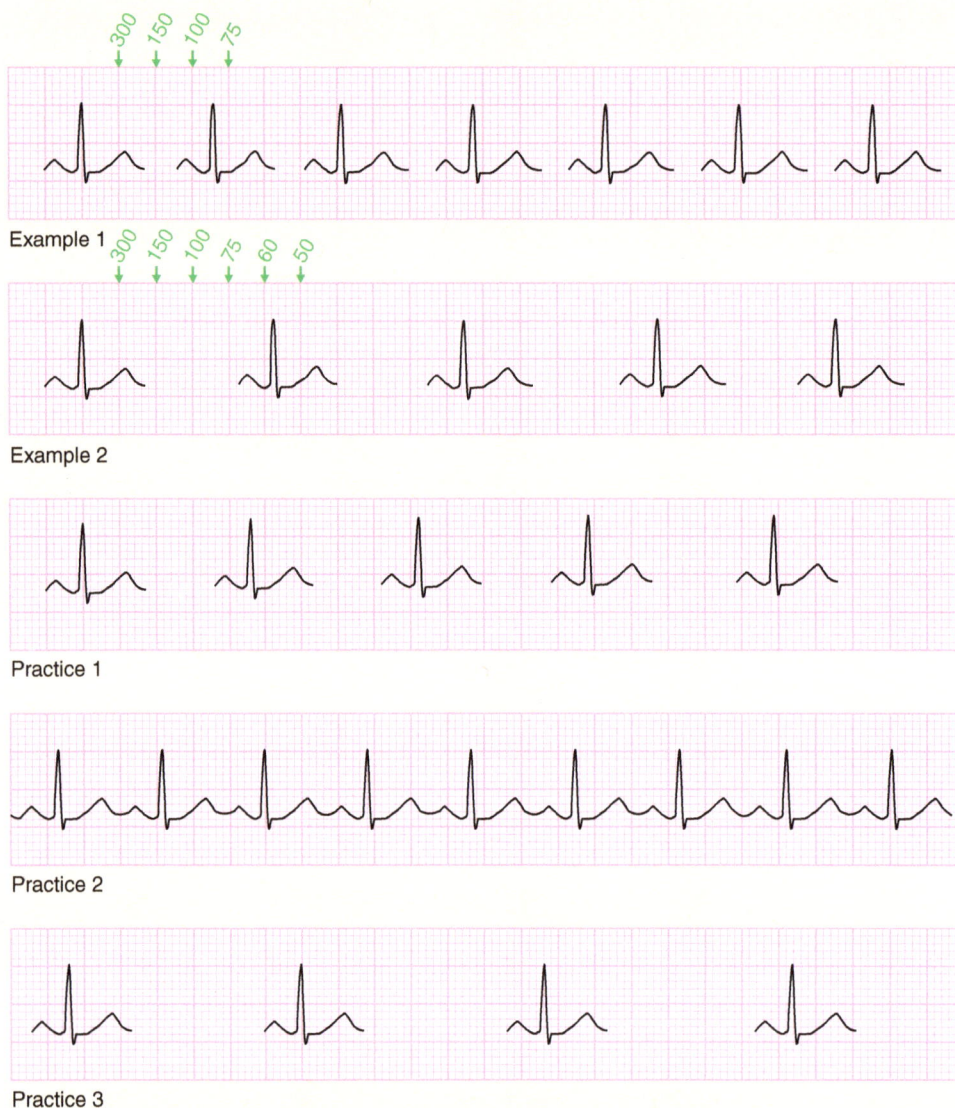

Figure 1.9 Countdown method examples and practice ECGs.

Practice ECG answers: Practice 1, roughly 65 beats per minute. Practice 2, roughly 110 beats per minute. Practice 3, roughly 45 beats per minute.

The 'Normal' ECG[15, 16]

It is time to bring together what has been learned so far and look at a standard lead II ECG rhythm strip showing sinus rhythm. The majority of ECGs you will assess in clinical practice will have no significant abnormalities and will show either sinus rhythm or sinus arrhythmia. Deciding that an ECG has no significant abnormalities carries a lot of responsibility, as missing a sinister change could lead to misdiagnosis, or worse, unexpected deterioration of a patient who was presumed to have no significant illness. For this reason, it is vitally important that you, as a paramedic, can confidently assess an ECG and reasonably exclude any significant abnormalities. Think of sinus rhythm as a diagnosis of exclusion; once you have ruled out any other presenting rhythm and found no significant abnormalities, you can diagnose sinus rhythm.

Using the 9-step ECG interpretation tool you can systematically analyse every ECG so that when you diagnose sinus rhythm, you can do so with confidence.

Normal ECG Values

- P-R interval: Between 0.12–0.20 seconds or 3–5 small squares.
- QRS complex: Under 0.12 seconds or up to 3 small squares.
- QT Interval corrected: Between 0.36–0.44 seconds or 9–11 small squares (0.44 seconds in men, 0.46 seconds in women). (See page 52 for more on QT interval correction).

Most ECG monitors will print out the calculated ECG values with the ECG.

Interpreting an ECG with the 9-step ECG Interpretation Tool

Let us now look at an ECG showing sinus rhythm using the first five ECG steps of the 9-step ECG interpretation tool.

ECG 1.1 – Sinus Rhythm

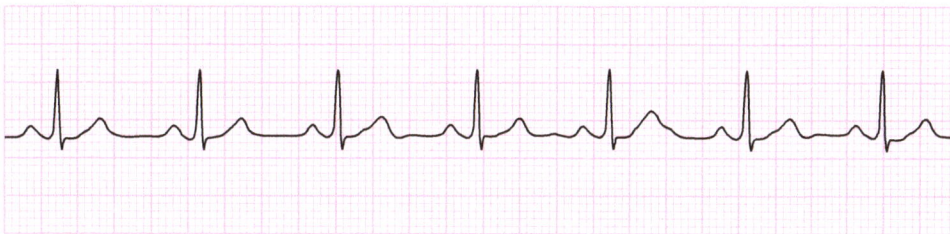

ECG 1.1	
ECG Steps	**Answers**
1 **What is the rate and rhythm?**	*The rate is around 80 beats per minute and the rhythm is regular.*
2 **Are there any P waves and what is their relationship with the QRS complex?**	*There are P waves before every QRS complex and there is a QRS complex after every P wave. The P-R interval is consistent and normal at 0.16 seconds (4 small squares). Between 0.12 and 0.20 seconds (3–5 small squares) is normal.*
3 **What is the duration and morphology of the QRS complex?**	*The QRS complex duration is 0.08 seconds (2 small squares). Under 0.12 seconds (3 small squares) is normal.*
4 **Is the ST segment isoelectric, depressed or elevated?**	*The ST segment is isoelectric, which is normal.*
5 **Are the QT intervals and T waves normal?**	*The T wave is of normal shape and the QT interval is 0.36 seconds (9 small squares). Between 0.35 and 0.45 seconds (9–11 small squares) is normal.*

ECG 1.2 – Sinus Arrhythmia

It is normal for the heart rate to vary slightly during breathing, becoming slower during exhalation and faster during inhalation; this is known as sinus arrhythmia. Sinus arrhythmia is a normal and common finding on ECGs and of no clinical significance. An example of sinus arrhythmia can be seen in ECG 1.2. Sinus arrhythmia can be an abnormal finding in elderly patients as it may indicate underlying disease.

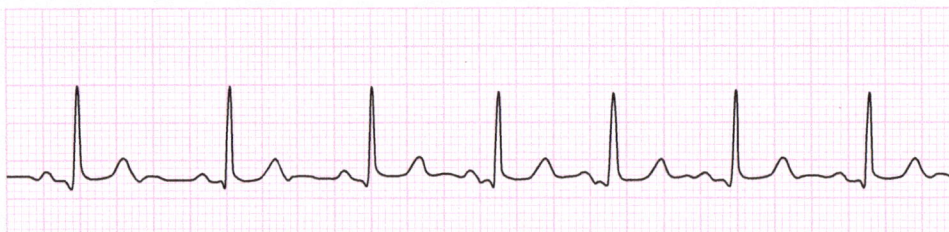

The only thing that stops this rhythm strip from being sinus rhythm is the variable rate, thus making it sinus arrhythmia.

The 12-lead ECG and Cardiac Axis[1, 15]

The 12-lead ECG is made up of 12 different directional views of the heart.

- A 'lead' is a tracing on the ECG that shows the electrical activity of the heart from a specific angle.
- 'Electrodes' are the 10 physical wires and sticky electrode pads that are attached to the patient (confusingly, people often incorrectly refer to the wires and electrodes as 'leads').
- The 12 lead views that make up the 12-lead ECG are recorded through the 10 physical electrodes.
- The first six lead views are recorded through the three electrodes attached to the patient's limbs. The other six lead views, V1–V6, are recorded through the six precordial electrodes attached to the patient's chest.
- During each heartbeat the electrical impulses spread and move in many directions, travelling forwards and back, up and down, to reach and depolarise every part of the atria and ventricles.
- Each of these millions of electrical impulses has its own vector (direction of travel). The prevailing vector of these electrical impulses at any one time dictates how it will appear on each of the ECG leads.
- When the overall sum of all the vectors is moving towards the positive electrode it will appear as a positive (upwards) deflection on that ECG lead.
- When the overall sum of all the vectors is moving away from the positive electrode it will appear as a negative (downwards) deflection on that ECG lead.
- Each wave on the ECG has its own vector; this is the overall net direction of the electrical impulse during that part of the heartbeat. There is a P wave vector, a QRS complex vector and a T wave vector.
- Cardiac axis is the term used for the QRS complex vector, representing depolarisation across the ventricles. In a normal heart, the cardiac axis is downward and towards the left side of the body, directly towards the positive electrode of lead II.

Limb Leads and the Hexaxial System

The limb electrodes attached to the Right Arm (RA), Left Arm (LA) and Left Leg (LL) together give rise to the first six ECG lead views: I, II, III, aVR, aVL and aVF. The Right Leg (RL) electrode is neutral and not used for recording measurements.

The first six ECG lead views are recorded along imaginary lines, each drawn between two points.

- Leads I, II and III are each recorded from lines drawn between two of the limb electrodes (Figure 1.10).
  - ▸ Lead I is recorded along the line between the RA and LA electrodes. The LA electrode is positive.
  - ▸ Lead II is recorded along the line between the RA and LL electrodes. The LL electrode is positive.
  - ▸ Lead III is recorded along the line between the LA and LL electrodes. The LL electrode is positive.
  - ▸ Together these three lines form Einthoven's Triangle.
- Leads aVR, aVL and aVF are each recorded between one of the limb electrodes and the calculated middle point between all three limb electrodes. All three limb leads record electrical activity and the ECG monitor calculates the mid-point; this is known as Wilson's Central Terminus (WCT). These three lead views are known as the 'augmented leads'.
  - ▸ Lead aVR is recorded along the line between the RA electrode and WCT. The RA electrode is positive.
  - ▸ Lead aVL is recorded along the line between the LA and WCT. The LA electrode is positive.
  - ▸ Lead aVF is recorded along the line between the LL electrode and WCT. The LL electrode is positive.
- The six lines drawn that form leads I, II, III, aVR, aVL and aVF together form the basis of the hexaxial system as seen in Figure 1.10.

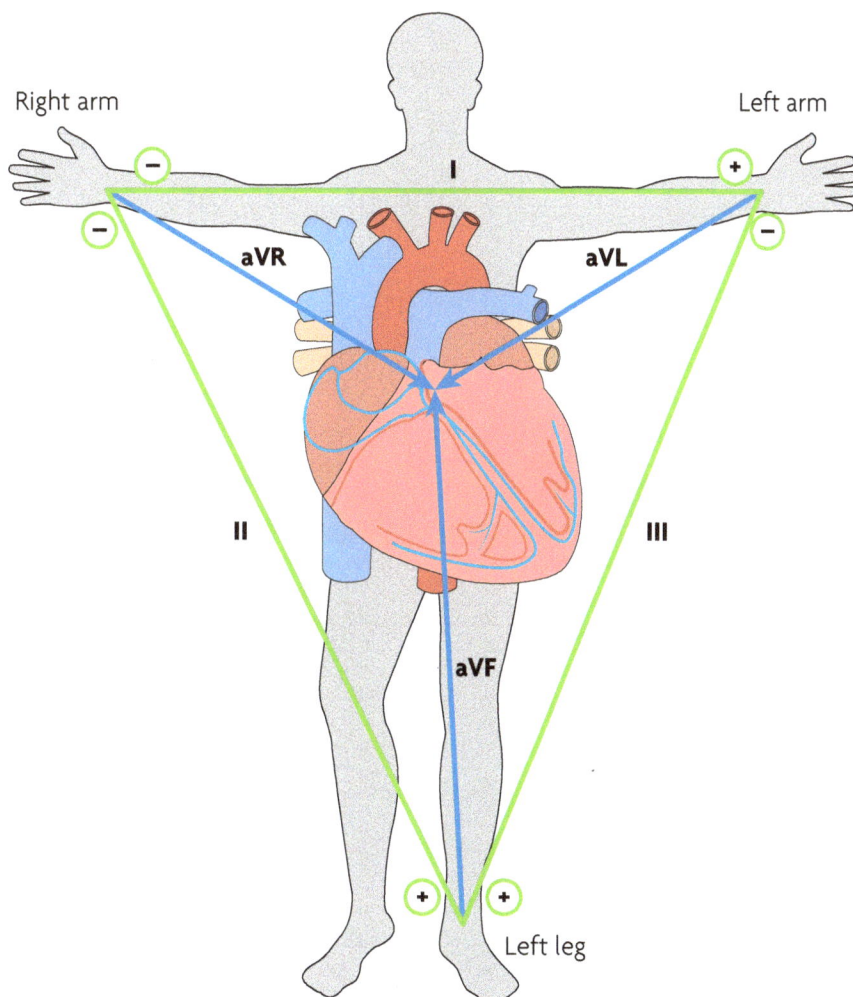

Figure 1.10 Limb leads forming Einthoven's triangle.

Put Simply!

This may seem rather confusing. To put it as simply as possible, each of the 12 lead views on the ECG look at the heart from a different direction; imagine each view as a camera. When the electrical impulse of each heartbeat moves towards that camera, it appears as upright on that ECG lead. If it moves away from that camera, it appears downwards on the ECG. Understanding which part of the heart each ECG lead is focused on (Figure 1.11) can tell us a lot about different arrhythmias and problems with the heart which we will discuss throughout this book.

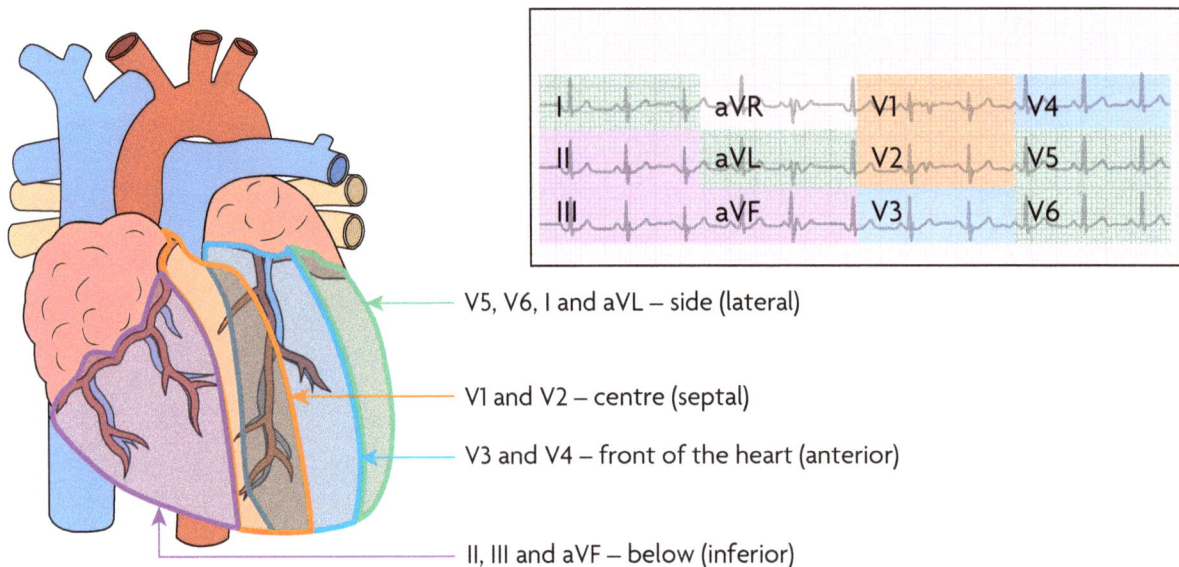

V5, V6, I and aVL – side (lateral)

V1 and V2 – centre (septal)

V3 and V4 – front of the heart (anterior)

II, III and aVF – below (inferior)

Figure 1.11 Lead views of the heart on the printed ECG.

The Precordial Leads

The remaining six ECG lead views are made up from the six precordial, or chest, leads. These leads are a little simpler as each electrode looks directly at the heart from where it is anatomically placed. The electrode is positive so it follows the same rule that electrical impulses moving towards the electrode are positive (upwards), and impulses moving away are negative (downwards), on the ECG. For each precordial lead, the WCT acts as the negative electrode.

- The precordial leads are termed 'V' leads (Figure 1.12).
  - ‣ Leads V1 and V2 look at the septal wall.
  - ‣ Leads V3 and V4 look at the anterior wall of the left ventricle.
  - ‣ Leads V5 and V6 look at the lateral wall of the left ventricle.

Cardiac Axis and Axis Deviation

Cardiac axis is the term used for the QRS complex vector, representing depolarisation across the ventricles. In a normal heart, the cardiac axis is downward and towards the left side of the body, directly towards the positive electrode of lead II.

As we can see from Figure 1.13, the cardiac axis is described using degrees using the hexaxial system. Each half-circle comprises 180 degrees; one half is positive, the other negative. Calculation of the cardiac axis in degrees is complex and unnecessary, as ECG monitors calculate this automatically and print the cardiac axis, written in degrees, along with the other numerical ECG values. Some monitors even print the hexaxial wheel with the cardiac axis.

What we do need to know is the normal range of the cardiac axis and how to identify whether left or right axis deviation is present.

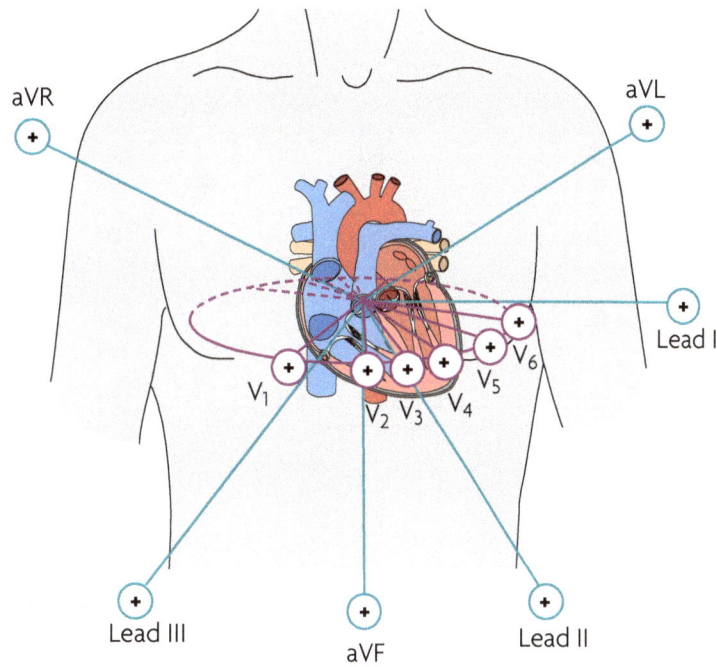

Figure 1.12 The heart with ECG lead views.

Axis deviation occurs when the cardiac axis shifts to either the left or the right within the frontal plane, beyond what is considered the normal range. This can be due to either changes in the mass of the cardiac muscle, or rotation of the heart within the chest. It can also occur if the electrical depolarisation travelling through the heart is disrupted and takes a different route (see bundle branch blocks, page 124).

A normal cardiac axis can range from −30 degrees to +90 degrees, as shown by the pink area in Figure 1.13.

Left axis deviation ranges from −90 degrees to −30 degrees, the purple area in Figure 1.13.

Right axis deviation ranges from +90 degrees to +/−180 degrees, the green area in Figure 1.13.

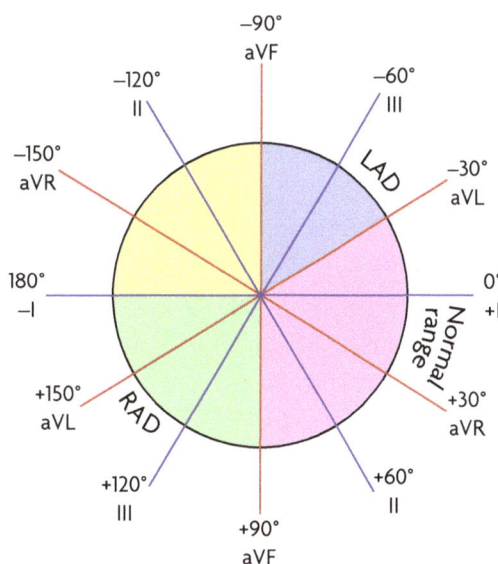

Figure 1.13 The hexaxial system wheel.

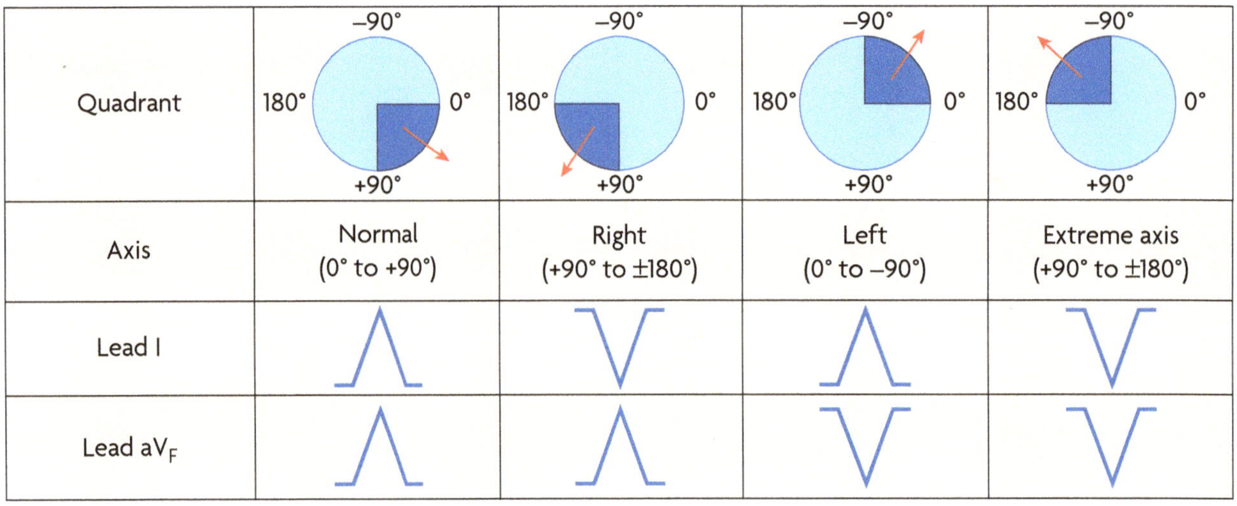

Quadrant	−90° 180° 0° +90°	−90° 180° 0° +90°	−90° 180° 0° +90°	−90° 180° 0° +90°
Axis	Normal (0° to +90°)	Right (+90° to ±180°)	Left (0° to −90°)	Extreme axis (+90° to ±180°)
Lead I	⋀	⋁	⋀	⋁
Lead aV$_F$	⋀	⋀	⋁	⋁

Figure 1.14 Axis deviation in relation to lead views and the hexaxial wheel.

We can identify the presence of right and left axis deviation on the ECG without relying on the calculations of the monitor. We know that if the net electrical activity, the vector, is moving towards an electrode it causes a positive deflection on the ECG. The more degrees away that the vector is pointing, the less the amplitude (height) of the QRS complex. This continues until the vector is more than 90 degrees away from the electrode. Once this occurs it appears as a negative (downward) deflection in that lead (when the electrical activity is at a 90-degree angle from the electrode the QRS becomes equiphasic, where it is as positive as it is negative). This allows us to compare two differently located electrodes and impose their fields over each other. This gives us the ability to 'narrow down' the rough direction of the vector and determine the cardiac axis.

To do this, we first look at ECG lead I. If lead I is positive we then look at ECG lead II. If lead I and lead II are both positive, there is a normal cardiac axis, seen as the purple area in Figure 1.13.

If lead I is positive but lead II is negative, there is left axis deviation, seen as the red segment in Figure 1.13. However, if lead I is negative, we look to lead aVF as our comparison. If lead I is negative and lead aVF is positive, there is right axis deviation, seen as the blue segment in Figure 1.13.

A useful analogy here is to imagine that in left axis deviation, lead I and aVF are 'Leaving' the page, as both are pointing towards the edge of the paper. Conversely, in right axis deviation, lead I and aVF are 'Reaching' for each other, pointing inwards towards each other.

It may help your understanding if we think of the leads that represent the vertical and horizontal 'force' of the electrical activity. Lead I represents the horizontal force, with the R wave showing the leftward force and the S wave showing the rightward force. Lead aVF represents the vertical force, the R wave being the downward force and S wave being the upward force. Knowing this, we can compare the two leads and their net electrical activity (positive or negative) and 'narrow down' the direction of the vector into a 90-degree quadrant (see Figure 1.14).

Clinical Information-Gathering and Formulating a Working Diagnosis

Throughout this book we will be considering the ECG as a diagnostic tool that forms part of a wider clinical picture of patient care. The majority of information needed for diagnosis comes from the verbal history taken from the patient during the patient care episode. In this section we will look at the importance of accurate, detailed and specific information gained from history-taking in the context of cardiac care.

Without clinical context, an ECG is of little use. However, combined with a thorough and comprehensive history, it can be a key contributor to the formation of a diagnosis and decision making.

Medical Model of Structured History-Taking

Each case scenario within this book will provide a medical history in the form of the medical model of structured history-taking. When approaching each scenario, try and consider all of the history alongside your interpretation of the ECG when answering clinical questions and making diagnostic decisions.

Medical Model of Structured History-taking[17, 18, 19]

- **Presenting complaint**: What the patient says is their primary concern or symptom.
- **History of presenting complaint**: Full and detailed information about presenting symptoms. Including recent illness and associated symptoms. Utilising OPQRST AS PN to explore symptoms.
- **Previous medical and surgical history**: Medical conditions formally diagnosed or suspected. Surgical procedures both previous and scheduled.
- **Drug history**: Prescribed medication and any self-medication with over-the-counter or alternative medicines. Concordance with medication – are they taking it as directed?
- **Allergies**: Presence of allergies and the previous severity of reactions.
- **Social history**: Living and working situation. Care packages or assisted living support. Lifestyle risk factors including alcohol consumption, smoking, body mass index and obesity, diet and recreational drug use.
- **Family history**: Potential genetic or familial risk factors from direct family, heart disease, cancer.
- **Review of systems**: Body system-based, catch-all questions to cover potentially missed symptoms.
- **Physical examination**: Physical examination based on history obtained.

- **OPQRST AS PN** is one of many medical mnemonics that can be used to help remember some of the questions we ask to explore each symptom.
  - **O – Onset** of symptoms. Was the onset gradual or sudden? What were they doing when it started?
  - **P – Provoking** and **Palliating** factors. Does anything make the symptom better or worse?
  - **Q – Quality** of the pain or feeling. How would the patient describe the symptom in their own words?
  - **R – Radiation**. Does the pain or sensation go to any other parts of the body?
  - **S – Severity** score. Can they rate the pain or discomfort on a scale of 0–10?
  - **T – Time** of onset. How long ago did it start?
  - **AS – Associated Symptoms**. Do they have any other symptoms?
  - **PN – Pertinent Negatives**. Key symptoms that the patient is *not* currently experiencing. The absence of a symptom can contribute as much to the working diagnosis as the presence of a symptom.

Differential and Working Diagnoses

In most cases, to formulate an appropriate, person-centred care plan for a patient, we need to first establish a working diagnosis. To do this we must consider the information we have gathered from the history-taking and physical assessment of the patient. Throughout the patient care episode, we will be adding and removing potential diagnoses from our mental list of differential diagnoses.

- Differential diagnoses: The list of possible diagnoses. Potential diagnoses will be added and removed from your list as you progress through the patient consultation.
- Working diagnosis: The most probable, or most serious, diagnosis that you conclude from your list of differential diagnoses after taking an appropriate history and physical assessment.

It is important to note that a working diagnosis is not the same as a diagnosis. Often, in the out-of-hospital setting, we do not have the time, resources or knowledge at our disposal to make a confirmed diagnosis. Sometimes our working diagnosis will be a potentially serious condition that it is unsafe and unreasonable for us to exclude (rule out) based on the patient's presentation.

As we formulate our list of differential diagnoses and move towards a working diagnosis, we need to consider the clinical context of the findings that are influencing our decision making.

The importance of clinical context can be highlighted in this example:

> 'A 78-year-old male patient has collapsed. He has not lost consciousness, but has been unable to stand since his collapse, feeling dizzy and faint. He is pale and clammy, with a low blood pressure'.

Based on the above information, would you expect this patient's pulse rate to be fast, slow or normal?

No matter what you answered, you are both right and wrong. With only this information available we cannot confidently predict what the heart rate might be, nor establish the cause of his collapse. But we can use the information we do have available to inform further questions and examinations.

- The heart rate could be very low. Let's imagine it is 30 beats per minute. This would explain the collapse and signs of low blood pressure; the heart rate is too low to sustain sufficient cardiac output.
- Alternatively, the heart rate could be very high. Hypothetically, the patient could be in ventricular tachycardia (page 49) with a heart rate of 180 beats per minute; this again would cause reduced cardiac output and low blood pressure.
- But, there is more: What if the patient has a non-cardiac cause for the collapse? He might have internal bleeding, a severe infection that has led to septic shock or perhaps a neurological event has occurred. In these cases we could expect the heart rate to be fast, but not too fast, let's say 110 beats per minute. This tachycardia is the heart's response to the reduced cardiac output.
- But wait, let's take it a step further, what if this patient has been prescribed beta blockers for high blood pressure? The medication limits the patient's heart rate to around 60 beats per minute and therefore renders the heart unable to speed up to compensate for the reduced cardiac output.
- Or, taking it even further, what if the patient has been taking an accidental overdose of his beta blocker medication? This can cause bradycardia, so this takes us back to the first possibility, maybe the heart rate is 30 beats per minute due to medication overdose ...

This all can seem very complex but that's what makes it interesting! We are performing detective work, being thorough, identifying clues so that we can make a good attempt at determining what is going wrong, and thus form a working diagnosis.

Cardiovascular Risk Factors[20, 21]

The prevalence of coronary heart disease is associated with many risk factors; these can be divided into modifiable risk factors and non-modifiable risk factors.
- Cardiovascular risk factors:
  - Modifiable:
    - Smoking.
    - Poor diet.
    - High cholesterol.
    - Obesity.
    - Hypertension.
    - Sedentary lifestyle (physical inactivity).
    - Stress.
  - Non-modifiable:
    - Family history of cardiovascular disease.
    - Diabetes.
    - Sex – greater risk to men than women.
    - Age – risk increases with increasing age.

- Ethnicity – people of African or Asian ethnic origin have a high risk compared to other groups.
- Socioeconomic status – poverty increases risk of heart disease and stroke.

The Cardiac Arrest Rhythms[22, 23, 24]

Cardiac arrest occurs when a person ceases to have palpable central pulses. This is the moment when the body becomes unable to sustain life on its own. It is important to understand the distinction between cardiac arrest and death. When cardiac arrest occurs, a person is in the final stage of dying. At this stage, depending on many factors, they may respond positively to resuscitation attempts and death can be averted, at least temporarily. But once a person has truly died, resuscitation is futile and inappropriate. Refer to the JRCALC Clinical Guidelines and local policies for more information on recognising life to be extinct and guidance on when not to commence resuscitation.[24]

When carrying out resuscitation, a lead II rhythm is rapidly assessed through the defibrillator pads and viewed on the monitor screen, alongside the checking of central pulse points, to determine which cardiac arrest rhythm the patient's heart is currently in. The patient's rhythm determines the specific treatment and resuscitation algorithm to be followed.

There are four cardiac arrest rhythms, which can be divided in two different ways. First, into shockable and non-shockable rhythms and second, by rhythms which are or are not compatible with a cardiac output (the rhythm is compatible with a pulse). These can be visualised best in Table 1.1.

Table 1.1 Cardiac arrest rhythms

	Shockable	Non-shockable
Compatible with pulse	Ventricular tachycardia	Pulseless Electrical Activity (PEA)
No pulse possible	Ventricular fibrillation	Asystole

Asystole

- Non-shockable, incompatible with life.
- Origins of the term: 'A' meaning absent, 'systole' meaning heartbeat. 'Asystole' thus meaning absent heartbeat.
- The famous 'flatline' rhythm, indicates that there is no electrical activity with in the ventricles. This is the clinical definition of asystole 'the absence of any ventricular activity'.
- Asystole is the final rhythm into which all hearts will eventually pass at the moment of death.
- Currently, in Advanced Life Support (ALS), adrenaline is given to try to stimulate the heart to produce some electrical activity.
- Defibrillation will have no effect on asystole as there is no electrical activity to stun.

ECG 1.3 – Asystole

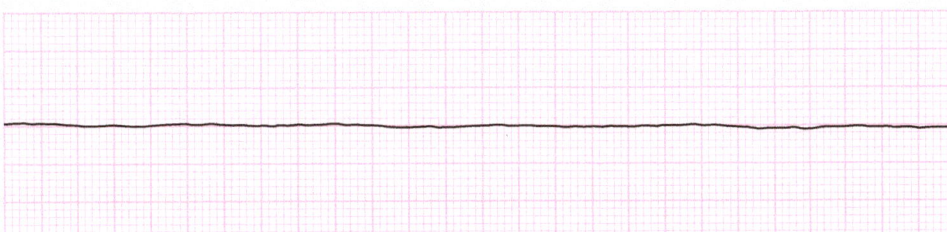

Pulseless Electrical Activity (PEA)

- Non-shockable, organised rhythm capable of producing a pulse, compatible with life.
- PEA is the 'catch-all' cardiac arrest rhythm. If the visualised rhythm on the monitor is one which could produce a pulse, but is currently not producing a pulse, and is not VT, then it must be PEA.
- PEA does not benefit from defibrillation as there is already an organised rhythm which could generate a pulse. Defibrillation could potentially have a negative effect and cause the heart to deteriorate into VF or asystole.
- PEA can be further divided into two groups:
  - ▸ Wide and slow PEA. This indicates that the heart is sick and is suggestive that the cause of cardiac arrest is cardiovascular in nature. This could also be caused by electrolyte abnormalities.
  - ▸ Fast and narrow PEA. This indicates that the heart's electrical pathways are working and that the cardiac muscle may be functioning and contracting. This should prompt the clinician to consider causes of cardiac arrest external to the heart itself; for example, hypovolaemic shock (page 14), pulmonary embolism or other forms of obstructive shock (page 15).

ECG 1.4 and ECG 1.5 – PEA

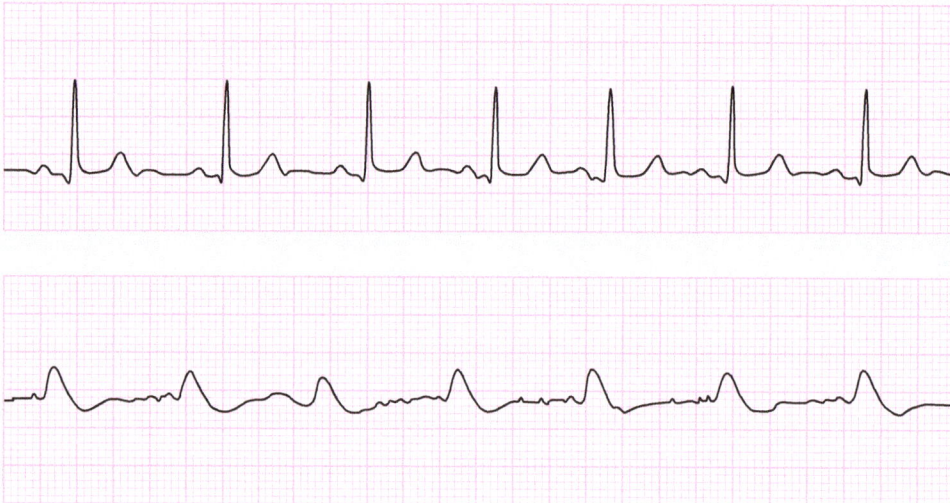

Both of these rhythm strips would be classed as PEA if the patient did not have a pulse. ECG 1.4 is an example of a fast and narrow PEA. ECG 1.5 is a wide and slow PEA.

Ventricular Fibrillation (VF)

- Shockable, incompatible with life.
- 'Ventricular' refers to the ventricles. 'Fibrillation' means shaking or quivering.
- The ventricular cardiac muscle cells are in a state of uncontrolled and disorganised polarisation and depolarisation, meaning they are unable to contract and generate a pulse.
- The SA node may still be functioning, but the impulses it generates are lost in the fibrillating ventricles.
- Defibrillation of the heart is intended to 'stun' all the cardiac muscle cells by depolarising them and thus give the impulses generated by the SA node a chance to take back control and restore an organised rhythm.

ECG 1.6 – Ventricular Fibrillation

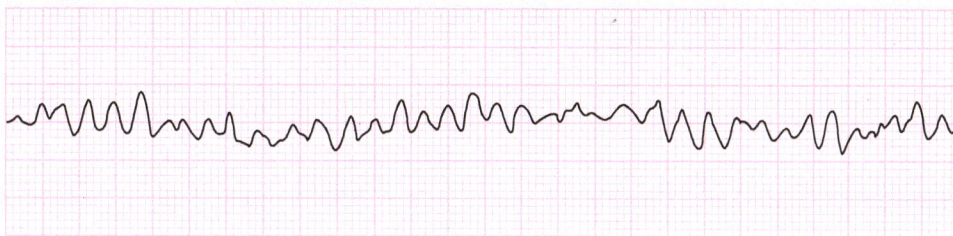

Ventricular Tachycardia (VT)

- Shockable, compatible with life.
- VT is a broad complex tachyarrhythmia.
- VT may have a pulse; if so, the patient is time critical as this is a peri-arrest rhythm, the heart will become fatigued and there is a high risk of the patient either losing their pulse or transitioning into VF.
- The heart is pumping continuously, with the cardiac cells depolarising and generating a beat the moment they are repolarised and ready to contract again.
- Defibrillation of the heart is intended to 'stun' the cardiac muscle cells by depolarising them all and thus give the impulses generated by the SA node a chance to take back control and restore an organised rhythm.

See page 49 for more on VT.

ECG 1.7 – Ventricular Tachycardia

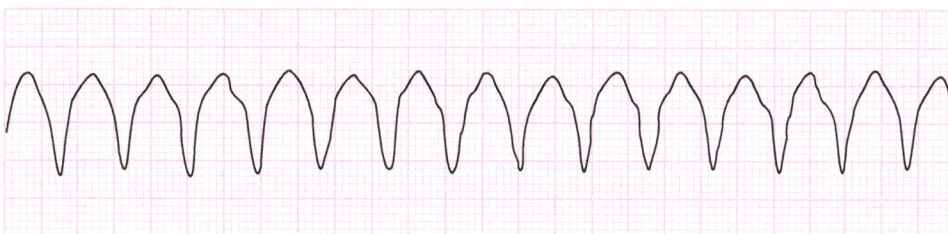

Section 1 Self-Test Questions

Questions

1 What are the normal values for the following?
  a) P-R interval
  b) QRS complex
  c) QT interval

2 Physical heart:
  a) Which two structures does the mitral valve sit between?
  b) Which valve sits between the right ventricle and the pulmonary artery?
  c) Which heart chamber pumps blood to the lungs?
  d) Which artery leaves the left ventricle and takes blood to the body?
  e) Which two blood vessels carry deoxygenated blood to and from the heart?

3 Cardiac cycle:
  a) What happens during atrial systole?
  b) What represents atrial systole on the ECG?

4 Coronary blood supply:
  a) Which parts of the heart are supplied by the Left Anterior Descending (LAD) artery?
  b) Which parts of the heart are supplied by the right coronary artery?

5 Cardiac output:
  a) What is the cardiac output when the heart rate is 42 beats per minute and the stroke volume is 60 ml?
  b) What effects does the sympathetic nervous system have on the heart to increase cardiac output?
  c) What is the difference between cardiogenic shock and hypovolaemic shock?

6 Use the first five ECG steps of the 9-step ECG interpretation tool to analyse Test ECG 1.1 below.

ECG Steps
Remember to look at every ECG lead, not just lead II

1 What is the rate and rhythm?

2 Are there any P waves and what is their relationship with the QRS complex?

3 What is the duration and morphology of the QRS complex?

4 Is the ST segment isoelectric, depressed or elevated?

5 Are the QT intervals and T waves normal?

Test ECG 1.1

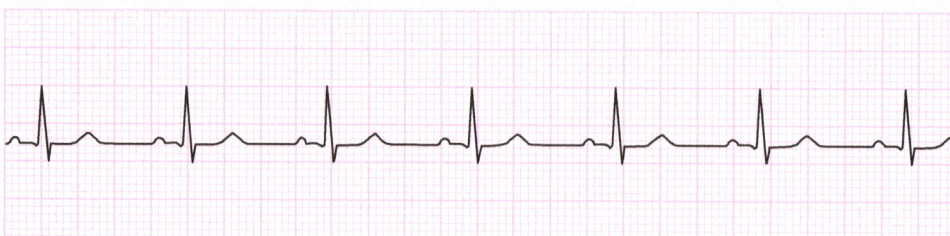

Section 1 Self-Test ECGs

Assess Test ECGs 1.2–1.5. These rhythm strips were all taken during rhythm checks in cardiac arrest; none are associated with a pulse.

Test ECG 1.2

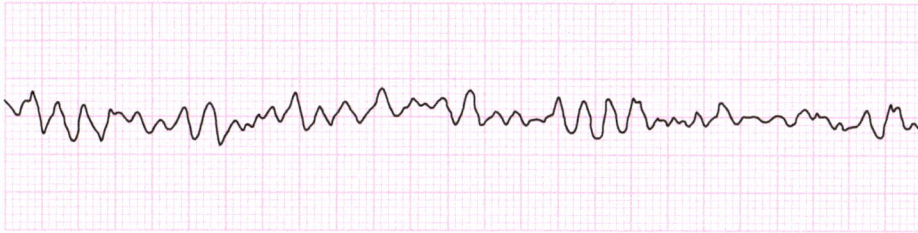

Test ECG 1.3

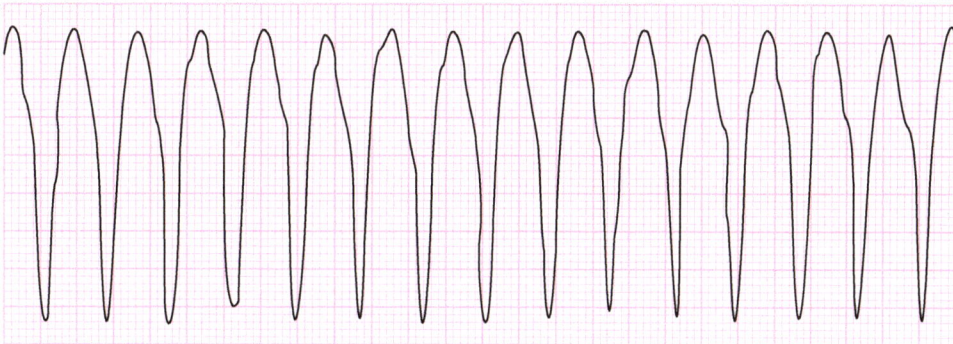

Test ECG 1.4

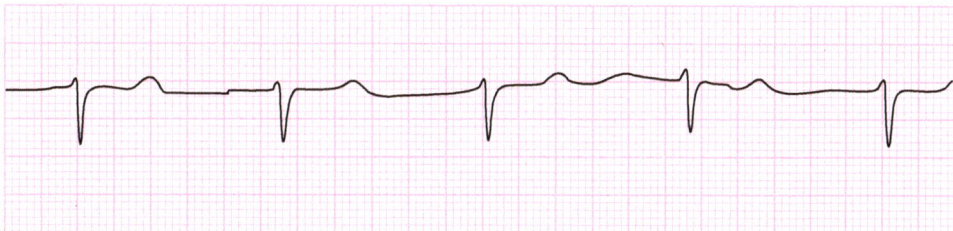

Test ECG 1.5

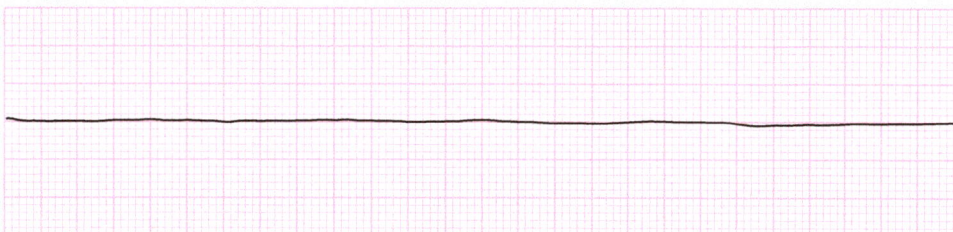

Section 1 Answers to Self-Test Questions

Answers		
1	What are the normal values for the following? a) P-R interval b) QRS complex c) QT interval	a) *P-R interval: Between 0.12–0.20 seconds (3–5 small squares).* b) *QRS complex: Under 0.12 seconds (under 3 small squares).* c) *QT interval: Between 0.35–0.43 seconds (9–11 small squares).*
2	Physical heart: a) Which two structures does the mitral valve sit between? b) Which valve sits between the right ventricle and the pulmonary artery? c) Which heart chamber pumps blood to the lungs? d) Which artery leaves the left ventricle and takes blood to the body? e) Which two blood vessels carry deoxygenated blood to and from the heart?	a) *The **mitral valve** (also known as the bi-cuspid valve) sits between the left atria and the left ventricle.* b) *The **pulmonary valve** sits between the right ventricle and the pulmonary artery.* c) *The right ventricle.* d) *The aorta.* e) *The vena cava and the pulmonary artery.*
3	Cardiac cycle: a) What happens during atrial systole? b) What represents atrial systole on the ECG?	a) *The SA node generates an electrical impulse which depolarises the atria as it travels towards the atrioventricular node (AV node). The atria contract and pump the remaining blood into the ventricles.* b) *The P wave.*
4	Coronary blood supply: a) Which parts of the heart are supplied by the Left Anterior Descending (LAD) artery? b) Which parts of the heart are supplied by the right coronary artery?	a) *The anterior wall of the left ventricle and anterior septum.* b) *The right atrium and parts of both ventricles. It also supplies the posterior side of the heart in 80% of people.*
5	Cardiac output: a) What is the cardiac output when the heart rate is 42 beats per minute and the stroke volume is 60 ml? b) What effects does the sympathetic nervous system have on the heart to increase cardiac output? c) What is the difference between cardiogenic shock and hypovolaemic shock?	a) *HR x SV = CO* *42 x 60 = 2,520 ml or 2.52 litres.* b) *Increasing heart rate, increasing contractility (increasing stroke volume), increasing AV node conduction.* c) *Cardiogenic shock occurs when the heart fails as a pump. Hypovolaemic shock occurs when fluid loss leads to an insufficient volume of blood to pump.*

Answers		
6	**Test ECG 1.1** **Use the first five ECG steps of the 9-step ECG interpretation tool to analyse Test ECG 1.1.**	***Test ECG 1.1 shows sinus rhythm.*** **1) *What is the rate and rhythm?*** *The rate is around 75 beats per minute and the rhythm is regular.* **2) *Are there any P waves and what is their relationship with the QRS complex?*** There are P waves before every QRS complex and there is a QRS complex after every P wave. The P-R interval is consistent and between 0.12 and 0.20 seconds (3–5 small squares).
		3) *What is the duration and morphology of the QRS complex?* The QRS complex is narrow with a duration under 0.12 seconds (under 3 small squares) and is of normal shape. **4) *Is the ST segment isoelectric, depressed or elevated?*** The ST segment is isoelectric. **5) *Are the QT intervals and T waves normal?*** The T wave is of normal shape and the QT interval is between 0.35 and 0.43 seconds (9–11 small squares).

Section 1 Self-Test ECG Answers

Test ECG 1.2: VF

Test ECG 1.3: VT

Test ECG 1.4: PEA

Test ECG 1.5: Asystole

References

1. T. Garcia, *12-Lead ECG: The Art of Interpretation*, 2nd edn. Burlington: Jones and Bartlett Learning, 2013.

2. S. J. Kovács, 'The heart as a pump: governing principles', in A. J. Camm et al., eds., *ESC CardioMed*, 3rd edn. Oxford: Oxford University Press, 2018.

3. D. E. Mohrman and L. J. Heller, *Cardiovascular Physiology*, 9th edn. New York: McGraw-Hill, 2018.

4. R. D. Evans et al., 'Cardiac physiology', in J. Firth, C. Conlon and T. Cox, eds., *Oxford Textbook of Medicine*, 6th edn. Oxford: Oxford University Press, 2020.

5. T. Matsuyama and H. Ishibashi-Ueda, 'Normal conduction system, coronary arteries, and coronary veins', in A. J. Camm et al., eds., *ESC CardioMed*, 3rd edn. Oxford: Oxford University Press, 2018.

6. M. Malik, 'Cardiac electrophysiology', in A. J. Camm et al., eds., *ESC CardioMed*, 3rd edn. Oxford: Oxford University Press, 2018.

7. J. Loscalzo, P. Libby and C. A. MacRae, 'Basic biology of the cardiovascular system', in *Harrison's Principles of Internal Medicine*. New York: McGraw-Hill, 2018.

8. V. Namana et al., 'Clinical significance of atrial kick', *Quarterly Journal of Medicine*, vol. 111, no. 8, 2018, pp. 569–570.

9. R. Kurapati, J. Heaton and D. R. Lowery, 'Atrial kick', *StatPearls* [Online], 2020. Available from: https://www.ncbi.nlm.nih.gov/books/NBK482421/.

10. J. S. Shahoud, M. Ambalavanan and V. S. Tivakaran, 'Cardiac dominance', *StatPearls* [Online], 2020. Available: https://www.ncbi.nlm.nih.gov/books/NBK537207/.

11. G. R. Nimmo and T. Walsh, 'Critical illness', in *Davidson's Principles and Practices of Medicine*. Edinburgh: Churchill Livingstone, 2014.

12. T. Standl et al., 'The nomenclature, definition and distinction of types of shock', *Continuing Medical Education*, vol. 115, no. 45, 2018, pp. 757–768.

13. F. G. Bonanno, 'Clinical pathology of the shock syndromes', *Journal of Emergency Trauma and Shock*, vol. 4, no. 2, 2011, pp. 233–243.

14. C. Vahdatpour, D. Collins and S. Goldberg, 'Cardiogenic shock', *Journal of the American Heart Association*, vol. 8, no. 8, 2019, pp. 1–12.

15. A. R. Houghton and D. Gray, 'Electrocardiography', in J. Firth, C. Conlon and T. Cox, eds., *Oxford Textbook of Medicine*, 6th edn. Oxford: Oxford University Press, 2020.

16. D. E. Newby, N. R. Grubb and A. Bradbury, 'Cardiovascular disease', in *Davidson's Principles and Practices of Medicine*, 22nd edn. Edinburgh: Churchill Livingstone, 2014.

17. J. Loscalzo, 'Approach to the patient with possible cardiovascular disease', in *Harrison's Principles of Internal Medicine*. New York: McGraw-Hill, 2018.

18. A. J. Innes, A. R. Dover and K. Fairhurst, eds., *Macleod's Clinical Examination*. Edinburgh: Elsevier, 2018.

19. J. Thomas and T. Monaghan, eds., *Oxford Handbook of Clinical Examination and Practical Skills*. Oxford: Oxford University Press, 2014.

20. World Heart Federation, 'Cardiovascular risk factors' [Online], 2017. Available: https://world-heart-federation.org/world-heart-day/cvd-causes-conditions/risk-factors/.

21. NHS, 'Cardiovascular disease' [Online], 2018. Available: https://www.nhs.uk/conditions/cardiovascular-disease/.

22. J. Soar, C. D. Deakin, J. P. Nolan et al. 'Adult advanced life support guidelines', *Resuscitation Council UK* [online], 2021. Available: https://www.resus.org.uk/library/2021-resuscitation-guidelines/adult-advanced-life-support-guidelines.

23. Resuscitation Council (UK), 'Prehospital resuscitation', in *Resuscitation Guidelines 2015*. London: Resuscitation Council (UK), 2015.

24. Joint Royal College Ambulance Liaison Committee and Association of Ambulance Chief Executives, *JRCALC Clinical Guidelines 2019*. Bridgwater: Class Professional Publishing, 2019.

Arrhythmias (Rate and Rhythm Problems)

In this section we will look at arrhythmias – problems that are associated with the rate or rhythm of the heartbeat. Rate and rhythm can be assessed from a lead II rhythm strip alone, although we will look at examples of rate and rhythm problems on 12-lead ECGs at the end of this section.

Rate-related Problems

A heart beating too fast or too slow can often cause symptoms which lead to an ambulance being called. This can be due to symptoms caused by the heart rate, such as palpitations or chest pain, or symptoms associated with low blood pressure due to reduced cardiac output (page 13), such as dizziness and loss of consciousness.

Key Definitions[1, 2]
- Bradycardia: A heart rate below 60 beats per minute.
- Absolute bradycardia: A heart rate below 40 beats per minute.
- Tachycardia: A heart rate above 100 beats per minute.
  - These definitions apply to adults only. Children have different physiological parameters. See page 266 for paediatric-specific information.

A heart which is beating too quickly can be associated with hypotension in two ways. Most commonly, a tachycardia is part of the body's response to correct hypotension by increasing cardiac output (page 13). Less commonly, extreme tachycardia may be the primary cause of hypotension due to a reduction in stroke volume caused by reduced ventricular filling time. Chest pain or discomfort may also be present due to the increased effort and strain on the heart associated with the sustained increase in rate.

When we are interpreting an ECG and identifying a rate-related issue, we need to consider the origin of the problem. Is the tachycardia originating in the atria or the ventricles? Is the bradycardia still a sinus rhythm or an escape rhythm originating further along the electrical pathway?

Bradycardia and Absolute Bradycardia

Bradycardia and absolute bradycardia are differentiated by rate, with bradycardia being a ventricular rate below 60 beats per minute and absolute bradycardia being a ventricular rate below 40 beats per minute. Sinus bradycardia is an ECG diagnosis in itself, though a bradycardic heart rate is often found when assessing an ECG and forms part of a different arrhythmia.

Definition of Bradycardia[1, 2, 3, 4, 5]

There is ongoing debate over the definition of bradycardia. The discussion focuses on whether bradycardia can be defined as either 50 or 60 beats per minute. Resuscitation Council (UK) and the JRCALC Clinical Guidelines state that 60 beats per minute remains the definition, with the emphasis on treatment decisions being based on whether the bradycardia is symptomatic or impacting perfusion rather than on rate alone. The argument for 50 beats per minute is based on the fact that some people will have a natural resting heart rate below 60 beats per minute.

ECG Identification of Bradycardia[1, 2, 5, 6]

- Sinus bradycardia:
  - Ventricular rate below 60 beats per minute.
  - Normal P-QRS-T complexes with no change to rhythm.
- Symptomatic bradycardia:
  - Ventricular rate below 60 beats per minute *and* clinically symptomatic with signs of impaired perfusion (hypotensive, reduced level of consciousness, other clinical signs of circulatory shock).
- Absolute bradycardia:
  - Ventricular rate below 40 beats per minute.

ECG 2.1 – Sinus Bradycardia

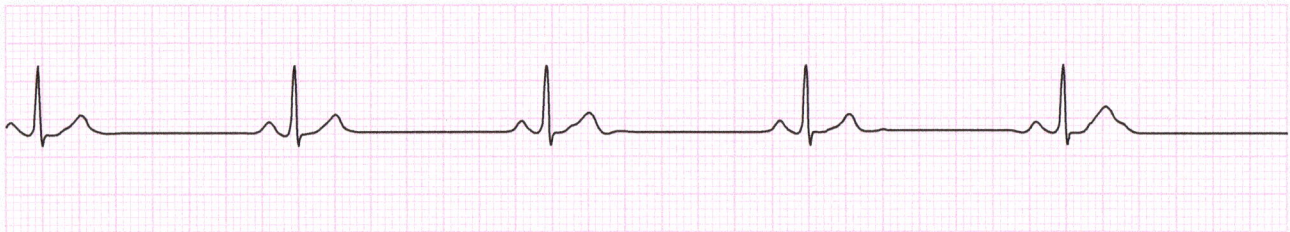

The only abnormality on this rhythm strip is the heart rate which is around 45 beats per minute. This EGC rhythm strip meets the criteria for sinus bradycardia. Remember to always consider the clinical criteria as well as the ECG criteria; this rhythm strip could be classified as symptomatic bradycardia if the patient were also showing signs of impaired perfusion.

ECG 2.2 – Absolute Bradycardia

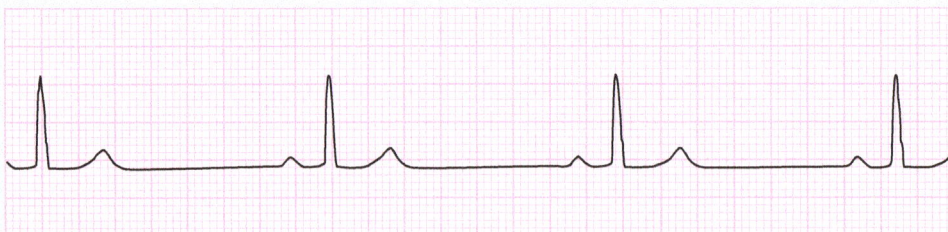

The only abnormality on this rhythm strip is the heart rate which is just above 30 beats per minute. This EGC rhythm strip meets the criteria for absolute bradycardia.

Clinical Presentation of Bradycardia[1, 7, 8, 9, 10]

Depending on the underlying cause of the bradycardia, the patient may present with:
- Chest pain, tightness or discomfort. Be alert for ischaemic ECG changes and signs of acute coronary syndrome (page 93).
- Shortness of breath.
- Signs and symptoms associated with circulatory shock (page 14), since bradycardia can reduce cardiac output:
  - Pale, cold and clammy skin.
  - Hypotension and weak or absent peripheral pulses.
  - Delayed capillary refill.
  - Tachypnoea.
  - Dizziness or near loss of consciousness.
  - Loss of consciousness or reduced level of consciousness.
  - Anxiety and confusion.

Causes of Bradycardia[4, 5, 6, 11, 12, 13, 14]

- Damage to the cardiac conduction system, through cardiac ischaemia, especially in right coronary artery occlusion (page 114).
- Sick sinus syndrome.
- Hypothermia.
- Cushing reflex.
- Hypoxia.
- Vagal nerve stimulation: Persistent vomiting, iatrogenic (suction, intubation).
- Drug overdoses, including:
  - Beta-adrenoceptor blocking drugs (beta blockers), including: atenolol, bisoprolol, metoprolol, propranolol.
  - Calcium channel blockers, including: amlodipine, nifedipine, diltiazem, verapamil.
  - Cardiac glycoside (digoxin).
  - Opioids, including: morphine, tramadol, codeine, methadone.
  - Cholinergic toxicity (organophosphates).

> In children, bradycardia is most commonly caused by hypoxia, requiring immediate oxygenation and management of airway, breathing and circulation. Atropine therapy for children is only indicated if the bradycardia is caused by vagal nerve stimulation.[1]

Management of Bradycardia[1, 2]

- The decision to provide treatment for bradycardia should be based on the patient's symptoms and if they are showing adverse clinical signs or signs of poor perfusion.
  - All patients with bradycardia should be monitored during transport. Bradycardia in the presence of 2nd degree type II (page 62) and 3rd degree heart blocks (page 64) carries an increased risk of asystole and should be monitored closely.
- Sinus bradycardia:
  - Sinus bradycardia alone does not require any specific clinical interventions, although you should be thorough in your assessment to identify any sinister underlying causes such as myocardial infarction (page 93).
  - Continuous monitoring and regular clinical observations during care and transport are important to allow early detection of deterioration.

- Symptomatic bradycardia and absolute bradycardia:
  - Consider oxygen therapy if signs of poor perfusion are present, following current oxygen administration guidelines.
  - Changes to the patient's positioning should be carefully considered; sitting up from a supine position or standing from a sitting position carry significant risk of postural hypotension which could potentially lead to loss of consciousness or cardiac arrest.
  - Gain IV access.
  - Atropine acts to increase heart rate by preventing the parasympathetic nervous system acting on the heart by blocking vagal activity, reversing vagal overdrive and enhancing A-V conduction. This in turn increases cardiac output, raising the patient's blood pressure. Depending on the underlying cause, some types of bradycardia will be resistant or unresponsive to atropine therapy or require several repeat doses before clinical improvement is seen. This is especially so if the bradycardia is caused by 3rd degree heart block (page 64).
    - Atropine is administered via intravenous or intraosseous routes and needs to be given as a rapid bolus. Repeat doses are given every 3–5 minutes if required to a maximum dose of 3 milligrams. Continuous ECG monitoring should take place during atropine therapy and a live ECG print-out obtained at the point of administration. This will provide a paper copy of any ECG changes or further arrhythmias that can occur during administration.
    - **Remember**: Always refer to and follow current national and local (employer) guidelines regarding drug administration.
  - Transcutaneous pacing by advanced care providers may be required if unresponsive to atropine therapy. If transcutaneous pacing is unavailable, percussion pacing (fist pacing) may be attempted.

Fluid Therapy in Cardiogenic Shock[1, 15]

A patient who is hypotensive due to cardiogenic shock is suffering from a relative drop in blood pressure due to pump failure causing a reduced cardiac output; the patient is not suffering from a decrease in blood volume due to fluid loss (hypovolaemia).

A healthy heart is not likely to enter into a state of cardiogenic shock; as such, there is a high likelihood that a patient suffering cardiogenic shock has significant underlying cardiac pathologies. In these patients, the smallest infusions of intravenous fluid may be enough to cause fluid overload, putting additional strain on the fragile heart and circulatory system and potentially leading to acute heart failure and pulmonary oedema.

In a hypotensive patient, a bolus of fluid will act to transiently raise blood pressure by increasing pre-load to the right side of the heart. If the patient is so hypotensive that end organ perfusion is compromised, then a fluid bolus may be the only immediate option to raise blood pressure to sufficiently protect the organs until definitive care is reached and the original cause of the hypotension is corrected. It should be noted that this would only serve as a transient increase in blood pressure, as it does not correct pump failure.

The decision to administer fluid therapy to a patient in apparent cardiogenic shock should be carefully considered and not taken lightly. The potential risks often outweigh the benefits and other methods to maintain blood pressure are often sufficient during transport to hospital.

The focus should first be to treat the reversible causes of the cardiogenic shock, such as the administration of atropine therapy for symptomatic bradycardia. Fluid therapy should only be considered if these treatments of the primary cause are ineffective and the clinical need is sufficient to outweigh the potential risks.

If the decision to administer fluid therapy is taken, doses should be titrated and kept to the minimum volume necessary to maintain end organ perfusion so as to minimise the risk of fluid overload and iatrogenic heart failure.

Relative Bradycardia[1]

Bradycardia is defined as a heart rate below 60 beats per minute, but a patient can be *relatively bradycardic* if their heart rate is inappropriately slow for their current physiological state. If an increased heart rate would be expected as part of the body's response to reduced cardiac output due to an emergent medical condition or traumatic injury, but the heart rate is not increased, this would be considered a relative bradycardia. This can occur when patients taking heart rate controlling medications, such as beta blockers, become unwell or injured.

Key Points: Bradycardia

- Bradycardia can be a diagnosis in itself or a result of other arrhythmias and cardiac conditions.
- The low heart rate associated with bradycardia can severely decrease cardiac output and cause cardiogenic shock.
- Atropine is used to treat absolute bradycardia. The administration of fluid therapy should be carefully considered and is often not appropriate. If administered, fluid should be used with caution to reduce the risk of fluid overload.

Narrow Complex Tachycardias

The terms 'narrow complex tachycardia' and 'Supraventricular Tachycardia' (SVT) are often used interchangeably as umbrella terms for any tachycardia originating above the ventricles. By originating above the ventricles, a tachycardia will normally have narrow QRS complexes (under 0.12 seconds, 3 small squares). The exception is if aberrant conduction (such as a bundle branch block, see page 124) is present within the ventricles, which makes the QRS complexes appear broad. Remember that 'tachycardia' means a rate above 100 beats per minute.

Settling for SVT or narrow complex tachycardia as a diagnosis should be avoided. Instead, identifying a narrow complex tachycardia should prompt you to consider the rhythms which fall under this umbrella as differential diagnoses to investigate further. A working diagnosis should be formed based on the ECG and the patient's presenting clinical signs and symptoms.[2, 16]

The term 'SVT' is widely, and incorrectly, used to describe a re-entrant tachycardia (see below). Usage of the term should be discouraged to avoid confusion. It is often simpler to avoid the term 'SVT' altogether and instead use 'narrow complex tachycardia' if unable to focus the diagnosis further.

Rhythms That Fall Under the Narrow Complex Tachycardia Umbrella

A narrow complex tachycardia can be either physiological or pathological in nature. The heart will naturally increase its rate to respond to physiological stresses within the body such as exercise, pain, infection or emotion. Pathological causes relate to when a problem has occurred within the electrical functioning of the heart leading to an increased heart rate.

Sinus Tachycardia

Sinus tachycardia is a physiological tachycardia and a common finding when assessing ECGs. Sinus tachycardia can be an ECG diagnosis in itself, but is often found alongside other ECG changes, especially when the tachycardia is present due to pain or cardiogenic shock (page 14) caused by myocardial infarction (page 93) or other emergent cardiac conditions. Sinus tachycardia is also a common ECG finding when a patient is suffering from a systemic illness that is not cardiac in origin.

ECG Identification of Sinus Tachycardia[1, 17, 18]

- Rate above 100 beats per minute. If above 140 beats per minute, consider possibility of re-entrant tachycardia (page 42).
- R-R variability. There is often a slight variability in the heart rate and the R-R interval for the same reasons as in sinus arrhythmia.
- QRS of normal duration and originating in the SA node, meaning:
  - P wave before each QRS complex.
  - QRS complex under 0.12 seconds, or 3 small squares.
  - If wide complex tachycardia is found, consider VT (page 49) or SVT with aberrant ventricular conduction (page 45).

ECG 2.3 – Sinus Tachycardia

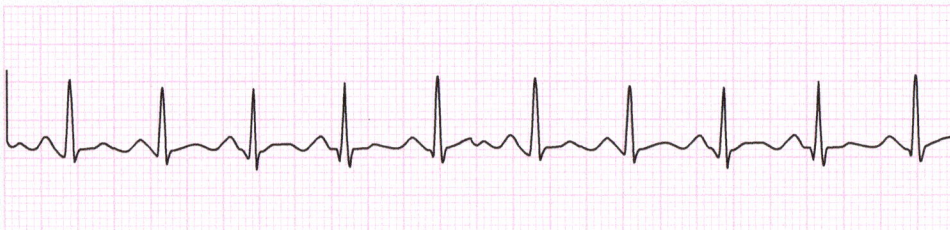

This rhythm strip meets the criteria for sinus tachycardia, as the heart rate is around 120 beats per minute. There is a slight variability between each R-R interval, further suggesting that the rhythm is sinus in origin.

Causes of Sinus Tachycardia[19, 20, 21]

- Increased demand for oxygen to the body:
  - Exercise.
  - Difficulty breathing or reduced lung function.
  - Increase in metabolic activity such as an inflammatory response to infection and sepsis.
- Compensation to increase cardiac output due to reduced stroke volume:
  - Circulatory shock (page 14).
  - Cardiomyopathy.

- Pharmacological:
  - ▸ Beta agonists (salbutamol).
  - ▸ Adrenaline.
  - ▸ Cocaine.
  - ▸ Caffeine.
  - ▸ Alcohol.
- Psychological and extreme emotion:
  - ▸ Fear.
  - ▸ Distress.
  - ▸ Anxiety.
  - ▸ Stress.
  - ▸ Pain.

Management of Sinus Tachycardia[1]

- Identify and treat the underlying cause. Sinus tachycardia is a reaction by the body to increase cardiac output (page 13) to meet physiological demand. All potentially sinister clinical physiological causes should be considered and excluded before assuming that sinus tachycardia is caused by psychological or emotional factors.
- Even when psychological factors are not the primary cause of sinus tachycardia, they can contribute to the increased heart rate through the patient's stress and anxiety associated with being ill and the perceived seriousness of their situation requiring an ambulance. This can be alleviated to some extent by providing appropriate reassurance and emotional support to the patient. The tachycardia may reduce or subside as they become calmer.
- Consider and exclude a re-entrant tachycardia (page 42).

Relative Tachycardia

Tachycardia is defined as a heart rate above 100 beats per minute. But a patient can be relatively tachycardic if their heart rate is normally low and is currently fast but not exceeding 100 beats per minute. For example, an athlete may have a documented resting heart rate of 40 beats per minute instead of the expected 60–80 beats per minute of a normal adult. If that athlete became unwell and had a heart rate of 90 beats per minute, it would appear as only a slight increase to a normal adult, but to this athlete it is actually over double their resting heart rate, making it of significant concern. This would be considered to be a relative tachycardia.

This is an important consideration when making clinical decisions. Tools such as the NEWS2 Score are based on the expected norm, and individual patient situations should be considered.

Hyperventilation Syndrome[1, 22, 23, 24]

Hyperventilation syndrome, also referred to as anxiety or panic attacks, can often present with symptoms that prompt the acquisition of an ECG. Around 25% of patients experiencing palpitations suffer from regular panic attacks, and chest pain and shortness of breath are common symptoms. It is common for tachycardia to be present during an episode of hyperventilation syndrome, driven by the associated anxiety and increased respiratory rate.

Hyperventilation syndrome is a diagnosis of exclusion; it shares key symptoms with ACS, pulmonary embolism and other potentially life-threatening conditions. As such, the safe diagnosis of hyperventilation syndrome relies on the appropriate exclusion of other sinister conditions, which is not always possible in the out-of-hospital environment. Although it is relatively common for a patient to be discharged from scene with a diagnosis of 'panic attack', great care should be taken by the attending clinician to thoroughly assess the patient and make sure the symptoms have resolved prior to discharge. Detailed and specific safety netting should be in place in these instances. Clinicians should hold a low threshold for conveyance or referral to onward care, especially if any discrepancy or uncertainty is present regarding the diagnosis of hyperventilation syndrome.

Re-entrant Tachycardias

Re-entrant tachycardia occurs when an electrical impulse wrongly re-enters the atria, or the AV node, via a re-entry pathway and prematurely triggers another heartbeat. This subsequent heartbeat also follows the re-entrant pathway, triggering another heart beat and so on. This prevents the SA node from maintaining a sinus rhythm. Because the re-entrant electrical impulse triggers the next heartbeat immediately, the heart rate increases to the maximum that the AV node will allow, ranging anywhere from 140 to 280 beats per minute depending on the specific patient.

The re-entrant pathway can be located within the AV node, known as an AV Nodal Re-entrant Tachycardia (AVNRT). The pathway can also be located outside of the AV node anywhere along the atrioventricular septum between the atria and the ventricles. This is called an AV Re-entrant Tachycardia (AVRT). Conditions such as Wolff-Parkinson-White syndrome (page 46) are precursors to AVRT and can be detected on an ECG when the heart is in sinus rhythm.[16]

It is difficult to differentiate between an AVNRT and an AVRT at the time of the arrhythmia. Often it is not possible or necessary for paramedics to differentiate between the two, thus it is sufficient to recognise the presence of a re-entrant tachycardia and provide appropriate management and transport.

ECG Identification of Re-entrant Tachycardia[2, 6, 21, 25, 26]

- Often the differentiation between a re-entrant tachycardia and sinus tachycardia can be challenging; see box (page 43) for more information.
- Rate above 140 beats per minute, can range from 140–280 beats per minute.
- Narrow QRS complex:
  - QRS complex under 0.12 seconds, or 3 small squares.
  - If wide complex tachycardia, consider VT (page 49) and narrow complex tachycardia with aberrant ventricular conduction (page 45).
    - Absent P waves.
    - Constant rate with little or no variability.

ECG 2.4 – Narrow Complex Tachycardia

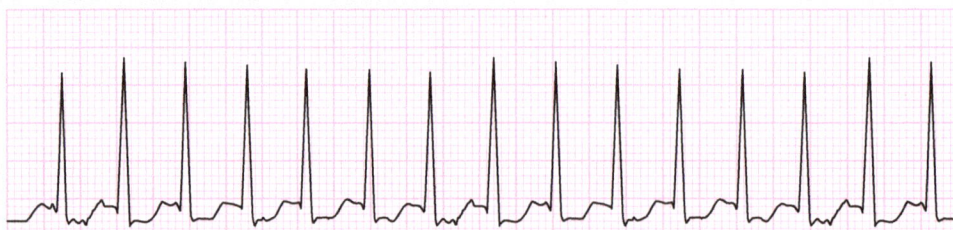

At first glance, we can establish that this is a narrow complex tachycardia. There are two indicators that suggest this rhythm is a re-entrant tachycardia. The rate of 180 beats per minute alone should make us consider re-entrant tachycardia as a differential. This rhythm is also very regular, with no rate variability, again suggesting it is not sinus in nature, but more likely a re-entrant tachycardia.

ECG 2.5 – Narrow Complex Tachycardia

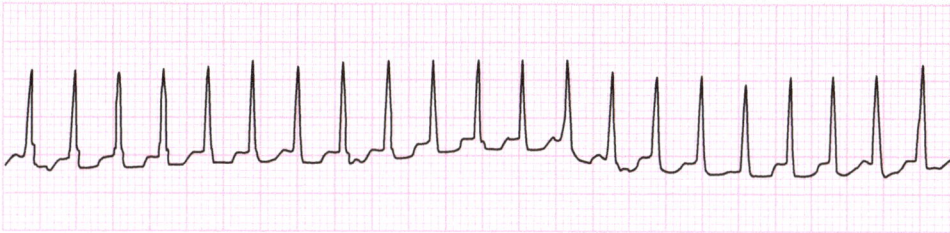

This narrow complex tachycardia has a rate of around 250 beats per minute. This is too fast for sinus tachycardia in an adult, immediately removing it as a differential. This rhythm is also regular, with no rate variability. This is a clear example of a re-entrant tachycardia. Once the arrhythmia resolved, this patient was found to have Wolff-Parkinson-White syndrome on their normal ECG.

Differentiating Sinus Tachycardia and Re-entrant Tachycardia[21, 25]

The following are all important considerations when trying to differentiate sinus tachycardia from re-entrant tachycardia:

- **History**: It cannot be overstated how important the history is in the differentiation between sinus tachycardia and re-entrant tachycardia. Patient experience may provide vital information if they have experienced these symptoms or have been diagnosed previously. If the symptoms were of sudden onset and without apparent cause, this might lead you towards a pathological re-entrant tachycardia, but if the patient has a physiological reason to be tachycardic, then sinus tachycardia is more likely. For example, a patient who experienced symptoms while at rest is more likely to have a pathological re-entrant tachycardia than if they had been exercising at the time of onset.
- **Rate**: Generally, the maximum sinus rate for a person is estimated using the formula of 220 beats per minute minus patient age (HRmax = 220 – age).[27] This means that a 25-year-old could be expected to show a sinus tachycardia up to a maximum of 195 beats per minute, whereas an 80-year-old would only be able to produce a sinus tachycardia rate at most of 140 beats per minute. Rates that go above this simple formula are unlikely to be sinus tachycardia. Equally, re-entrant tachycardia is unlikely if the rate is below 140 beats per minute.
- **Rate changes and variability**: In sinus tachycardia, the rate should increase and decrease gradually through physiological changes. If the rate varies with the patient's position, breathing or relaxation, it is strongly suggestive of sinus tachycardia. Re-entrant tachycardia usually starts and stops suddenly and remains at the same fixed rate when present.
- **Absent P waves**: The presence or absence of P waves is an unreliable differentiator; a re-entrant tachycardia will not have P waves due to the re-entry pathway. But sinus tachycardia can show the apparent absence of P waves with increased heart rates (usually above 150 beats per minute) due to the P wave being hidden or obscured by the preceding T wave or QRS complex.
- **Reaction to vagal stimulation**: In sinus tachycardia a gradual slowing may be seen. A sudden reduction to a slower rate or no effect at all is suggestive of re-entrant tachycardia.

Clinical Presentation of Re-entrant Tachycardia[18, 21, 25, 28]

- Palpitations, often uncomfortable and felt as sudden onset, regular and rapid.
- Loss of consciousness or near loss of consciousness due to reduced blood pressure caused by reduced cardiac output (page 13).
- Dizziness.
- Chest pain or tightness, especially if underlying coronary artery disease is present.
- Shortness of breath.
- Anxiety due to experiencing symptoms.
- Nausea.
- Diaphoresis.

Paroxysmal Re-entrant Tachycardia[21, 25, 29]

Paroxysmal re-entrant tachycardia, also known as Paroxysmal Supraventricular Tachycardia, or 'PSVT', describes episodes of re-entrant tachycardia which occur intermittently and start and end suddenly. They can often prove a challenge to diagnose as they can be difficult to capture on an ECG due to their intermittent occurrence and short duration. Patients may be given portable and wearable ECG recorders that they activate when experiencing symptoms. If you are called to a patient who is experiencing palpitations and is under investigation for PSVT, take an ECG tracing at the earliest opportunity to try and capture the arrhythmia before it self-terminates.

Management of Re-entrant Tachycardia[1, 2, 15, 16, 21]

- Consider oxygen therapy if signs of poor perfusion are present, following current oxygen administration guidelines.
- The patient is likely to be anxious or distressed due to the symptoms, so appropriate reassurance and a calm approach are beneficial.
- Assess for adverse or time-critical features, such as shock, loss of consciousness, myocardial ischaemia, heart failure.
- Consider gaining IV access if there are signs of haemodynamic compromise.
- The patient is unlikely to be haemodynamically unstable, but the faster the heart rate, the more likely they are to have a reduced cardiac output. As such, an extremely tachycardic patient may present with hypotension. As this is a relative hypotension due to reduced cardiac output, fluid therapy is normally not required and should be considered with great caution and only if signs of poor perfusion are present and after vagal manoeuvres and positional attempts to increase blood pressure have been attempted. See page 38 fluid therapy in cardiogenic shock.
- Unstable patients in re-entrant tachycardia may require synchronised cardioversion. This should only be carried out by appropriately qualified clinicians and where local protocols exist. This is currently beyond the scope of practice of the majority of frontline paramedics in the UK.
- Vagal manoeuvres may be attempted with the aim of ceasing a re-entrant tachycardia; however, these may be of limited effectiveness.

Modified Valsalva Manoeuvre and Vagal Manoeuvres[1, 2, 16, 21]

Vagal manoeuvres are attempts made by a clinician to stimulate the vagus nerve and cause an increase in parasympathetic drive in the hopes of slowing the heart rate.

The modified Valsalva manoeuvre (forced expiration against a closed glottis): With the patient in a semi-recumbent position, have them blow into a 20 ml syringe for 15 seconds. Follow immediately by repositioning the patient to a supine position with passive leg raise (to 45-degree angle) for a further 15 seconds. Monitor the patient's ECG rhythm during the attempt and where possible also continuously print a rhythm strip. Monitor for small reductions in heart rate which are suggestive of sinus tachycardia.

Aberrant Ventricular Conduction and Narrow Complex Tachycardia[2, 21, 25, 30]

If a patient has a new or pre-existent ventricular conduction abnormality (aberrant conduction), such as right or left bundle branch block (page 124), their ECG QRS complexes will be wider than 0.12 seconds (3 small squares). This can cause a narrow complex tachycardia to appear as a Ventricular Tachycardia (VT) (page 49).

Unless it is possible to establish a previous diagnosis of a bundle branch block or other form of aberrant conduction, or to confidently identify the presence of a bundle branch block, we must treat for the worst-case scenario and assume the patient is in VT. Even if the patient has a history of aberrant conduction it may be safer to treat and transport them as though the rhythm is VT.

The likelihood of VT increases if the patient has a family history of sudden cardiac death, is aged over 35 years or is in the presence of structural heart disease.

The likelihood of narrow complex tachycardia with aberrant conduction increases if the patient has had a previous diagnosis of Wolff-Parkinson-White syndrome (page 46), a bundle branch block (page 124) or re-entry tachycardias.

Rate-related aberrancy: A sudden increase in heart rate can cause the QRS complex to widen; this is due to the cardiac conduction system not being able to accommodate sufficiently by shortening its refractory periods. Once the refractory period has adapted, the QRS complex usually narrows. Depending on the heart rate, this aberrancy can appear as either a right or left bundle branch block.

Key Points: Narrow Complex Tachycardia
- Narrow complex tachycardia and SVT are umbrella terms which should prompt further differentiation to identify the specific rhythm.
- Sinus tachycardia is a common ECG finding, often co-existing alongside other arrhythmias.
- It may not be possible to determine the exact cause of a narrow complex tachycardia and the priority should be to manage the patient's clinical presentation and provide transport to further care.

Wolff-Parkinson-White Syndrome

In Wolff-Parkinson-White (WPW) syndrome there is an additional pathway for electrical activity to travel between the atria and the ventricles. Additional pathways are referred to as 'accessory pathways'; in the case of WPW syndrome the pathway is known as the bundle of Kent.[31] This accessory pathway allows electrical activity to bypass the AV node and move directly between the top and bottom of the heart through the atrioventricular septum (Figure 2.1). The most common location for the accessory pathway is within the fibrous tissue surrounding the mitral or tricuspid valves. Unlike the AV node, accessory pathways have no ability to control the rate of their electrical conduction; this is what can lead to tachycardias developing.

The accessory pathway may allow electrical activity to travel in both directions. When travelling from the atria to the ventricles, this causes an area of ventricular muscle to depolarise prematurely. A re-entrant pathway is present if electrical activity can travel 'up' from the ventricles into the atria. This can lead to a re-entrant tachycardia (page 42).[16, 31]

When residing in sinus rhythm, the only clue to the presence of an accessory pathway is the presence of a delta wave, seen at the beginning of the QRS complex. This delta wave occurs due to early depolarisation of a portion of the ventricles as electrical activity moves through the accessory pathway from the atria. This majority of the ventricular muscle depolarises normally as the electrical activity passes through the AV node, the delta wave ends as the normal depolarisation takes over and the R wave sharply increases its angle and amplitude. This makes the QRS complex a fusion beat between the normal depolarisation and the depolarisation from the accessory pathway.[16]

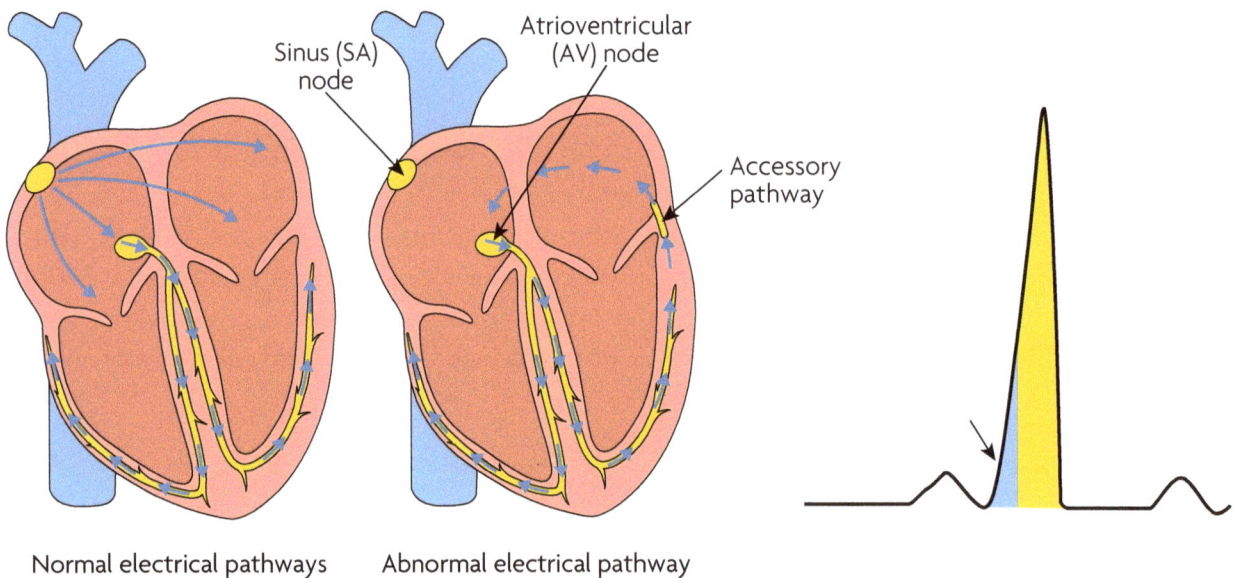

Figure 2.1 Normal conduction pathway (left) and accessory pathway causing pre-excitation and re-entry (right).

ECG Identification of Wolff-Parkinson-White Syndrome[16, 17, 31]

- A delta wave is present in the initial phase of the QRS complex. It is seen as a widening and slurring of the first upstroke of the R wave.
- This causes the QRS to be wide, greater than 0.10 seconds.
- A short PR interval will also be present.
- There may also be an increased QRS complex amplitude, T wave abnormalities and Q waves. These are caused by the fusion beat between the accessory pathway and normal depolarisation.

ECG 2.6a – Wolff-Parkinson–White syndrome

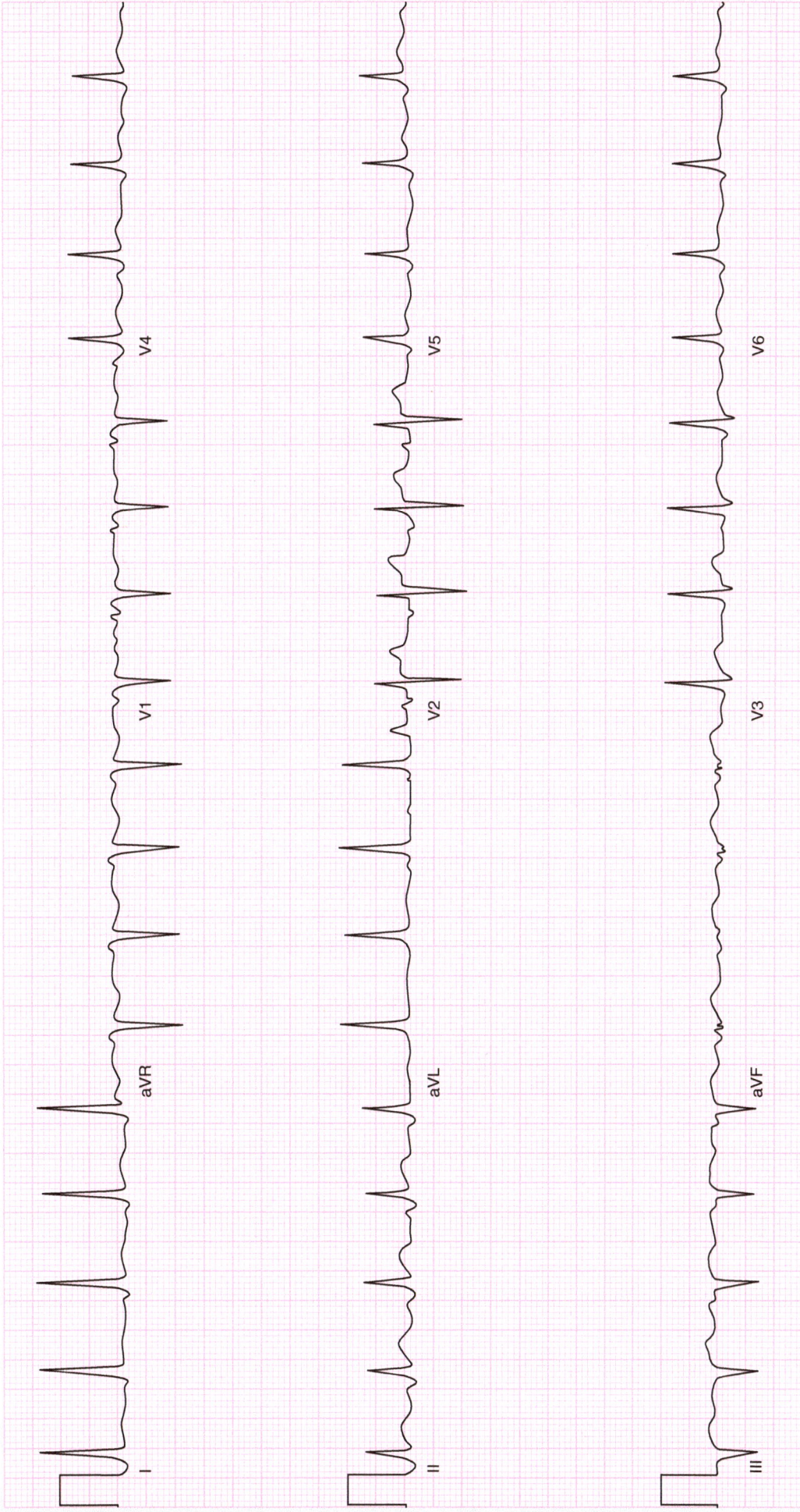

Initially, this ECG may appear normal, but on closer inspection we can see it meets the criteria for WPW syndrome. The QRS complexes are on the wider side of normal, at around 0.11 seconds. The delta waves can be difficult to spot in some lead views. They can be seen in leads I and II, but they are most clearly seen in leads V4, V5 and V6. There is also a short PR interval.

ECG 2.6b – AVRT

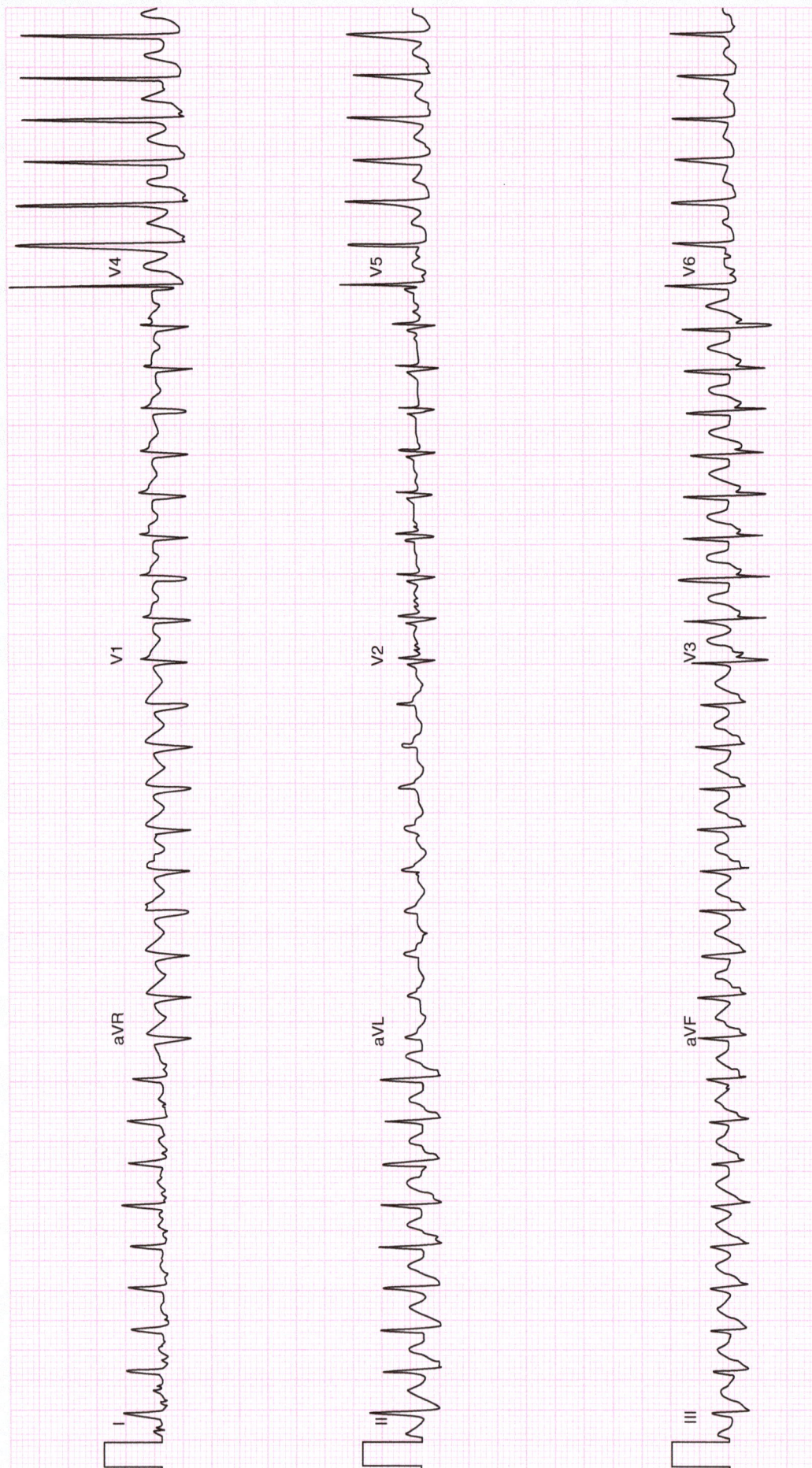

This ECG is from the same patient as ECG 2.6a; it was taken during a symptomatic episode of AVRT. The rate is around 220 beats per minute and there is no rate variability; combining this with the patient's history of WPW syndrome, the diagnosis of AVRT/re-entrant tachycardia is clear.

Clinical Presentation of Wolff-Parkinson-White Syndrome[16, 31]

- In WPW syndrome, the accessory pathway on its own does not create any clinical signs or symptoms.
- It may be that you are called to a patient who has experienced symptoms in keeping with a re-entrant tachycardia (page 42) that has now resolved. It may be the case that the patient has WPW syndrome and has experienced a self-limiting episode of re-entrant tachycardia. Having resolved, the only likely abnormal finding on the ECG will be a delta wave as described above.

Causes of Wolff-Parkinson-White Syndrome[16, 31]

- WPW syndrome is a congenital condition which develops during fetal development and is present at birth. It can become symptomatic at any age, though most commonly between the ages of 30 and 40 years old.

Management of Wolff-Parkinson-White Syndrome[1, 16]

- WPW itself is not immediately dangerous and as such there is no out-of-hospital treatment aside from recognition and appropriate referral.
- See page 44 for treatment of the re-entrant tachycardias which may result from WPW syndrome.
- If a patient with previously diagnosed WPW syndrome is found to be in atrial fibrillation, rapid transport with pre-alert message and continuous ECG monitoring is required as there is an imminent risk of ventricular fibrillation and cardiac arrest.

> !
> If atrial fibrillation occurs in the presence of an accessory pathway, it conducts a rapid and irregular rhythm to the ventricles causing a wide QRS complex and carrying a high risk of deteriorating into ventricular fibrillation or ventricular tachycardia.[32]

Broad Complex Tachycardia[1, 2, 21]

The term broad complex tachycardia is used to describe any tachycardia where the QRS complex is wider than 0.12 seconds (3 small squares). The vast majority of broad complex tachycardias are VT; as such all broad complex tachycardias should be considered to be VT until proven otherwise. Another less common cause of broad complex tachycardia is a supraventricular tachycardia with aberrant conduction (page 45).

Ventricular Tachycardia

Ventricular Tachycardia (VT) is a tachyarrhythmia which originates in the ventricles and is dissociated from any underlying atrial activity. The most common cause of VT is a re-entrant circuit formed after cardiac muscle damage occurs within the ventricles. In VT, the ventricular muscle cells continuously depolarise due to a re-entrant pathway, allowing the electrical impulse to continuously circulate within and around the ventricles.

VT causes a reduction in cardiac output and can lead to cardiac arrest, particularly at faster rates above 200 beats per minute or if underlying structural heart disease is present.[33, 34]

ECG Identification of Ventricular Tachycardia[2, 6, 17, 18, 33]

- Three or more ectopic ventricular complexes in a row with a heart rate above 100 beats per minute.
- Rate greater than 100 beats per minute (usually between 120–300 beats per minute).
- Wide and bizarre QRS complex.
- Regular rhythm with complete loss of baseline.
- Fusion and capture beats may be seen if there is still underlying atrial activity. They occur because the sinus beat partially depolarises the ventricles alongside the re-entrant pathway. P waves may be seen as notching on the ventricular QRS complexes.

Remember! Broad complex tachycardia is considered VT until proven otherwise.

!

ECG 2.7 – Ventricular Tachycardia

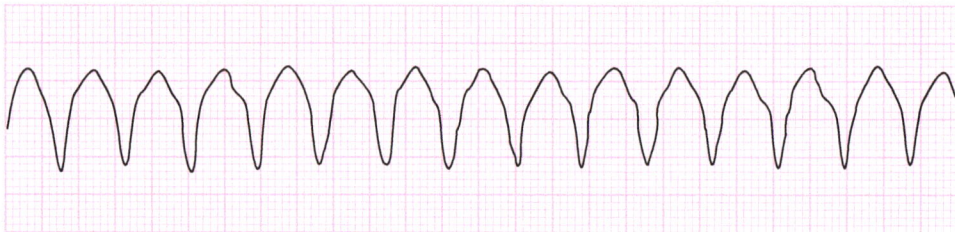

This is a classic example of VT. The regular, wide and bizarre QRS complex sits at a rate of around 200 beats per minute.

Classification of Ventricular Tachycardia[18]

- Monomorphic VT: The morphology (shape) of all the QRS complexes is the same. Often described as 'sawtooth' in appearance.
- Polymorphic VT: The morphology of the QRS complexes continuously changes from beat to beat and appears to 'twist and turn' along the central axis. Torsade de pointes is a form of polymorphic VT.

Clinical Presentation of Ventricular Tachycardia[6, 7, 8, 9, 10, 18, 33]

- The patient may present in cardiac arrest.
- VT reduces cardiac output, so the patient will likely present with signs and symptoms associated with circulatory shock (page 14):
    - Pale, cold and clammy skin.
    - Hypotension and weak or absent peripheral pulses.
    - Delayed capillary refill.
    - Tachypnoea.
    - Dizziness or near loss of consciousness.
    - Loss of consciousness or reduced level of consciousness.
    - Anxiety and confusion.

- Palpitations.
- Chest pain or discomfort.
- Shortness of breath.
- Fatigue.
- Diaphoresis.
- Abrupt or sudden onset of symptoms.

Causes of Ventricular Tachycardia[6, 33, 34]

- VT most commonly occurs when the ventricular cardiac muscle has become damaged and a re-entrant pathway has formed within the scar tissue. Common causes of cardiac muscle damage include:
  - Myocardial infarction (page 93).
  - Ischaemic heart disease.
  - Cardiomyopathy (page 122).
  - Cardiac surgery.

Management of Ventricular Tachycardia[1, 15, 34, 35, 36]

- All classifications of VT require the same out-of-hospital management.
- Cardiac arrest:
  - Resuscitate following national and local guidelines for shockable rhythms.
- If not in cardiac arrest, the patient is in an unstable peri-arrest state and requires rapid transport with hospital pre-alert and support of ABCs en route.
- Consider oxygen therapy if signs of poor perfusion are present, following current oxygen administration guidelines.
- Commence ventilatory support if required.
- Gain IV access.
- Consider fluid therapy to address hypotension (page 38).
- Be prepared for imminent cardiac arrest and the need for immediate defibrillation.
- Patients in sustained pulsed VT may require synchronised cardioversion. This should only be carried out by appropriately qualified clinicians and where local protocols exist. This is currently beyond the scope of practice of the majority of frontline paramedics in the UK.

Polymorphic VT and Torsade de Pointes[2, 33]

In clinical practice, Torsade de Pointes (TdP) and polymorphic VT are often thought of as the same rhythm but there are actually some variations between them. The only way to distinguish between the two is on review of the patient's ECG when, and if, it has returned to a sinus rhythm. TdP is diagnosed in the presence of Long QT syndrome. It is caused by 'R on T', a phenomenon which occurs when the ventricles begin to depolarise whilst parts of them are still repolarising; on an ECG this is seen as an R wave on top of a T wave, thus giving the term 'R on T'.

ECG 2.8 – Torsade De Pointes

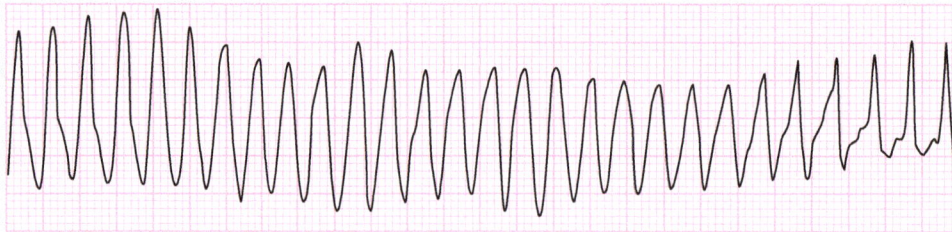

An example of torsade de pointes, a form of polymorphic VT. We can see that the amplitude of the waves increases and decreases in a cyclic fashion, helping to distinguish it from monomorphic VT.

Long QT Syndrome

When the QT interval prolongates and exceeds the maximum normal duration, the patient has Long QT Syndrome (LQTS). Normal QT interval duration differs according to the patient's sex. Long QT syndrome is present if the QT interval is greater than 0.46 seconds in females and greater than 0.44 seconds in males.[37] Because 0.44 seconds is represented by 11 small squares on an ECG, this is commonly used as the upper 'normal' QT interval; any QT interval greater than this prompts further investigation or calculation.

A prolonged QT interval is associated with the development of potentially fatal tachyarrhythmias such as torsade de pointes and is responsible for many of the sudden cardiac deaths seen in young people.

In a normally functioning heart, the QT interval shortens as heart rate increases and lengthens as heart rate decreases. Because of this, a corrected QT interval needs to be used to determine if long QT syndrome is actually present. There are multiple formulas used to calculate the QT corrected (QTc) value and many websites provide a calculator. Fortunately, most ECG monitors automatically calculate and print out the QTc value with each 12-lead ECG. This allows a rapid check to determine whether the QTc is within normal parameters or is prolonged. An obvious and extreme elongation of the QT segment can be detected on the ECG and give rise to suspected Long QT syndrome without calculating QTc.[37, 38, 39]

ECG 2.9 – Long QT Syndrome

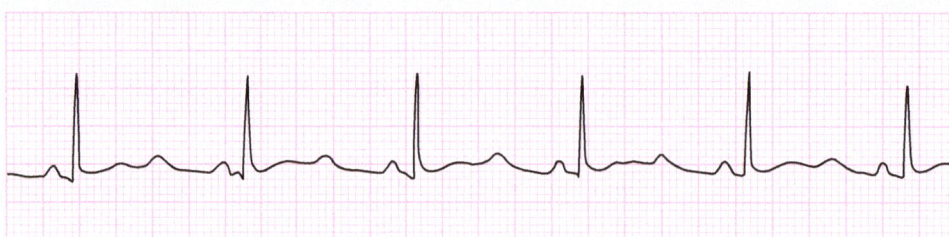

This ECG shows sinus rhythm with a rate of around 68 beats per minute. We can clearly see that the QT interval is just over 0.52 seconds (13 small squares), well above the 0.46 second upper limit for QT interval in this female patient.

Bazett Formula for Calculating QT Corrected[37, 38, 39, 40]

Bazett Formula allows the 'correction' of a QT interval to the value of a heart rate of 60 beats per minute, providing a QT corrected (QTc) theoretical value for the patient. It is not normally necessary to calculate QTc as most ECG monitors do this automatically and print the QTc value with each 12-lead ECG.

Bazett Formula: $QTc = QT$ interval in seconds $/ \sqrt{}$ cardiac cycle in seconds.

For example: A QT interval of 0.32 seconds and a heart rate of 120 beats per minute (cardiac cycle = 0.5 seconds) would fit into the formula as [0.32/√0.5 = 0.32/0.7 = QTc 0.45].

$$QTc = \frac{QT \text{ interval in seconds}}{\sqrt{\text{cardiac cycle in seconds}}}$$

Clinical Presentation of Long QT Syndrome[41]

- Long QT syndrome in itself is not symptomatic. Frequently, it is only detected when a patient has received an ECG for an unrelated reason, for cardiac screening or after they have suffered an episode of torsade de pointes or transient loss of consciousness.

Causes of Long QT Syndrome[6, 34, 42]

Long QT syndrome can be either inherited or acquired. Acquired Long QT syndrome may resolve when the cause no longer affects the heart. Multiple causes of Long QT syndrome can be accumulative and result in an even longer QT interval. This can further increase the risks of an associated arrhythmia occurring.

- Causes of Long QT syndrome may be:
  - Inherited.
  - Acquired:
    - Electrolyte imbalances (page 143).
    - Myocardial infarction/ischaemia (page 93).
    - Neurological conditions (page 148).
    - HIV.
    - Hypothermia
    - Pharmacologically induced:
      - Ondansetron.
      - Metoclopramide.
      - Cocaine.
      - Methadone.
      - Tricyclic anti-depressants.
      - Anti-psychotics.
      - Selective Serotonin Reuptake Inhibitors (SSRIs).
      - Anti-arrhythmics such as amiodarone.
      - Many antibiotics.
      - Some non-sedating anti-histamines.

Bundle branch blocks (page 124) also lengthen the QT Interval on the ECG, but this is not true Long QT syndrome as it is the QRS width that causes the increased length. As such, the associated risks of Long QT syndrome are not present.

Management and Risk of Long QT Syndrome[1]

- There are no specific out-of-hospital management priorities when Long QT syndrome has been detected.
- If the patient has not previously been diagnosed with Long QT syndrome, your detection and referral may prevent them suffering a potentially fatal arrhythmia in the future.
- The patient may have associated signs and symptoms of an acquired cause of Long QT syndrome; these should be managed as per clinical practice guidelines.
- Use extreme caution when considering the administration of any QT-lengthening medications such as ondansetron or metoclopramide.

Risk

Torsade de pointes is caused by the 'R on T' phenomenon which occurs when the ventricles begin to depolarise while parts of them are still repolarising. On an ECG this will be seen as an R wave on top of a T wave, thus the term 'R on T'. In a normally functioning heart the QT interval shortens as the heart rate increases and prevents an 'R on T' from occurring. But in Long QT syndrome there is a risk that 'R on T' will occur when the heart rate increases. This can lead to torsade de pointes during exercise and exertion, which may result in syncope during exercise or cardiac arrest.[1, 38, 43]

All patients who suffer transient loss of consciousness, near-syncope or palpitations during exercise or exertion should receive a 12-lead ECG and have it assessed for the possible presence of Long QT syndrome.[41, 43]

Rhythm Problems

Atrial Fibrillation

Atrial fibrillation, usually referred to as 'AF', is the most common sustained arrhythmia.[44] An estimated one million people in the UK are living with AF at any given time, with around 7% of people aged over 65 years suffering from the condition.[45] Every year, between 10–40% of patients with AF are admitted to hospital.[46]

In clinical practice, the majority of times a clinician will encounter AF is in patients where it has been previously diagnosed and may not be directly related to the patient's current clinical presentation. Despite this, it is important to always consider if AF is affecting the patient or their current clinical presentation.

In atrial fibrillation, the SA node does not have control of the atria; rather, the atria are fibrillating, or 'shaking'. There are no P waves present and instead the isoelectric line shows constant fibrillation of the atria. There is no organised contraction and as such no active cardiac output from the atria to the ventricles.[6, 17]

Atrial Kick[6, 46, 47, 48, 49, 50]

The ventricles receive around 20–30% of the blood for each heartbeat from atrial contraction; this is known as the 'atrial kick'. The other 70–80% of blood the ventricles receive is from passive filling, where blood flows through the atria into the ventricles during diastole (page 10). Thus, when the atria are not functioning effectively, such as in AF, the heart continues to function effectively, maintaining blood pressure and circulation, albeit with a reduced cardiac output due to the lost 20–30% from the atrial kick. This can also lead to worsening signs and symptoms of heart failure in patients with poor left ventricular function. Twenty to thirty per cent of AF patients are found to have left-sided heart failure.

ECG 2.10 – Atrial Fibrillation

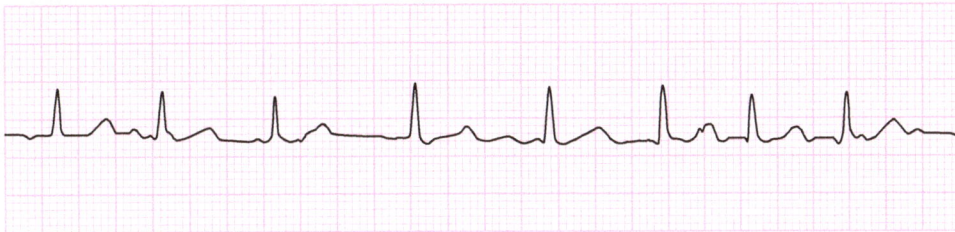

This is a classic example of AF. The ventricular rate is irregularly irregular, there are no P waves and the baseline is fibrillating.

Atrial Fibrillation with Rapid Ventricular Response[51]

If untreated, atrial fibrillation normally has a rapid ventricular response with a ventricular rate above 110 beats per minute. This is called atrial fibrillation with rapid ventricular response (previously, and sometimes still, referred to as 'fast atrial fibrillation'), or uncontrolled atrial fibrillation, and is a form of supraventricular tachycardia (page 39). When drug therapy is commenced to control the rate by slowing the ventricular response, the heart rate should stay below 110 beats per minute. This is referred to as controlled atrial fibrillation, or often simply atrial fibrillation. The majority of patients you will encounter with diagnosed atrial fibrillation will be medicated and in a controlled state of atrial fibrillation.

ECG 2.11 – Atrial Fibrillation with Rapid Ventricular Response

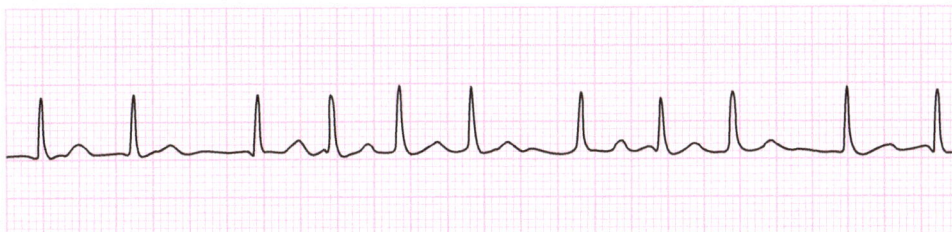

This example of AF with rapid ventricular response has a coarse, fibrillating baseline. Taken in isolation, some of the fibrillation waves can appear as P waves, creating a misleading diagnosis. There is an irregularly irregular ventricular rate at around 130 beats per minute; coupled with the absent P waves and fibrillating baseline, this meets the criteria for AF with rapid ventricular response.

Clinical Presentation of Atrial Fibrillation[6, 46]

- AF can be symptomatic or asymptomatic. It may be that the patient is presenting with signs and symptoms either of the condition that has led to them develop AF, or of a condition, medication or event that is the result of AF.

- Symptoms of AF are more likely at the onset of the rhythm and in paroxysmal atrial fibrillation, which can cause a reduced cardiac output and associated symptoms (page 13).
  - Symptoms of AF include:
    - Palpitations.
    - Fatigue.
    - Shortness of breath.
    - Symptoms of angina.
  - AF often progresses from short and infrequent episodes that spontaneously terminate, to longer and more sustained episodes that can become permanent.
  - Often when a patient is diagnosed with atrial fibrillation, their heart will remain in this rhythm as permanent AF and they will be prescribed preventative medications.
  - 'Silent AF' is asymptomatic, is often undetected and can lead to serious complications such as stroke and death.

Causes of Atrial Fibrillation[46, 49, 50]

- Hypertension.
- Myocardial infarction.
- Ischaemic heart disease.
- Chronic lung disease.
- Advanced age.
- Hypoxia.
- Hypothermia.
- Left atrial enlargement.
- Heart valve disease.
- Cardiac surgery.
- Excessive alcohol consumption.
- Thyroid disease.
- Respiratory disease.
- Chronic kidney disease.
- Smoking.

Management of Atrial Fibrillation[1, 6, 29, 44, 46, 52]

- If a patient has not previously been diagnosed with AF, history should be obtained with a focus on trying to detect a potential cause for the new onset atrial fibrillation and their clinical presentation should be managed as appropriate.
- The fibrillating atria create an increased risk of blood clot formation, putting the patient at increased risk of stroke and pulmonary embolism. AF is thought to account for 14% of all strokes and is associated with increased mortality, with 20–30% of patients with ischaemic stroke having previously been diagnosed with AF during or after the event.
- Up to 25% of stroke patients have AF on their pre-hospital ECG. If a patient is FAST-positive, transport should not be delayed in order to obtain a 12-lead ECG as it is unlikely to have any additional diagnostic value and is associated with worse outcomes in these patients.
- In previously diagnosed AF, the patient is likely to be prescribed preventative medication; be alert to potential side-effects that may relate to the current presenting complaint.
- Paroxysmal atrial fibrillation may cause the patient to become haemodynamically unstable due to the body's compensatory mechanisms not having had a chance to take effect. Support ABCs and initiate rapid transport.
- Remember that AF with a ventricular rate above 100 beats per minute is a form of narrow complex tachycardia (page 39).
- If a patient with heart failure has developed AF, their heart failure symptoms may have worsened depending on their left ventricular function.

Classifications of Atrial Fibrillation[6, 46, 50]

AF is classified depending on the frequency and duration of its occurrence.

- Paroxysmal AF: Self-terminating within seven days of onset. Often terminating within 48 hours. More likely to be symptomatic than other forms of AF.
- Persistent AF: Does not self-terminate and lasts longer than seven days or until treatment.
- Permanent or accepted AF: Not terminated or restarting after termination is attempted. Lasting longer than one year.

Atrial Flutter

Atrial flutter occurs when an area of cardiac muscle tissue within the right atrium becomes scarred or enlarged, causing electrical impulses to travel more slowly through this area than via surrounding, healthy tissue.[6] This forms a re-entry circuit within the atria, leading to electrical impulses circling the atria and causing them to constantly depolarise and repolarise. This typically occurs at their maximum rate (in adults) of 300 beats per minute. The atria contract marginally, with little strength due to the high rate, thus reducing the amount of blood actively pumped into the ventricles from the atria, as is the case with AF (page 54). Atrial flutter is a transient rhythm that can last from minutes to days; it can self-resolve back into sinus rhythm or deteriorate into atrial fibrillation.

ECG Identification of Atrial Flutter[2, 17, 18, 26, 32]

- Atrial rate of 300 beats per minute (can be between 250–350, most often around 300).
- 'Saw tooth' F waves (P waves), with a loss of baseline (no isoelectric segments).
- Regular and rapid ventricle response at a rate of 100–150 beats per minute.
  - The ventricular rate is determined by the ratio of atrial beats that are conducted by the AV node.
  - If every second atrial beat is conducted, then the ventricular rate would be 150 (300/2 =150) with a 2:1 conduction ratio.
  - If every third atrial beat is conducted, the ventricular rate would be 100 (300/3=100) with a 3:1 conduction ration.
  - Other conduction ratios are possible, but 2:1 is the most common.

ECG 2.12 – Atrial Flutter

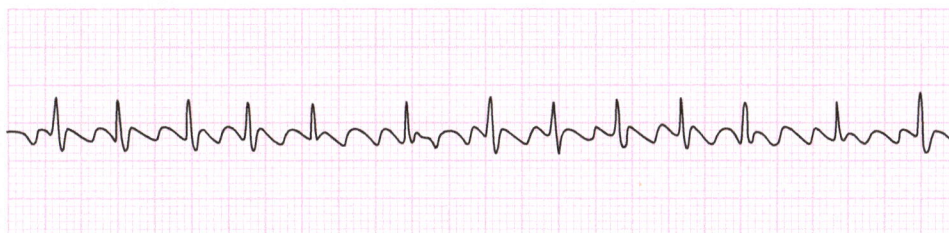

This is an example of atrial flutter with variable conduction. The majority are 2:1 conduction but there are occasional QRS complexes with 3:1 conduction. The atrial rate is around 300 beats per minute, with the ventricular rate sitting around 150 beats per minute. These findings should guide us to diagnosing this 'SVT' as atrial flutter.

Clinical Presentation of Atrial Flutter[18]

- Tachycardia.
- Palpitations.
- Shortness of breath.
- Fatigue.
- Chest pain or discomfort.
- Dizziness, syncope or near-syncope.

Causes of Atrial Flutter[18, 32, 53]

The risks of developing atrial flutter increase with age and the presence of co-morbidities, particularly heart failure (3.5 times more likely) and COPD (1.9 times more likely). Sex also affects incidence, with atrial flutter being 2.5 times more common in men.

- Heart failure.
- COPD.
- Myocardial infarction.
- Digoxin toxicity.
- Excessive alcohol consumption.
- Thyrotoxicosis.
- Pulmonary embolism.
- Pericarditis.
- Atherosclerosis.
- Right middle lobe pneumonia.
- Previous heart surgery.

Management of Atrial Flutter[1, 46]

- In the out-of-hospital environment there are no specific treatments for atrial flutter. Recognition and appropriate onward referral are key.
- If the patient is haemodynamically unstable, support ABCs and initiate rapid transport.
- Search for clues to a sinister underlying cause of the atrial flutter; does the patient have signs of myocardial infarction or other cardiac risk?
- Patients with atrial flutter share similar risk of stroke from thrombus formation as those with AF (page 54).

Atrial Flutter Mimics

- Atrial fibrillation can resemble atrial flutter in ECG lead V1.
- Parkinson's disease tremors may mimic flutter waves on the ECG.

Wandering Atrial Pacemaker

A Wandering Atrial Pacemaker (WAP) rhythm occurs when three or more ectopic pacemaker cell groups within the atria are consistently producing conducted electrical impulses. Each of these ectopic pacemaker cell groups will produce different morphologies of P waves.

ECG Identification of Wandering Atrial Pacemaker[17]

- Irregularly irregular rhythm.
- Three or more P wave morphologies each with their own PR interval duration.
- Rate less than 100 beats per minute.

Causes of Wandering Atrial Pacemaker

Causes include:
- Lung disease.
- Enhanced vagal stimulation.

ECG 2.13 – Wandering Atrial Pacemaker

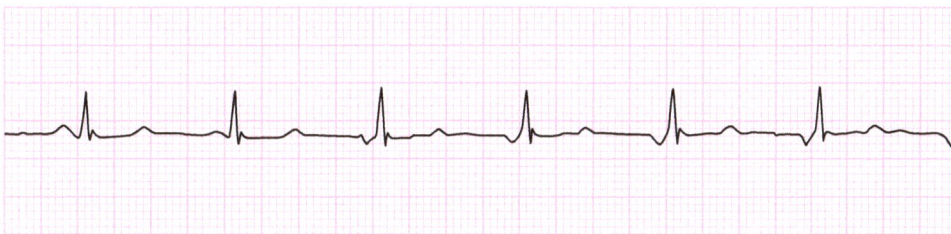

If you were to look at any one of these heartbeats in isolation you might struggle to find any abnormality. But analysing the rhythm as a whole shows us that there are multiple, different P wave morphologies. The rhythm is subtly irregularly irregular and the PR interval is variable. These findings together give us a diagnosis of WAP.

Multifocal Atrial Tachycardia

Multifocal Atrial Tachycardia (MAT) occurs when a wandering atrial pacemaker rhythm exceeds 100 beats per minute. This difference in rate is the only differentiating factor between WAP and MAT on an ECG. Patients may experience symptoms including palpitations and fatigue.[18, 21]

ECG 2.14 – Multifocal Atrial Tachycardia

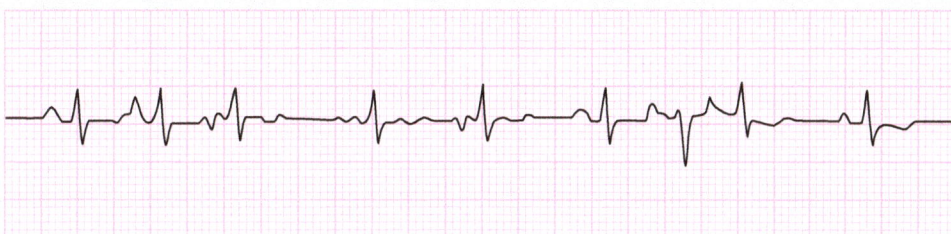

This is an example of MAT. With an irregularly irregular rate of around 115 beats per minute, this rhythm strip has several different P wave morphologies and meets the criteria for WAP, but as the rate is above 100 beats per minute it is a MAT.

Heart Blocks

The term 'heart block' refers to a disruption or block in the normal electrical conduction pathway of the heart where the electrical impulse is either delayed or blocked from reaching the ventricles. There are several types of heart block, all with varying degrees of severity and associated clinical risks.[54]

Heart blocks fall into two distinct groups:

- Atrioventricular (AV) blocks which occur at the AV node or within the bundle of His and cause rhythm abnormalities. AV blocks are seen on the ECG through the relationship between the P waves and QRS complexes.
- Vesicular blocks which occur below the level of the AV node, in the electrical pathways within the ventricles, and cause intra-ventricular conduction abnormalities. Vesicular blocks affect the morphology (shape) of the QRS complex as the block occurs below the level of the AV node and within the ventricles. As vesicular blocks do not cause rhythm disturbances and require a 12-lead ECG for identification, they are covered further in Section 3 on page 124.

When an AV block occurs alongside certain combinations of vesicular blocks it is known as a trifascicular block (page 135).

Atrioventricular (AV) Blocks

AV blocks are caused by degeneration of, or damage to, the AV node or the bundle of His and cause a disruption (delay or complete block) of the electrical impulse as it travels from the atria to the ventricles.[38, 54] This means we can identify the different AV blocks by looking at the pattern and relationship between the P waves and QRS complexes on the ECG rhythm strip.

There are three degrees of AV block, with 2nd degree AV block further divided into two types, leaving a total of four different AV blocks:[54]

- 1st degree AV block.
- 2nd degree type 1 AV block.
- 2nd degree type 2 AV block.
- 3rd degree AV block.

The clinical presentation of patients will vary widely depending on which AV block their heart is currently in as well as their overall health state and ability to compensate for the resulting degree of reduced heart rate.

They may have symptoms relating to another cardiac presentation which has led to an AV block developing, such as myocardial ischaemia (page 93).[55]

The prevailing presentation of the patient will reflect the ventricular rate which is resulting from the AV block. The more severe the bradycardia, the more hypotensive and haemodynamically unstable the patient is likely to be.

AV blocks are progressive in nature, often with a 1st degree block eventually leading to one of the 2nd degree blocks, and a 2nd degree block leading to a 3rd degree block. A 3rd degree AV block carries the risk of deterioration and cardiac arrest, usually due to ventricular standstill leading to asystole. It is important that patients presenting with AV blocks, especially those that are symptomatic, are monitored for possible deterioration en route to hospital.

Causes of AV Blocks[11, 12, 13, 38, 54, 55, 56]

The risk of AV block occurrence increases with age. There is no significant difference in occurrence between the sexes.
- Fibrosis of the cardiac conduction system.
- Acute myocardial ischaemia.
- Increased vagal tone.

- Congenital heart block.
- Aortic stenosis.
- Cardiomyopathy.
- Post-cardiac surgery or catheter ablation.
- Hypoxia.
- Acidosis.
- Medications:
  - Beta-adrenoceptor blocking drugs (beta blockers), including: atenolol, bisoprolol, metoprolol, propranolol.
  - Calcium channel blockers, including: amlodipine, nifedipine, diltiazem, verapamil.
  - Cardiac glycoside (digoxin).

Management of AV Blocks[1, 2, 54]

- Attempt to identify the underlying cause of the AV block and manage clinical presentation as necessary.
- 1st degree AV block alone does not require any specific clinical interventions.
- 2nd and 3rd degree AV blocks may cause decreased cardiac output due to the reduced ventricular rate (page 14) and require atropine therapy. This is managed as per the management of bradycardia (page 37) following clinical practice guidelines for bradycardia and hypotension.
- 2nd degree type 2 and 3rd degree heart blocks carry an increased risk of cardiac arrest (usually asystole) and should be monitored closely for deterioration.

1st Degree AV Block

ECG Identification of 1st Degree AV Block[17, 38, 54]

A consistent increase in PR interval of greater than 0.20 seconds (5 small squares).
- The PR interval is consistently prolonged, with no variation or change between each beat.

Clinical Presentation of 1st Degree AV Block

- In itself, 1st degree heart block is asymptomatic, though the underlying cause of the heart block may affect the patient's clinical presentation.

ECG 2.15 – 1st Degree AV Block

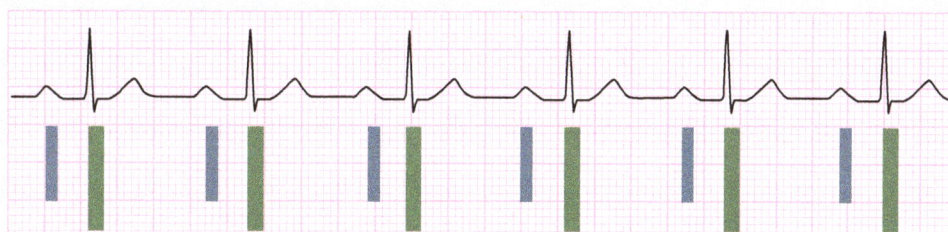

1st degree AV block can be easily overlooked. This rhythm strip shows a clearly prolonged PR interval of over 0.24 seconds (6 small squares), but otherwise this strip would meet the criteria for sinus rhythm.

2nd Degree AV Blocks

2nd degree AV heart blocks are further divided into two subgroups, 2nd degree heart block type 1 and 2nd degree heart block type 2. They share similarities in clinical presentation and management as both can cause hypotension and produce signs of reduced cardiac output due to the reduced ventricular rate and relative bradycardia (page 35).

Clinical Presentation of 2nd Degree AV Blocks[2, 7, 8, 9, 10, 54]

- In acute cases there may be signs and symptoms associated with the underlying cause of the heart block.
- If the ventricular rate is bradycardic, cardiac output may be reduced and the patient may present with signs and symptoms associated with circulatory shock (page 14):
  - Pale, cold and clammy skin.
  - Hypotension and weak or absent peripheral pulses.
  - Delayed capillary refill.
  - Tachypnoea.
  - Dizziness or near loss of consciousness.
  - Loss of consciousness or reduced level of consciousness.
  - Anxiety and confusion.

2nd Degree Type 1 AV Block (Wenckebach/Mobitz Type I)

ECG Identification of 2nd Degree Type 1 AV Block[17, 38, 54]

- In 2nd degree type 1 AV block, the AV node conducts each impulse with an increasing delay until it fails to conduct an impulse. The delay then resets and the AV node starts conducting impulses again with the same increasing delays.
- The PR interval lengthens with each beat until there is a 'dropped' QRS complex. This will be seen as a P wave that is not followed by a QRS complex, instead there will be a gap before a second P wave which will conduct into a QRS complex. This forms the first P-QRS of the next sequence, the PR interval will have returned to the original duration and again start to lengthen and so the pattern continues.

ECG 2.16 – 2nd Degree AV Block Type 1

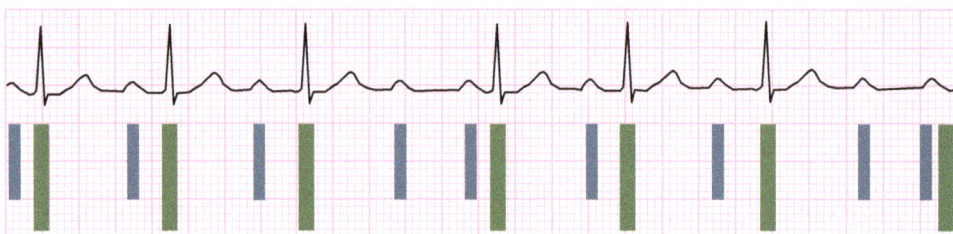

It is important to remember that 2nd degree type I AV block (Mobitz Type 1) can have a variable number of conducted P waves before each dropped beat. In this rhythm strip there are three conducted P waves before the fourth is dropped. We can see that the PR interval is significantly prolonged in the third conducted P wave compared to the first. This gives us the diagnosis of 2nd degree type 1 AV block. Taking a step back from the ECG and looking at the pattern lines we can see the gradual increase in PR interval until the dropped beat occurs. It is sometimes worth using pen and paper to draw our own lines from a patient's ECG to help recognise any subtle patterns.

2nd Degree Type 2 AV Block (Mobitz Type II)

ECG Identification of 2nd Degree Type 2 AV Block[17, 38, 54]

- Unlike in 2nd degree type 1 AV block, the PR interval in 2nd degree type 2 AV block will remain constant. The duration may also meet criteria for 1st degree AV block.
- In 2nd degree type 2 AV block some P waves are not conducted to the ventricles, leading to 'dropped' QRS complexes. These dropped QRS complex may occur randomly, or form a pattern.
- If the dropped QRS complexes form a pattern, it will be described in the form of a ratio. For example, if every second P wave is conducted, the ECG will have two P waves before every QRS, so this would be termed a 2:1 block or a 'two to one block' because there are two P waves for every QRS complex.
- Following this convention, if there were three P waves before every QRS complex, meaning there were two dropped QRS complexes for every one that was conducted, this would be termed a 3:1 block ('three to one block').

ECG 2.17 – 2nd Degree AV Block Type 2

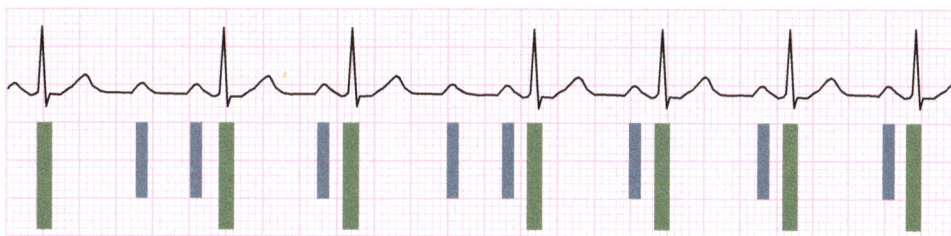

The non-conducted P waves randomly occur without pattern, and the PR intervals are consistent in the conducted beats. This gives us a 2nd degree AV block type 2. The lack of pattern can be seen in the pattern lines below the ECG.

ECG 2.18 – 2nd Degree AV Block Type 2

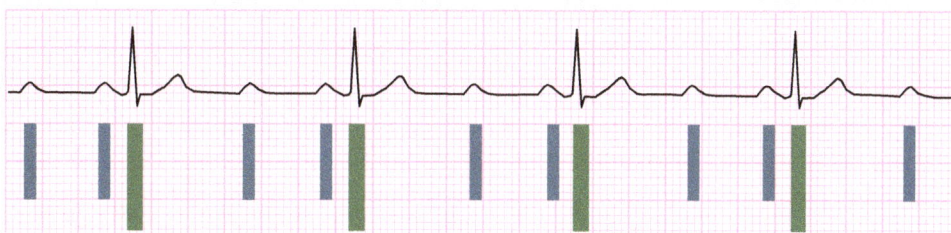

In this example there is a consistent 2:1 ratio present, with two P waves for every QRS complex. This is also a 2nd degree AV block type 2, the only difference between this and ECG 2.17 is that we can see a clear pattern between the P waves and QRS complexes. This is particularly easy to see when we look at the pattern strips.

The less frequently that a P wave is conducted through the AV node to the ventricles, the slower the resulting physical pulse rate will be. As such the patient is likely to present with a relative bradycardia compared to the rate being produced by the SA node.

For example, if the SA node is trying to produce a heartbeat at a rate of 90 beats per minute, but there is a 3:1 block, only one in three of these 90 beats will result in ventricular contraction and manifest as a physical pulse, meaning that the relative pulse rate for this patient in the context of cardiac output and blood pressure would be 30 beats per minute. This will reduce cardiac output and is a form of cardiogenic shock (page 14).

3rd Degree AV Block/Complete Heart Block

Third degree heart block, also referred to as complete heart block, occurs when there is no electrical connection between the atria and the ventricles, meaning that no impulse is conducted through the AV node at all.

ECG Identification of 3rd Degree AV Block[4, 17, 38, 54]

- The only ventricular activity present will be either a:
  - ▶ Ventricular escape rhythm (page 67), meaning that the QRS complexes will be wide, due to the inability of the impulse to follow the normal conduction pathway. The rate of these ventricular escape beats varies widely but will usually fall between 15 and 40 beats per minute, with a tendency towards the lower end of this range, or a
  - ▶ Junctional escape rhythm (page 66) meaning the QRS complexes will be narrow, as the impulse originates from within the AV node (note: This is not the same as the conduction of impulses through the AV node from the atria). The rate of a junctional escape rhythm is usually between 40–60 beats per minute.
- Due to the complete disassociation between the atria and ventricles, P waves will not have any relationship with the QRS complexes.
- This leads to 'inappropriate P waves', P waves which fall in inappropriate places in the cardiac cycle. There may be a P wave between a QRS complex and the following T wave. There may be notching or abnormal shaping of the T waves due to a P wave occurring at the same time.

ECG 2.19 – 3rd Degree AV Block

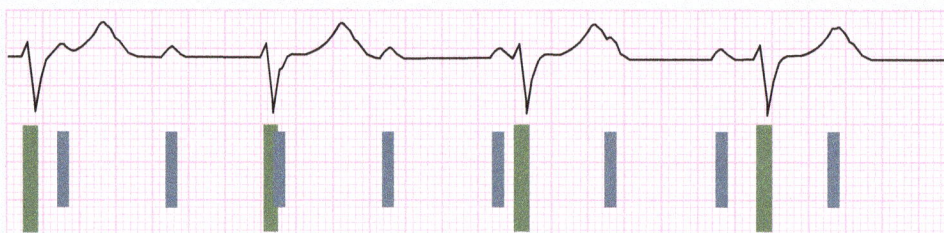

There is no relationship between the P waves and QRS complexes in this rhythm strip. The atrial rate is regular at around 100 beats per minute. The ventricular rate is also regular, with a rate of around 45 beats per minute. The blue lines indicate each P wave, notice how some of them fall in inappropriate places, there is one between the first QRS complex and its T wave. The final blue line indicates where a P wave is completely obscured by the T wave. There is no relationship between the P waves and QRS complexes, making this rhythm a 3rd degree AV block.

Clinical Presentation of 3rd Degree AV Block[2, 7, 8, 9, 10, 54]

- The patient is likely to present with a reduced cardiac output due to the slow ventricular rate and is also likely to exhibit signs and symptoms associated with circulatory shock (page 14):
  - Pale, cold and clammy skin.
  - Hypotension and weak or absent peripheral pulses.
  - Delayed capillary refill.
  - Tachypnoea.
  - Dizziness or near loss of consciousness.
  - Loss of consciousness or reduced level of consciousness.
  - Anxiety and confusion.

Key Points: AV Blocks

- AV blocks are progressive in nature and are at risk of deterioration. 2nd degree type 2 and 3rd degree AV blocks are at risk of deterioration and cardiac arrest.
- 2nd and 3rd degree AV blocks can cause a reduced cardiac output and cardiogenic shock.
- Treatment should be guided by the ventricular heart rate and any clinical signs of poor perfusion and cardiogenic shock (page 14).

Escape Rhythms

Throughout the cardiac conduction pathway, there are groups of pacemaker cells which act as back-up ectopic pacemakers should the SA node fail.

If the SA node ceases to function and stops producing electrical impulses, the next group of ectopic pacemaker cells will start to produce their own impulses and take on the role of ectopic pacemaker for the heart.

These back-up ectopic pacemaker sites are not connected with the rest of the body and are not influenced by the sympathetic and parasympathetic nervous system (page 11); therefore, the heart rate they set is not variable. This means the heart is not able to react to changes in blood pressure as it cannot increase cardiac output through increasing heart rate. Each group of ectopic pacemaker cells has a set heart rate which decreases the further down the cardiac conduction pathway the cells are located. Escape rhythms can also occur when the rate of impulses arriving from further up the cardiac conduction pathway are slower than the set rate of the ectopic pacemaker, causing the ectopic pacemaker to take over primary pacing of the heart despite the SA node being functional.

Clinical Presentation of Escape Rhythm[7, 8, 9, 10]

- The rate of the escape rhythm may be slow enough to cause a reduced cardiac output. The severity of the circulatory shock (page 14) and the associated symptoms is dictated by the rate of the escape rhythm. Symptoms associated with reduced cardiac output include:
  - Pale, cold and clammy skin.
  - Hypotension and weak or absent peripheral pulses.
  - Delayed capillary refill.
  - Tachypnoea.
  - Dizziness or near loss of consciousness.
  - Loss of consciousness or reduced level of consciousness.
  - Anxiety and confusion.
- Additional symptoms will depend on the underlying cause of the escape rhythm.

Causes of Escape Rhythms[4, 11, 12, 13, 38, 54]

The causes of escape rhythms are not direct, as we know an escape rhythm occurs to act as a back-up pacemaker when the SA node fails. The causes listed below are situations where an escape rhythm is likely to occur.
- 3rd degree heart block (page 64).
- Sinus arrest.
- Severe bradycardia (page 35).
- Drugs (by means of precipitating AV blocks):
  - Beta-adrenoceptor blocking drugs (beta blockers), including: atenolol, bisoprolol, metoprolol, propranolol.
  - Calcium channel blockers, including: amlodipine, nifedipine, diltiazem, verapamil.
  - Cardiac glycoside (digoxin).

Management of Escape Rhythm[1, 3, 35, 36]

- Treatment depends on the severity of the clinical presentation and degree of cardiogenic shock.
  - Cardiac arrest: Resuscitate following local guidelines for PEA/non-shockable rhythm.
  - If the patient is symptomatic they are time-critical and require rapid transport with hospital pre-alert and support of ABCs en route.
  - High-flow oxygen with ventilatory support if indicated.
  - Escape rhythms may cause decreased cardiac output due to the reduced ventricular rate and require atropine therapy or the administration of intravascular fluid therapy. This is managed as per the management of bradycardia and absolute bradycardia (page 37) following clinical practice guidelines for bradycardia and hypotension. It should be noted that atropine may have limited effectiveness depending on the cause of the escape rhythm. It is not often possible to determine the exact cause of an escape rhythm and as such the likelihood of the effectiveness of atropine.

Escape Beats and Sinus Arrest[3, 19]

Escape beats follow the same principles as escape rhythms, the only difference being that the SA node remains as the pacemaker for the heart following the escape beat. The single escape beat occurs during sinus arrest. Escape beats can also occur as the first beat following a PVC (page 69).

Sinus arrest, also known as sinus pause, occurs when the SA node intermittently fails to generate an electrical impulse, causing a period of asystole to appear on the ECG. Sinus arrest usually lasts for only a few seconds but may persist for several minutes. Often, an escape beat will interrupt a sinus arrest, or an escape rhythm will maintain cardiac output until the SA node recommences production of regular electrical impulses.

Junctional Escape Rhythm

A junctional escape rhythm, or just junctional rhythm, is the escape rhythm that originates from the AV node.

ECG Identification of Junctional Escape Rhythm[4, 17]

- Rate between 40–60 beats per minute and a regular rhythm.
- Narrow QRS complexes, under 0.12 seconds (3 small squares). Unless aberrant conduction is also present (page 45).
- P wave changes:
  - **Inverted**: The P wave may be inverted (upside down) due to the reversed direction of depolarisation across the atria.
  - **Absent**: The P wave may be hidden behind the QRS complex on the ECG due to occurring at the same time, or there may be no atrial depolarisation at all.
  - **Disassociated**: In 3rd degree heart block there is no relationship between the P wave and the QRS complex (page 64).

ECG 2.20 – Junctional Rhythm

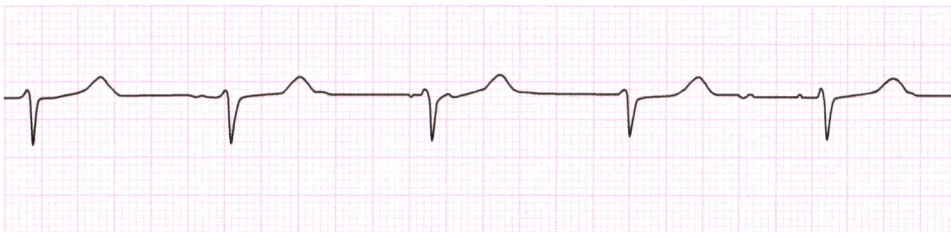

The absence of P waves should be the first indicator of a junctional rhythm. The regular rate of around 58 beats per minute and the narrow QRS complexes are the additional findings needed to confirm the diagnosis.

Accelerated Junctional Rhythms and Junctional Tachycardia

Occasionally junctional rhythms can occur at increased rates. They share the same identifying characteristics as a junctional rhythm except for the different rate:
- **Accelerated junctional rhythms** have a rate between 60–100 beats per minute.
- **Junctional tachycardia** has a rate of above 100 beats per minute.

Ventricular Escape Rhythm

Ventricular escape rhythms, also known as idioventricular rhythms, are the escape rhythm; that occur within the ventricles, below the bundle of His.

ECG Identification of Junctional Escape Rhythm[4, 17]

- Rate between 15–40 beats per minute and a regular rhythm.
- Wide, bizarre QRS complexes which may have right or left bundle branch block morphology.
- P wave changes:
  - **Absent**: There may be no atrial activity at all.
  - **Disassociated**: In third degree heart block there is no relationship between the P wave and the QRS complex (page 64).

ECG 2.21 – Ventricular Escape Rhythm

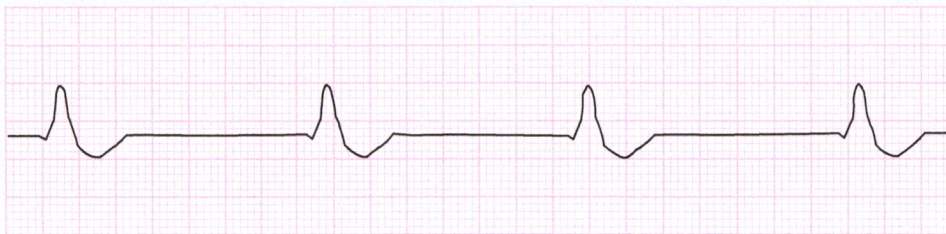

The wide and bizarre QRS complexes in conjunction with the absences of P waves and consistent but slow rate make this a ventricular escape rhythm.

Accelerated Idioventricular Rhythm[17, 25]

Accelerated idioventricular rhythm is a rapid idioventricular rhythm with a rate ranging from 40 to 100 beats per minute. This rate is above that typically expected of a ventricular ectopic pacemaker cell. The patient may present as haemodynamically stable if the increased rate is sufficient to maintain cardiac output (page 13). If the rate were above 100 beats per minute it would become ventricular tachycardia (page 49).

ECG 2.22 – Accelerated Idioventricular Rhythm

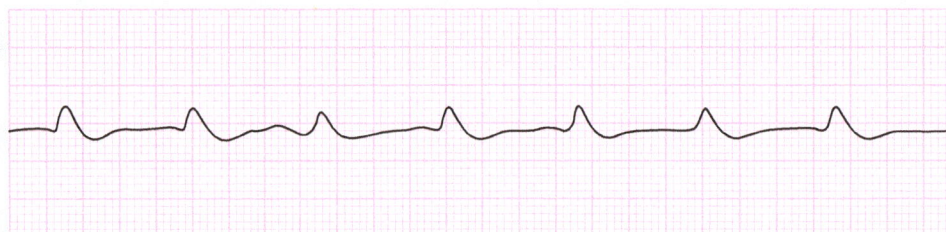

The wide QRS complexes combined with the absence of P waves tell us that this is likely to be a ventricular escape rhythm of some kind. The rate is consistently around 80 beats per minute which tells us this is an accelerated idioventricular rhythm.

Agonal Rhythm

When all other electrical activity in the heart has stopped, the final rhythm often seen prior to asystole is an agonal rhythm. With a rate of under 20 beats per minute, these wide and bizarre QRS complexes are unlikely to produce any cardiac output and are treated as a form of asystole; treatment follows the non-shockable advanced life support guidelines.[38]

Ectopic Beats

Ectopic beats are additional heartbeats that come from outside the normal electrical pathway of the cardiac conduction system. When present, ectopic beats are an additional finding alongside the primary diagnosis of an ECG rhythm. They also often make the interpretation of an ECG more difficult, at least until you realise that ectopics are present and can then attempt to analyse the underlying rhythm.

Ectopic beats occur when a cardiac muscle cell, or group of cells, generates an electrical impulse which triggers depolarisation of the cardiac muscle. These ectopic pacemaker cells can be generated by any normal cardiac muscle cell. Normally, rogue impulses generated by ectopic pacemaker cells are supressed and lost within the normal cardiac conduction cycle, but if they occur at the right time they can trigger depolarisation of the cardiac muscle and lead to an ectopic beat.

All ectopic beats fall outside the regular P QRS T pattern for their ECG and are usually followed by a compensatory pause before the next normal heartbeat.

Premature Atrial Contractions

Premature Atrial Contractions (PACs), atrial ectopic beats, originate within the atria. They appear on the ECG as an abnormally shaped P wave; the morphology (shape) of the P wave is dependent on the location of the ectopic pacemaker cells within the atria.[19] The P-R interval will likely also be of a different duration than normal, and reflect the proximity of the ectopic pacemaker location in relation to the AV node. If the PAC reaches the AV node and travels to the ventricles, the subsequent QRS complex should appear normal, as it is following the normal, conduction pathway once it travels below the AV node.[19]

Not all PACs are conducted by the AV node, meaning that only the abnormal P wave will be visible on the ECG.

ECG 2.23 – Premature Atrial Contractions

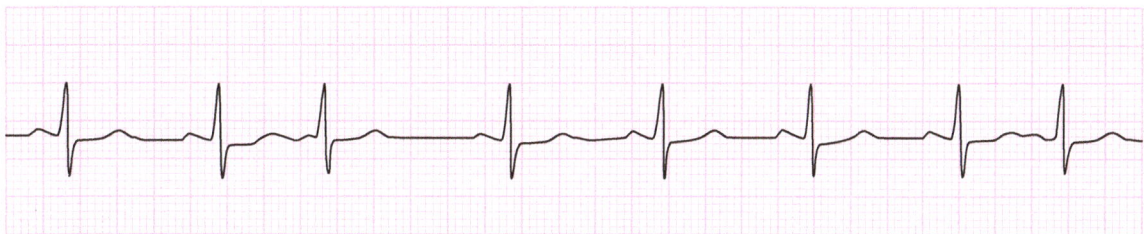

This ECG shows a sinus rhythm with PACs, the third and eighth beats (subtle inverted P waves precede the QRS complexes in these beats). There is a compensatory pause after both of the PACs before the normal heartbeat returns.

Premature Junctional Contractions

Premature Junctional Contractions (PJCs), junctional ectopic beats, occur when the AV node independently generates an electrical impulse. These appear with the same morphology as a junctional rhythm (page 66) except that they occur in isolation as a single ectopic beat on an ECG showing different underlying rhythm.

ECG 2.24 – Premature Junctional Contractions

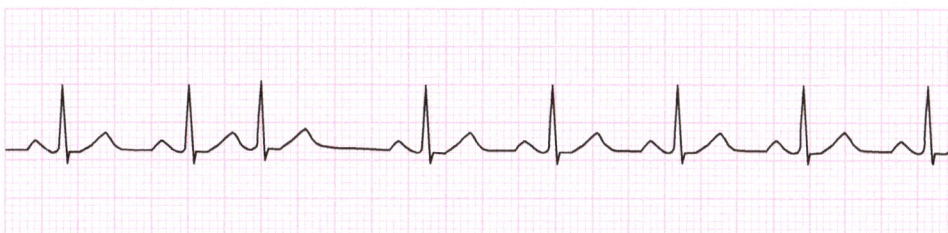

The third QRS complex on this rhythm strip is a premature junctional contraction. It occurs without a preceding P wave and there is a compensatory pause before the next normal beat. The fact that this premature beat has a narrow QRS complex tells us it originates from above the ventricles.

Premature Ventricular Contractions

Premature Ventricular Contractions (PVCs), also called ventricular extrasystoles (VEs) or ventricular ectopic beats, are the most common abnormality of heart rhythm in adults. They appear on the ECG as a wide, abnormal QRS complex, usually of greater magnitude than the underlying normal QRS complexes in the same lead. Usually, they show fixed coupling; the interval after the last beat is constant. These do not arise in the ventricles as much of the literature claims[19] and as the shape might suggest. Rather, they are a re-entry phenomenon.[57]

As the previous sinus beat passes through the Bundle of His and below, it travels through a relatively fast pathway but also a slow pathway. The ventricle is depolarised by the first impulse and may have already recovered (repolarised) by the time of the emergence of the second wave which can then cause a second depolarisation which is the extrasystole. Because of this PVC complexes may have right or left bundle branch block morphology.[19]

A second much less common type of ventricular extrasystole does arise within the ventricular myocardium and does not show fixed coupling. They tend to occur at their own intervals when the ventricle is not refractory and permits the depolarisation. These are called parasystolic beats and do have some danger if they fall on the peak of the previous T wave which is known as the vulnerable period; torsades de pointes may occur and can degenerate into ventricular fibrillation.

ECG 2.25 – Premature Ventricular Contractions

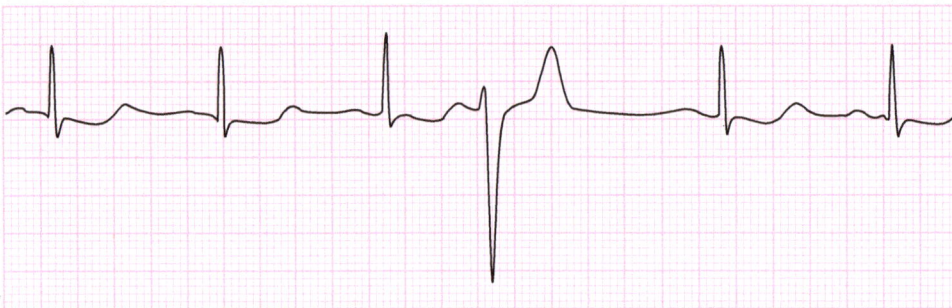

The fourth beat on this rhythm strip is a premature ventricular contraction, as described above. The short interval after the previous beat is compensated by a long interval known as a 'compensatory pause'. This occurs because the underlying sinus rhythm continues at its usual rate, but there is a blocked wave generally hidden within the T wave of the premature beat.

Causes of Ectopic Beats

The causes of ectopic beats are wide ranging, from sinister to benign. The frequency and type of ectopic beat can give an indication as to the level of concern warranted. Ectopic beats are a frequent normal variant in 1% of ECGs and almost everyone will have occasional ectopic beats. PVCs can trigger ventricular arrhythmias if underlying structural heart disease is present. Increased numbers of PVCs during and after myocardial infarction are associated with a poorer prognosis. In most cases your diagnosis and treatment will depend on the overall clinical presentation of the patient.

There are many causes of ectopic beats, including:[19]
- Myocardial infarction (page 93).
- Hypertension.
- Cardiomyopathy (page 122).
- Pharmacological:
  - Digoxin.
  - Tricyclic antidepressants.
  - Cocaine.
  - Alcohol.
- Stimulants such as caffeine and energy drinks.
- Electrolyte and metabolic imbalances:
  - Sepsis.
  - Diabetic ketoacidosis.
  - Hyperkalaemia (page 143).
- Stress, anxiety and fatigue.

Types of Premature Ventricular Contractions[17, 38]

When more than one PVC occurs on an ECG they are further categorised by their shape in comparison to each other and the pattern they may form.

- **Unifocal PVCs** occur when all the PVCs have the same morphology, meaning they all originate by the same mechanism.
- **Multifocal PVCs** occur when there are two or more morphologies of PVC. This indicates that there are multiple ectopic pacemaker sites as each site will create a different shape of PVC.

ECG 2.26 – Multifocal Premature Ventricular Contractions

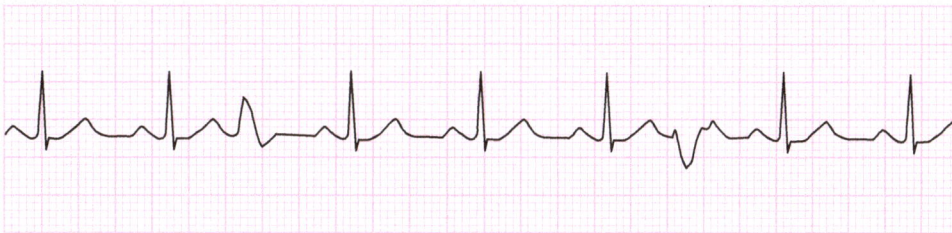

The different morphologies of the ventricular ectopic beats (the third and seventh beats on this strip) tell us that they have followed different pathways through the ventricle.

Bigeminy, Trigeminy and Quadgeminy[19, 38]

Bigeminy, trigeminy and quadgeminy occur when PVCs form a recurrent pattern with the underlying sinus rhythm.

- Bigeminy occurs when every second beat is a PVC, trigeminy when every third beat is a PVC and quadgeminy when every fourth beat is a PVC.
- PVCs may or may not generate a physical pulse. In cases were PVCs do not conduct a physical pulse, cardiac output may be proportionally decreased (page 13).
- If bigeminy is producing PVCs that do not generate a pulse, this effectively reduces the physical pulse rate by half of the rate set by the SA node. The same principle applies to trigeminy and quadgeminy, with the physical pulse rate being reduced by one third or one quarter respectively.

ECG 2.27 – Bigeminy

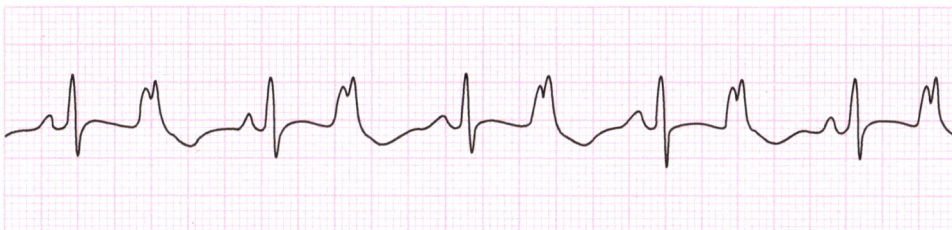

The ventricular ectopic beats occurring every second beat are easily identified by their wide and bizarre morphology. As every second beat is an ectopic beat, this rhythm is bigeminal.

ECG 2.28 – Trigeminy

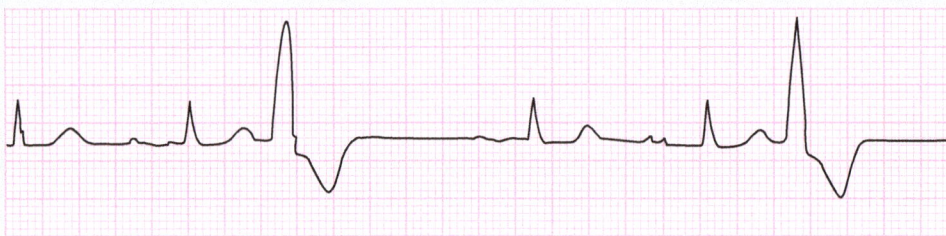

Every third beat is ectopic, making this a trigeminal rhythm. In this case, the ectopic beats are ventricular in nature because of their wide and bizarre morphology.

Couplets

Couplets are the most concerning of the different types of ectopic beats. They occur when two PVCs are 'coupled' together, with no gap or normal beat between them. This ECG finding is of concern and should alert you that the patient is at risk of rapid deterioration into an unstable tachyarrhythmia or cardiac arrest rhythm (page 27). The definition of VT is three or more ventricular ectopic beats in a row. Couplets are only one ectopic beat away from VT.[19]

ECG 2.29 – Couplets

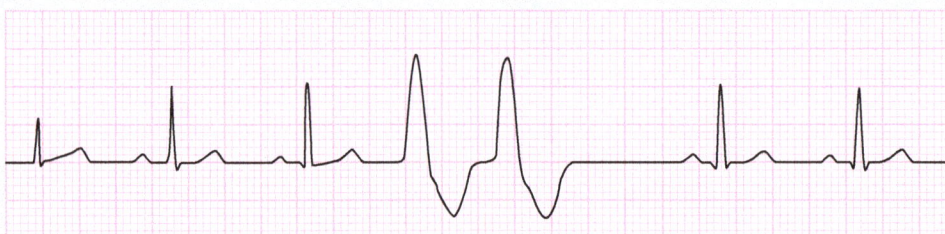

The third, fourth, eighth and ninth beats on this strip are all premature ventricular contractions. But being in pairs they are 'coupled' together. Imagine if the whole rhythm strip looked like beats three and four: It would then be VT.

> Any ectopic beats in an ischaemic ECG indicate an increased risk of cardiac arrest; couplets indicate a high risk of cardiac arrest. The patient should be continuously monitored, and you should be ready to commence resuscitation and rapid defibrillation. **!**

Section 2 Practice ECGs

You can now test yourself with these practice ECGs before continuing to the case scenarios. Remember to use the structured approach to ECG interpretation so you don't miss anything.

Test ECG 2.1

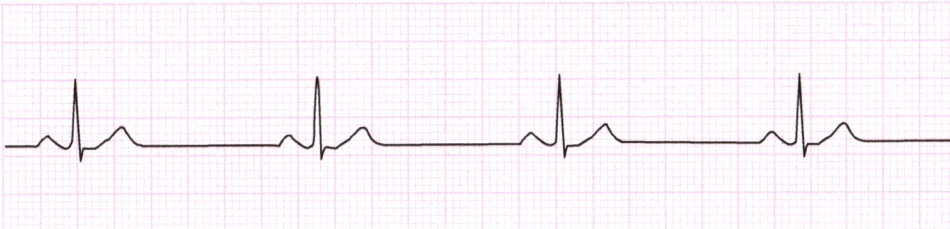

Test ECG 2.2

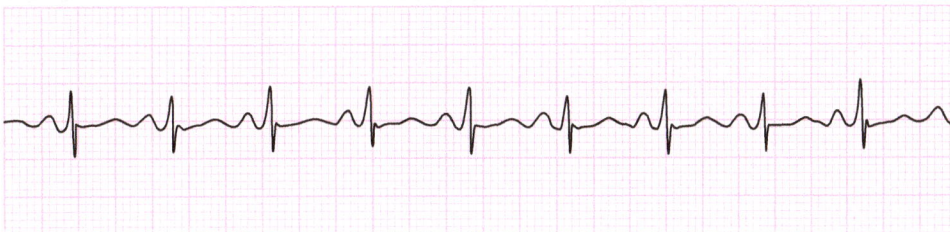

Test ECG 2.3

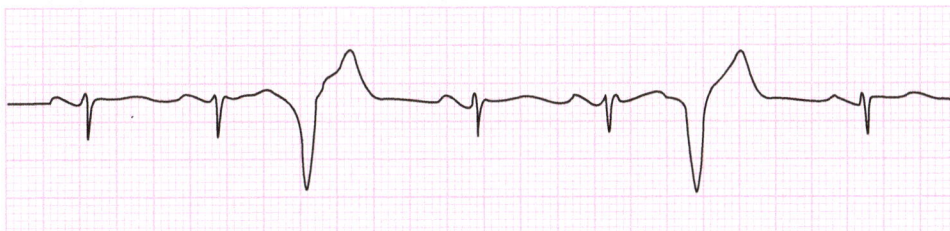

Test ECG 2.4

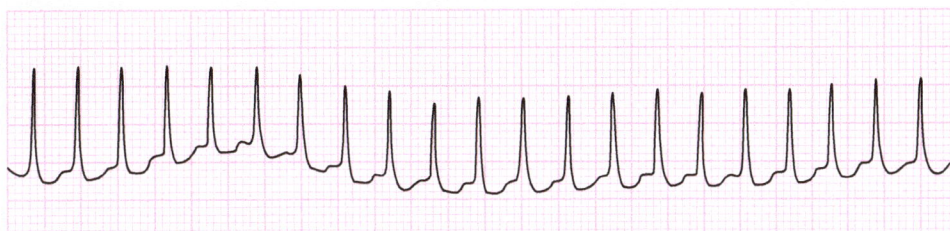

Test ECG 2.5

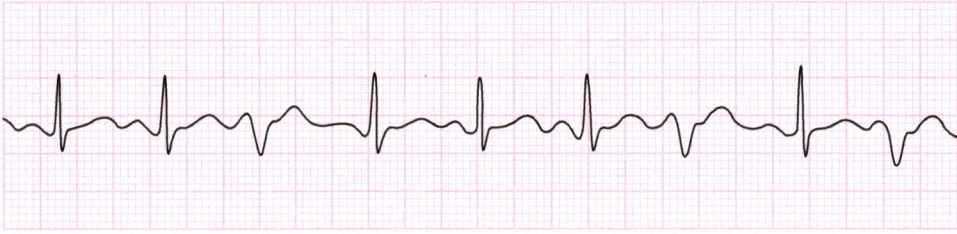

Test ECG 2.6

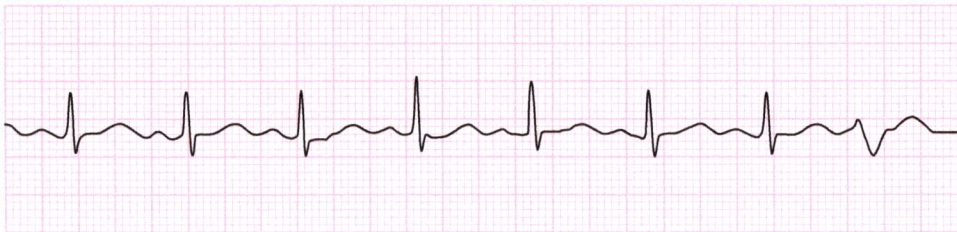

Test ECG 2.7

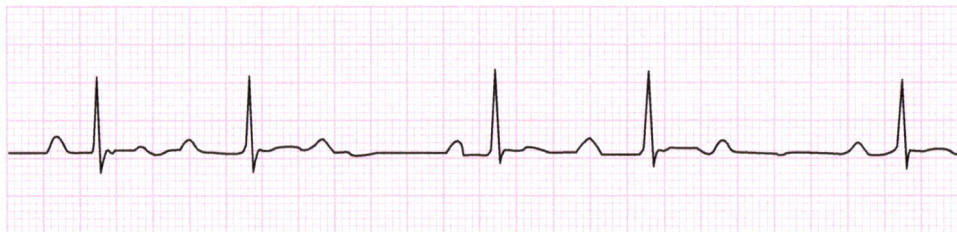

Test ECG 2.8

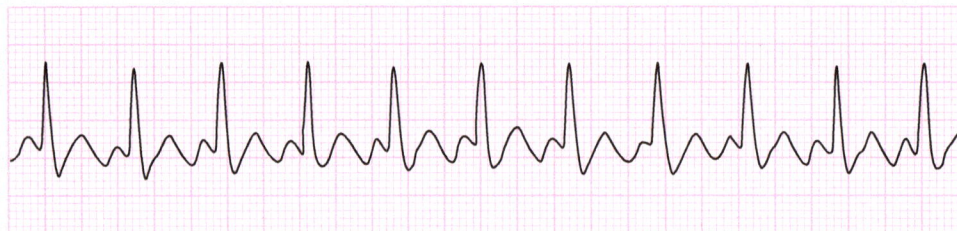

Test ECG 2.9

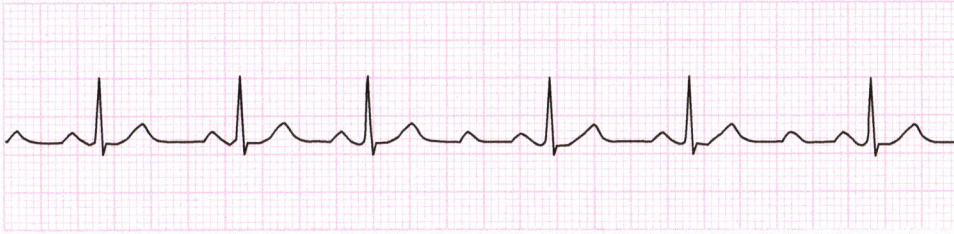

Test ECG 2.10

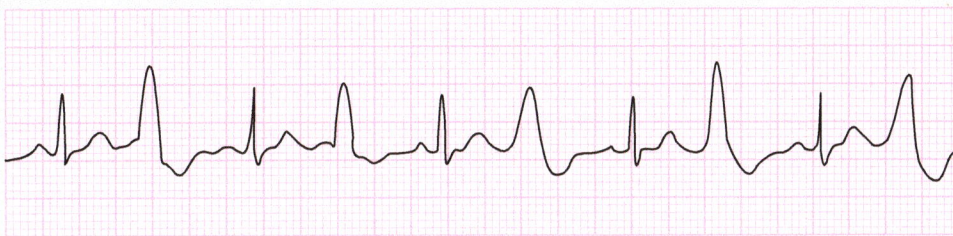

Section 2 Case Scenarios

These case scenarios will help you combine ECG knowledge gained from this chapter with your clinical knowledge and experience. In the following cases we will look at some 12-lead ECGs showing arrhythmias. Remember, it is easy to get distracted when looking at a 12-lead ECG; arrhythmias are usually most easily identified in lead II, so look for them in that lead primarily. The case scenario answers include additional learning points so be sure to read them after you have attempted the questions.

Case Scenario 2.1	34-year-old male with palpitations

Ross was sitting at his desk in the library when, around 15 minutes ago, he suddenly felt that his 'heart was beating really fast and going to jump out of his chest'. He also feels slightly out of breath, anxious and a little light-headed and dizzy. He has no pain and has not lost consciousness.

Past medical history: *Tonsils removed at 13 years old. Hay fever.*

Medication: *None.*

Allergies: *None.*

Social history: *Lives with partner. Does not smoke or use recreational drugs. Drinks 1–2 glasses of wine with dinner a couple of times a week. Average level of fitness with occasional exercise.*

Family history: *Parents and older sister in good health. Not aware of any medical problems.*

Review of systems: *Nothing identified.*

Examination: *Rapid, weak and regular radial pulse.*

Clinical Observations

SpO₂	%	EtCO₂	kPa	NIBP	mmHg	T°	Blood Glucose	GCS
	97		4.7		108	36.4°C	5.2 mmol/l	15
		RR	22	9730	56			(E4 / S5 / M6)

Questions

a) **What are your differential diagnoses for Ross?**
b) **Use the 9-step ECG interpretation tool to assess Ross's ECG.**
c) **What rhythm is the ECG?**
d) **What is your working diagnosis?**

ECG Steps	Remember to look at every ECG lead view, not just lead II
1	What is the rate and rhythm?
2	Are there any P waves and what is their relationship with the QRS complex?
3	What is the duration and morphology of the QRS complex?
4	Is the ST segment isoelectric, depressed or elevated?
5	Are the QT intervals and T waves normal?

Clinical Steps	
6	Is the heart generating a palpable pulse of appropriate rate and providing adequate perfusion?
7	Is the rhythm unstable and at risk of deterioration?
8	Does the presenting rhythm support or change your working diagnosis?
9	Are any clinical interventions required?

Case Scenario ECG 2.1

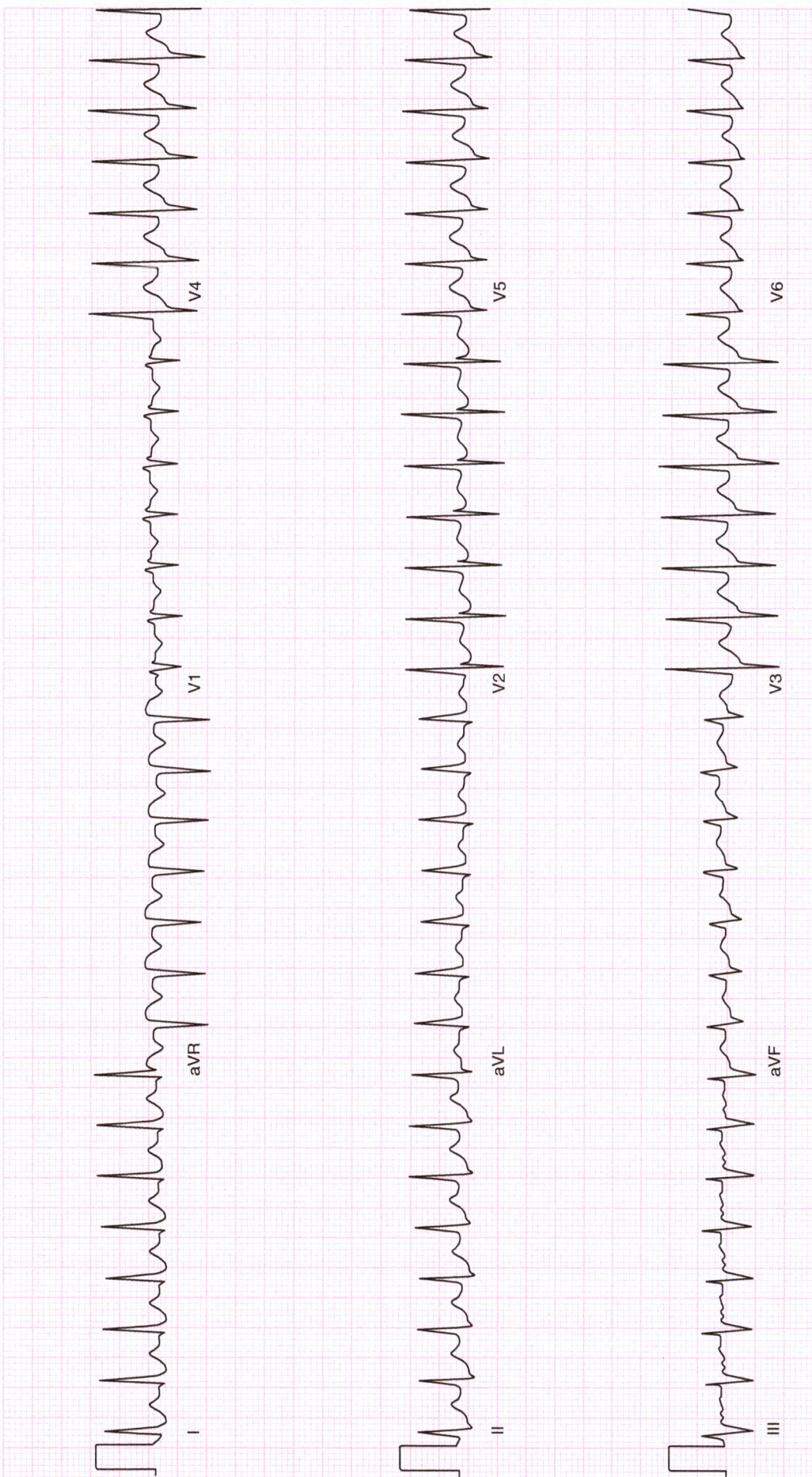

I aVR V1 V4

II aVL V2 V5

III aVF V3 V6

Case Scenario 2.2	84-year-old female fallen – cannot get up

Patricia is an 84-year-old woman living in warden-controlled accommodation. She has been found on her bedroom floor by the warden during his morning check-in. Patricia says she tripped on her slippers whilst getting out of bed about two hours ago. She had tried to get up but when she moved she experienced pain in her left hip. Her pain score is 3/10 when trying to stand but she is pain free at rest.

Past medical history: *Hypertension, osteoporosis, right knee replacement six years ago.*

Medication: *Bisoprolol, calcium and vitamin D supplements.*

Allergies: *None.*

Social history: *Lives independently in warden-controlled accommodation, active in the social groups within the facility. Never smoked, drinks small glass of sherry most evenings. Well supported by three adult children who all live locally and visit regularly.*

Family history: *No known hereditary conditions, she is the last living sibling having had three sisters and two brothers.*

Review of systems: *Episodes of dizziness in recent weeks when standing up from bed or chair.*

Examination: *Radial pulse present, regular and strong. Heart sounds are normal with no additional sounds. Lung sounds are clear with equal air entry. Tenderness over the left neck of femur and possible shortening of the left leg.*

Clinical Observations

SpO$_2$	%	EtCO$_2$	kPa	NIBP	mmHg
	98		5.8		132
		RR	14	91010	86

T°	Blood Glucose	GCS
36.7°C	6.2 mmol/l	15 (E4 / S5 / M6)

Questions

a) **What reasons have you identified to transport Patricia to hospital?**
b) **Use the 9-step ECG interpretation tool to assess the ECG.**
c) **What rhythm is the ECG?**

ECG Steps	Remember to look at every ECG lead view, not just lead II
1	What is the rate and rhythm?
2	Are there any P waves and what is their relationship with the QRS complex?
3	What is the duration and morphology of the QRS complex?
4	Is the ST segment isoelectric, depressed or elevated?
5	Are the QT intervals and T waves normal?

Clinical Steps	
6	Is the heart generating a palpable pulse of appropriate rate and providing adequate perfusion?
7	Is the rhythm unstable and at risk of deterioration?
8	Does the presenting rhythm support or change your working diagnosis?
9	Are any clinical interventions required?

Case Scenario ECG 2.2

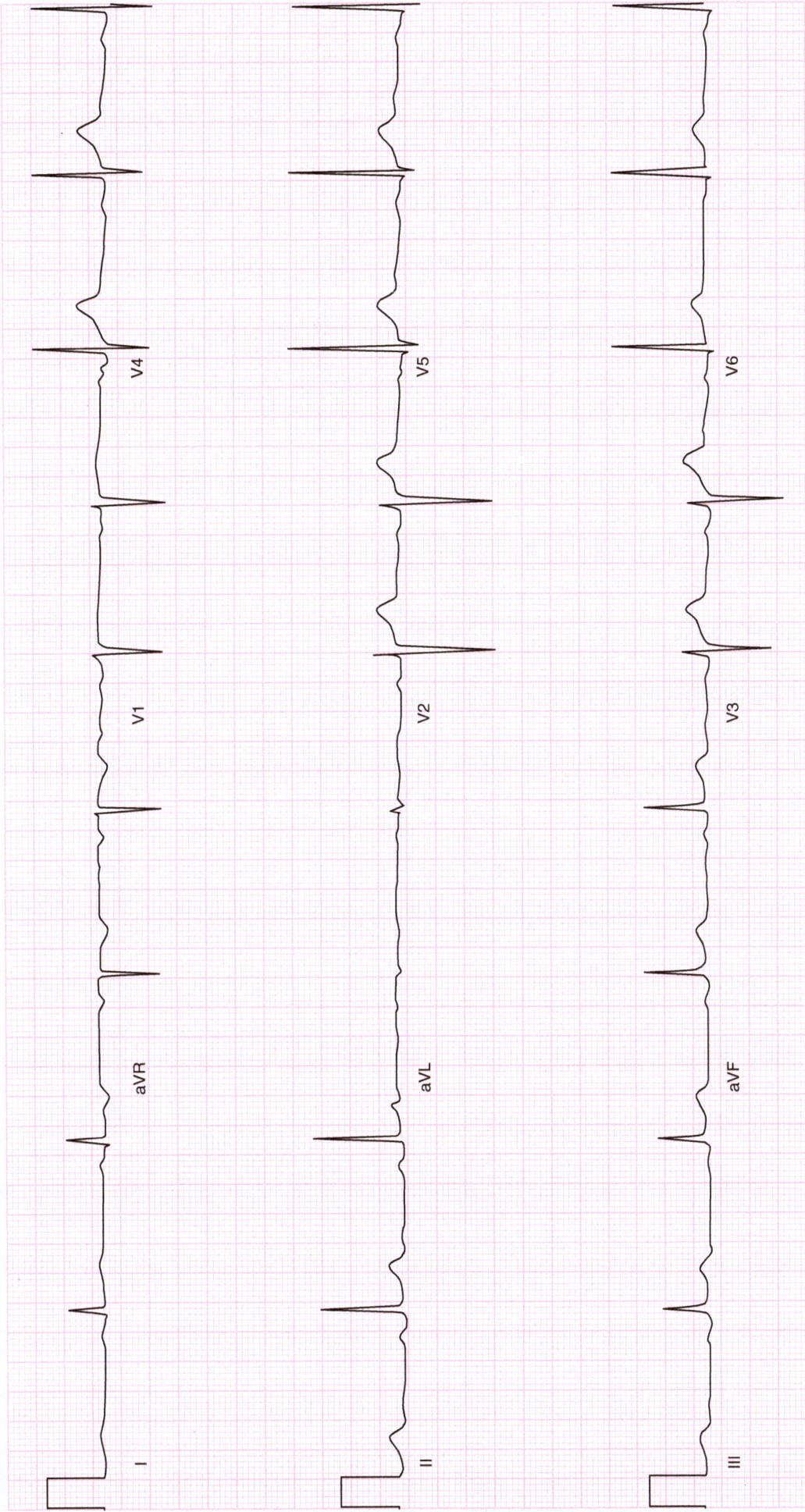

I
II
III
aVR
aVL
aVF
V1
V2
V3
V4
V5
V6

Case Scenario 2.3	47-year-old male with breathing problems

Martin works as a security guard. For the last four days he has had a productive cough, sore throat and has been feeling feverish. He has also been feeling more tired than usual. Today he has started to feel short of breath, with a sharp 'rubbing' pain on the right side of his chest each time he breathes.

Past medical history: *None.*

Medication: *None.*

Allergies: *None.*

Social history: *Lives alone. He drinks one or two pints several times a week. He stopped smoking cigarettes five years ago. He smoked cannabis as a teenager but has not used any other illicit drugs.*

Family history: *Parents are in good health.*

Review of systems: *He has been experiencing some general muscle aches and pains and a mild headache for the last two days.*

Examination: *Radial pulse present, regular and strong. Heart sounds are normal with no additional sounds. Lung sounds indicate some congestion to his right lung.*

Clinical Observations

SpO$_2$	%	EtCO$_2$	kPa	NIBP	mmHg	T°	Blood Glucose	GCS
	96		4.9		142	38.2°C	7.3 mmol/l	15
		RR	20	(109)	92			(E4 / S5 / M6)

Questions

a) **What are your differential diagnoses for Martin?**
b) **Use the 9-step ECG interpretation tool to assess Martin's ECG.**
c) **What rhythm is the ECG?**
d) **What is your working diagnosis?**

ECG Steps	Remember to look at every ECG lead view, not just lead II
1	What is the rate and rhythm?
2	Are there any P waves and what is their relationship with the QRS complex?
3	What is the duration and morphology of the QRS complex?
4	Is the ST segment isoelectric, depressed or elevated?
5	Are the QT intervals and T waves normal?

Clinical Steps	
6	Is the heart generating a palpable pulse of appropriate rate and providing adequate perfusion?
7	Is the rhythm unstable and at risk of deterioration?
8	Does the presenting rhythm support or change your working diagnosis?
9	Are any clinical interventions required?

Case Scenario ECG 2.3

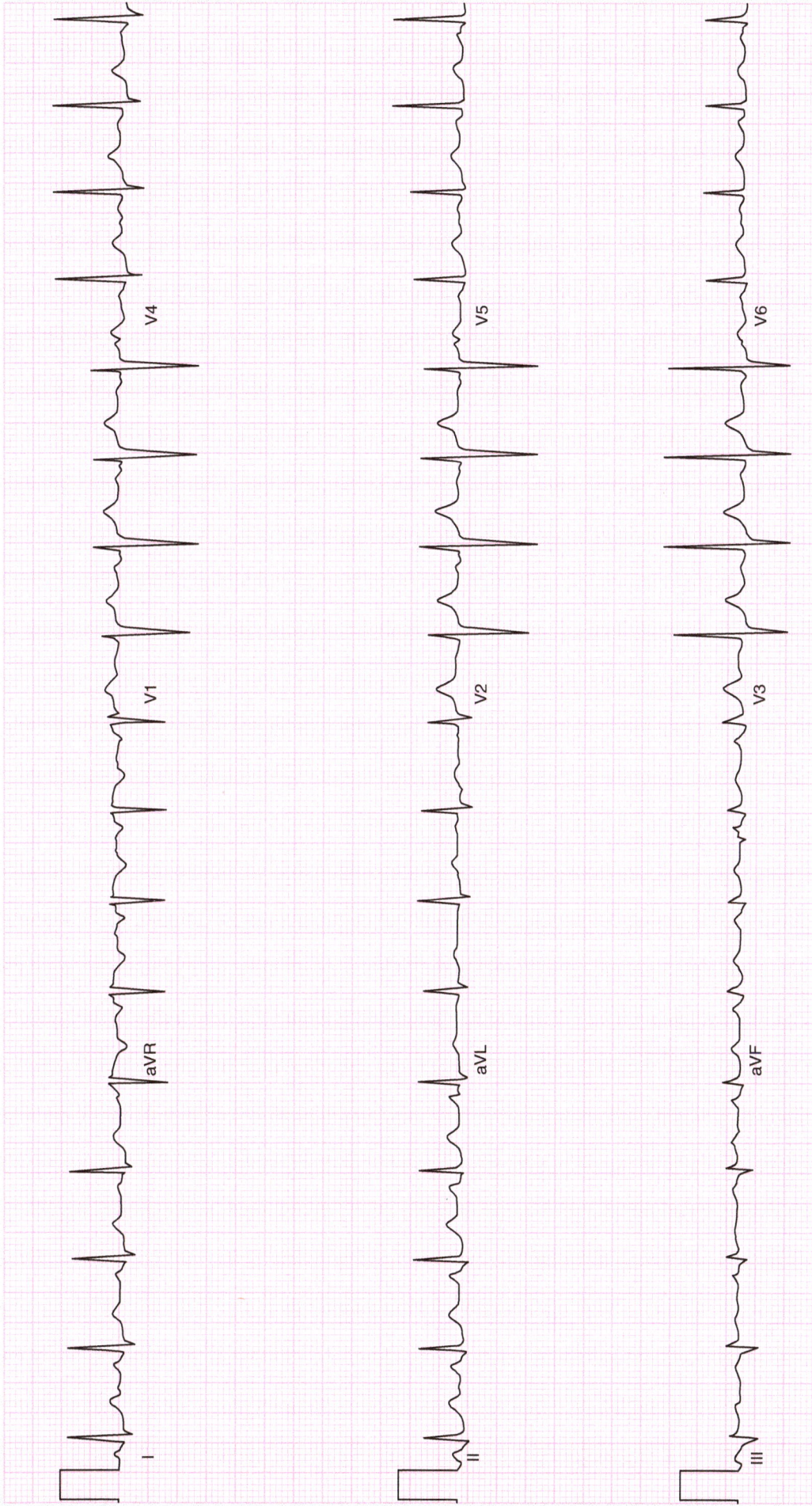

Case Scenario 2.4   66-year-old female, shortness of breath

66-year-old Sheila has been feeling fatigued and short of breath for three days. Today she has felt dizzy and as though she were about to pass out while sitting in her armchair.

Past medical history: *None.*

Medication: *None.*

Allergies: *None.*

Social history: *Lives alone, retired three months ago. Has been drinking 1–2 bottles of wine most days since retirement. Does not smoke or use illicit drugs.*

Family history: *Parents died in old age. An older brother has COPD due to heavy smoking.*

Review of systems: *Has been feeling occasional palpitations when lying in bed over recent days.*

Examination: *Rapid and regular radial pulse.*

Clinical Observations

SpO$_2$	%	EtCO$_2$	kPa	NIBP	mmHg
			5.7		121
	97	RR	18	(79)	58

T°	Blood Glucose	GCS
36.6°C	7.2 mmol/l	15 (E4 / S5 / M6)

Questions

a) **What are your differential diagnoses for Sheila?**
b) **Use the 9-step ECG interpretation tool to assess Sheila's ECG.**
c) **What rhythm is the ECG?**
d) **What is your working diagnosis?**

ECG Steps   Remember to look at every ECG lead view, not just lead II

1	What is the rate and rhythm?
2	Are there any P waves and what is their relationship with the QRS complex?
3	What is the duration and morphology of the QRS complex?
4	Is the ST segment isoelectric, depressed or elevated?
5	Are the QT intervals and T waves normal?

Clinical Steps

6	Is the heart generating a palpable pulse of appropriate rate and providing adequate perfusion?
7	Is the rhythm unstable and at risk of deterioration?
8	Does the presenting rhythm support or change your working diagnosis?
9	Are any clinical interventions required?

Case Scenario ECG 2.4

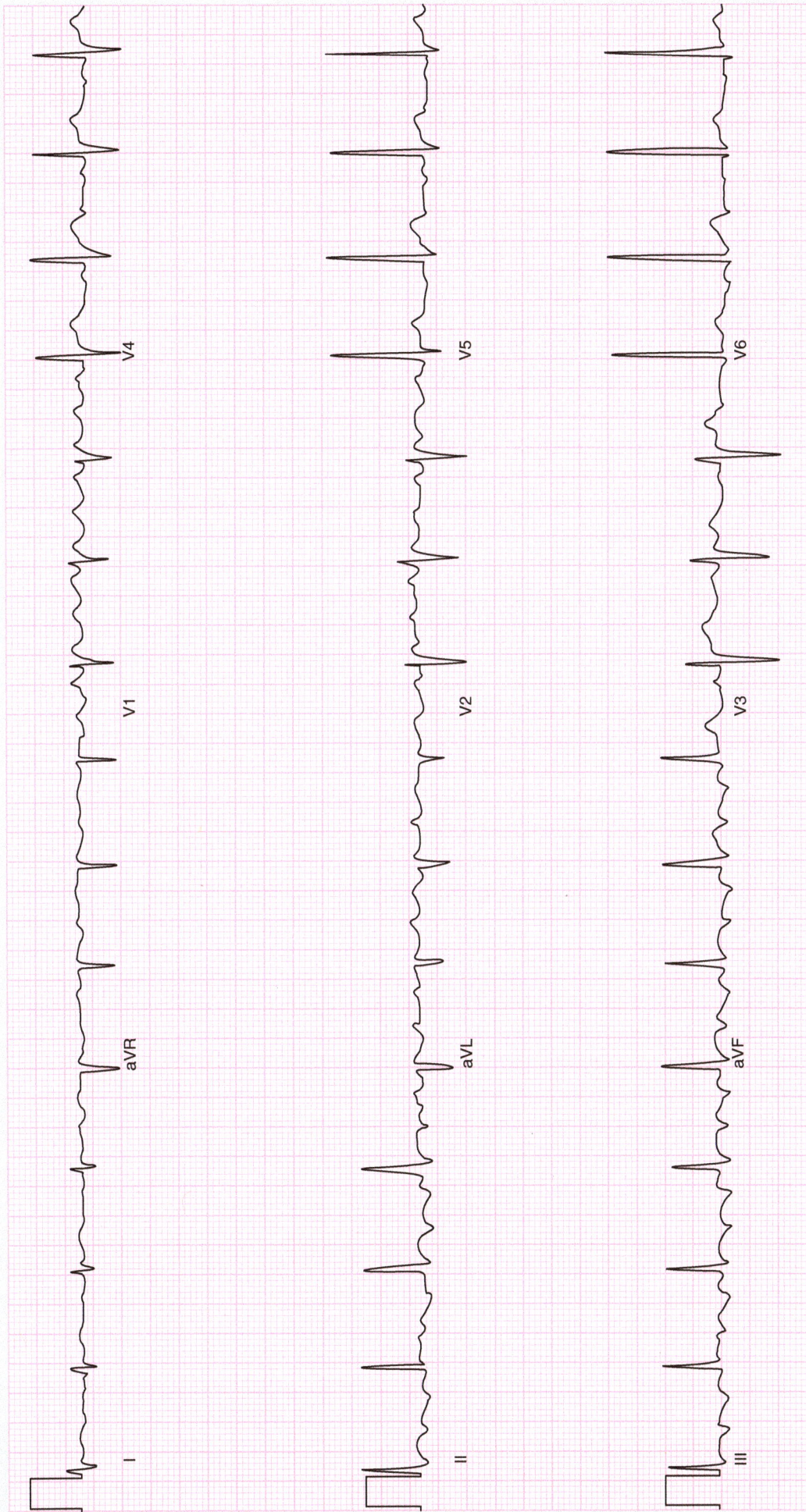

I   aVR   V1   V4

II   aVL   V2   V5

III   aVF   V3   V6

Case Scenario 2.5 — 71-year-old male collapsed, not alert

71-year-old Brian has collapsed on the living room floor. His wife has been unable to wake him and dialled 999. When you arrive on the scene Brian is still on the floor and not fully alert. You obtain the history from his wife as you assess Brian further. She says he was fine today before he collapsed. He came back from the kitchen and just a few seconds before the collapse he said he was feeling 'a bit off'. He had not complained of any pain or discomfort. Brian's wife also tells you that he has recently been diagnosed with 'mild heart failure'. He has been prescribed some new medication for the condition. The hospital appointment was arranged by the GP because Brian had been experiencing some shortness of breath while walking.

Past medical history: *Heart failure, hypertension, high cholesterol, aortic stenosis.*

Medication: *Simvastatin. Atenolol and ramipril were both started two weeks ago for heart failure.*

Allergies: *None.*

Social history: *Lives with his wife, both are retired. Takes a gentle daily walk for exercise. Does not smoke or use illicit drugs.*

Family history: *Parents died in old age. No siblings.*

Review of systems: *Unable.*

Examination: *Slow and weak radial pulse.*

Clinical Observations

SpO$_2$	%	EtCO$_2$	kPa	NIBP	mmHg	T°	Blood Glucose	GCS
	97		6.1		82	36.4°C	6.9 mmol/l	9
		RR	12	(66)	47			(E2 / S3 / M4)

Questions

a) **What are your differential diagnoses for Brian?**
b) **Use the 9-step ECG interpretation tool to assess Brian's ECG.**
c) **What rhythm is the ECG?**
d) **What is your working diagnosis?**

ECG Steps — Remember to look at every ECG lead view, not just lead II

1	What is the rate and rhythm?
2	Are there any P waves and what is their relationship with the QRS complex?
3	What is the duration and morphology of the QRS complex?
4	Is the ST segment isoelectric, depressed or elevated?
5	Are the QT intervals and T waves normal?

Clinical Steps

6	Is the heart generating a palpable pulse of appropriate rate and providing adequate perfusion?
7	Is the rhythm unstable and at risk of deterioration?
8	Does the presenting rhythm support or change your working diagnosis?
9	Are any clinical interventions required?

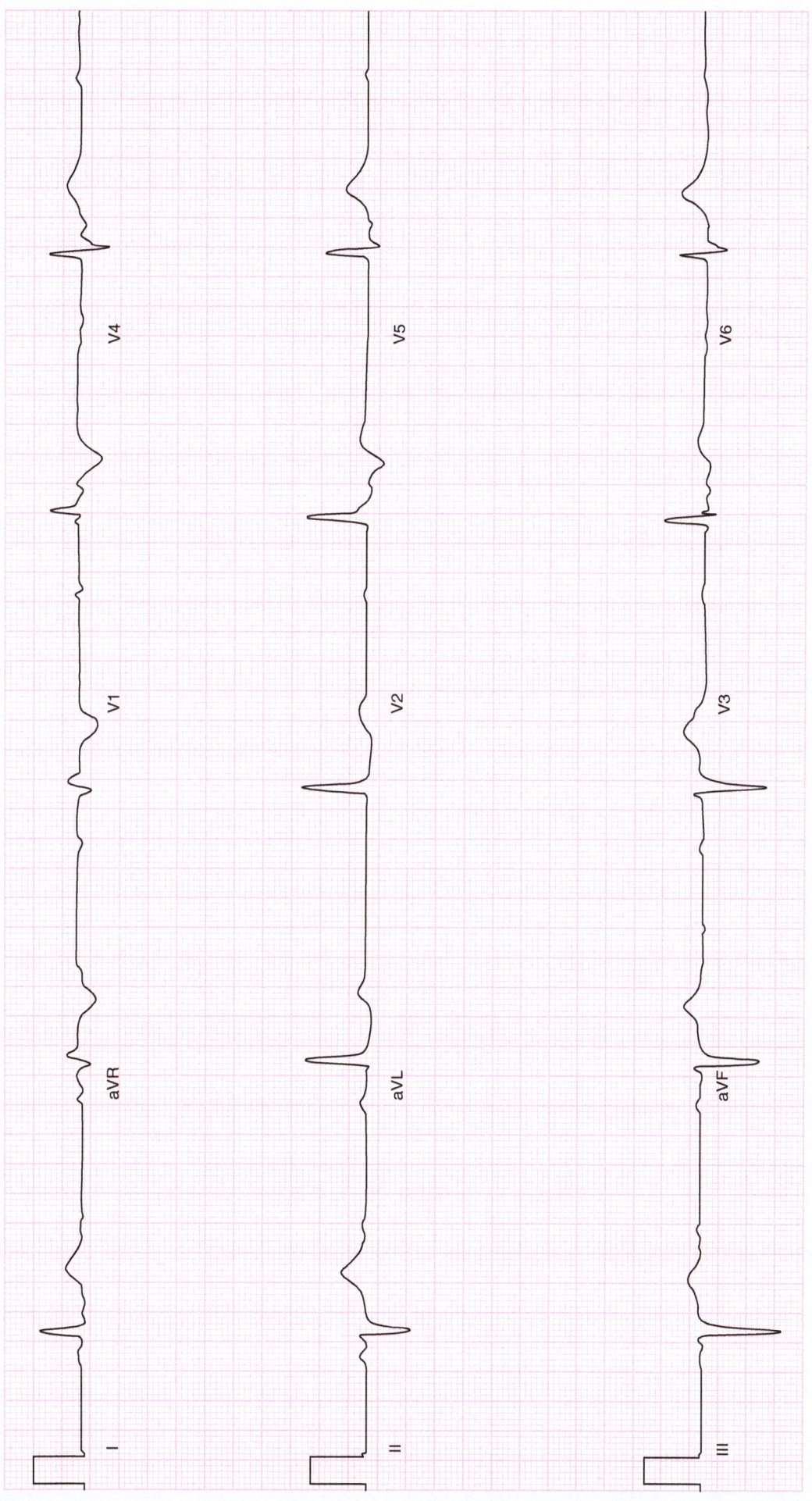

Case Scenario ECG 2.5

Section 2 Practice ECG Answers

Test ECG 2.1 Sinus bradycardia.

Test ECG 2.2 Sinus tachycardia.

Test ECG 2.3 Trigeminy.

Test ECG 2.4 Re-entrant tachycardia (AVRT/AVNRT).

Test ECG 2.5 Sinus rhythm with PVCs.

Test ECG 2.6 AF.

Test ECG 2.7 2nd degree AV block type 1 (Wenckeback/Mobitz Type I).

Test ECG 2.8 Atrial flutter.

Test ECG 2.9 2nd degree AV block type 2.

Test ECG 2.10 Bigeminy.

Section 2 Case Scenario Answers

Case Scenario 2.1 Answers
a) **What are your differential diagnoses for Ross?** *Differentials should include: re-entrant tachycardia, AF with rapid ventricular response, VT, pulmonary embolus, hyperventilation syndrome, use of drugs or stimulants (caffeine, energy drink) or overdose.* b) **Use the 9-step ECG interpretation tool to assess Ross's ECG.** c) **What rhythm is the ECG?** *Re-entrant tachycardia.* d) **What is your working diagnosis?** *Re-entrant tachycardia.*
Discussion: *Ross is presenting with the classic signs and symptoms of a re-entrant tachycardia. We are guided towards this working diagnosis as the alternative differentials are less likely. Pulmonary embolus would cause a sinus tachycardia, but to cause a rate of 180 beats per minute other signs and symptoms would be expected. Anxiety could induce a heart rate of 180 beats per minute, but Ross appears relatively calm with his symptoms. Anxiety is a diagnosis of exclusion and the history suggests re-entrant tachycardia, meaning that it is not appropriate to place anxiety as a working diagnosis in this case.*

ECG Steps		
1	What is the rate and rhythm?	*The rate is around 180 beats/minute and the rhythm is regular.*
2	Are there any P waves and what is their relationship with the QRS complex?	*There are no P waves visible.*
3	What is the duration and morphology of the QRS complex?	*The QRS complex is of normal shape and the duration is under 0.12 seconds (3 small squares).*
4	Is the ST segment isoelectric, depressed or elevated?	*There is ST segment depression in leads I, II, V3, V4, V5, V6.*
5	Are the QT intervals and T waves normal?	*The T wave is of normal shape and the QT interval is 0.25 seconds, which is appropriate for the rate (QTc 0.44 seconds).*

Clinical Steps		
6	**Is the heart generating a palpable pulse of appropriate rate and providing adequate perfusion?**	*They are generating a palpable pulse but the rate is inappropriately fast. The weak radial pulse and BP of 108/56 suggests that perfusion is reduced but currently adequate.*
7	**Is the rhythm unstable and at risk of deterioration?**	*Yes.*
8	**Does the presenting rhythm support or change your working diagnosis?**	*Supports re-entry tachycardia.*
9	**Are any clinical interventions required?**	*Consider vagal manoeuvres.*

Case Scenario 2.2 Answers

a) **What reasons have you identified to transport Patricia to hospital?** *She has signs of potential fracture to the neck of the femur.*
b) **Use the 9-step ECG interpretation tool to assess Patricia's ECG**.
c) **What rhythm is the ECG?** *Sinus bradycardia.*

Discussion: *Patricia is prescribed beta blocker medication which we know slows the heart rate. A finding of sinus bradycardia with a rate of around 50 beats per minute is therefore not surprising due to this medication. We would want to establish if there had been a recent change in her medication or dosage and if she has been taking it correctly. There is the potential that the dizziness she has been experiencing when standing is due to her heart not being able to increase its rate, and thus its cardiac output, to compensate for a change in posture, especially if she has been standing up quickly.*

ECG Steps		
1	**What is the rate and rhythm?**	*The rate is just above 50 beats per minute and the rhythm is regular.*
2	**Are there any P waves and what is their relationship with the QRS complex?**	*There is a P wave before every QRS complex and a QRS complex after every P wave.*
3	**What is the duration and morphology of the QRS complex?**	*The QRS complex is of normal shape and the duration is under 0.12 seconds (3 small squares).*
4	**Is the ST segment isoelectric, depressed or elevated?**	*The ST segment is normal.*
5	**Are the QT intervals and T waves normal?**	*The T wave is of normal shape and the QT interval is 0.44 seconds, which is appropriate for the rate (QTc 0.42 seconds).*
Clinical Steps		
6	**Is the heart generating a palpable pulse of appropriate rate and providing adequate perfusion?**	*Yes.*
7	**Is the rhythm unstable and at risk of deterioration?**	*No.*
8	**Does the presenting rhythm support or change your working diagnosis?**	*No.*
9	**Are any clinical interventions required?**	*No.*

Case Scenario 2.3 Answers

a) **What are your differential diagnoses for Martin?** *Differentials should include: bronchitis, pneumonia, sepsis, heart failure.*

b) **Use the 9-step ECG interpretation tool to assess Martin's ECG.**

c) **What rhythm is the ECG?** *Sinus tachycardia.*

d) **What is your working diagnosis?** *Pneumonia.*

Discussion: *Martin is presenting with signs and symptoms in keeping with a chest infection; specifically, his symptoms are more suggestive of pneumonia than bronchitis. His ECG shows a sinus tachycardia; this is an expected finding in keeping with the infection. The problem is not with his heart, but his heart is beating faster than normal due to the infection.*

ECG Steps		
1	What is the rate and rhythm?	*The rate is just above 100 beats per minute and the rhythm is regular.*
2	Are there any P waves and what is their relationship with the QRS complex?	*There is a P before every QRS complex and a QRS complex after every P wave.*
3	What is the duration and morphology of the QRS complex?	*The QRS complex is of normal shape and the duration is under 0.12 seconds (3 small squares).*
4	Is the ST segment isoelectric, depressed or elevated?	*The ST segment is normal.*
5	Are the QT intervals and T waves normal?	*The T wave is of normal shape and the QT interval is normal.*
Clinical Steps		
6	Is the heart generating a palpable pulse of appropriate rate and providing adequate perfusion?	*Yes.*
7	Is the rhythm unstable and at risk of deterioration?	*No.*
8	Does the presenting rhythm support or change your working diagnosis?	*Supports infection due to increased rate.*
9	Are any clinical interventions required?	*No.*

Case Scenario 2.4 Answers

a) **What are your differential diagnoses for Sheila?** *Differentials should include: atrial flutter, atrial fibrillation with rapid ventricular response, infection, heart failure, lung cancer.*

b) **Use the 9-step ECG interpretation tool to assess Sheila's ECG.**

c) **What rhythm is the ECG?** *Atrial flutter.*

d) **What is your working diagnosis?** *Atrial flutter potentially caused by the degree of Sheila's recent alcohol consumption.*

Discussion: *With a regular ventricular rate of just under 150 beats per minute and regular flutter waves with a rate just under 300 beats per minute, this is a good example of atrial flutter with 2:1 conduction. The cause of the atrial flutter may be Sheila's recent sustained increase of alcohol consumption. Her presenting symptoms of fatigue and shortness of breath are potentially a result of the atrial flutter. But we must also consider the possibility that the atrial flutter and her presenting symptoms are all the result of an underlying problem we cannot identify with the information available.*

ECG Steps		
1	What is the rate and rhythm?	*The rate is around 150 beats/minute and the rhythm is regular.*
2	Are there any P waves and what is their relationship with the QRS complex?	*There are P(F) waves visible. There are two P(F) waves before every QRS. The atrial rate is 300 beats per minute.*
3	What is the duration and morphology of the QRS complex?	*The QRS complex is of normal shape and the duration is under 0.12 seconds (3 small squares).*
4	Is the ST segment isoelectric, depressed or elevated?	*The ST segment appears to have ST depression in the inferior leads. This is most likely pseudo ST depression caused by the P(F) waves superimposed on the ST segment.*
5	Are the QT intervals and T waves normal?	*The T wave is of normal shape and the QT interval is appropriate for the rate.*
Clinical Steps		
6	Is the heart generating a palpable pulse of appropriate rate and providing adequate perfusion?	*Yes.*
7	Is the rhythm unstable and at risk of deterioration?	*Yes, could deteriorate into atrial fibrillation.*
8	Does the presenting rhythm support or change your working diagnosis?	*Atrial flutter.*
9	Are any clinical interventions required?	*No.*

Case Scenario 2.5 Answers

a) **What are your differential diagnoses for Brian?** *Differentials should include: stroke, subarachnoid haemorrhage, bradyarrhythmia, tachyarrhythmia, seizure.*

b) **Use the 9-step ECG interpretation tool to assess Brian's ECG.**

c) **What rhythm is the ECG?** *3rd degree heart block (complete heart block).*

d) **What is your working diagnosis?** *3rd degree heart block, potentially caused by the beta blocker he recently started taking or his aortic stenosis.*

Discussion: *A sudden collapse with few preceding symptoms can pose a tricky diagnosis, especially with the limited range of assessments available in the out-of-hospital environment. Brian had not recovered when we arrived; this suggests a more serious cause, as a simple faint should have resolved rapidly. Neurological and cardiac events can both cause sudden collapse. In this case, the complete heart block has caused an extreme bradycardia, which in turn has significantly reduced Brian's blood pressure, causing him to collapse. Identifying the certain cause of the heart block is not possible or necessary as we treat him at home. He is in a time-critical and life-threatening state so our priorities should be to correct any ABCDE problems we can and rapidly transport Brian to definitive care at the emergency department.*

ECG Steps		
1	**What is the rate and rhythm?**	*The rate is around 30 beats/minute and the rhythm is regular.*
2	**Are there any P waves and what is their relationship with the QRS complex?**	*There are P waves visible. The P waves have no connection to the QRS complexes. In some isolated beats they may appear to precede the QRS complex but this is by chance. There are inappropriate P waves present; some are between the QRS and T waves, others are on or just after the T waves.*
3	**What is the duration and morphology of the QRS complex?**	*The QRS complexes are over 0.12 seconds (3 small squares) in duration. They are wide and slurred, suggesting they are originating below the level of the AV node or bundle of His.*
4	**Is the ST segment isoelectric, depressed or elevated?**	*The ST segment is normal. There are some points where slurring of the terminal wave of the QRS complex could be mistaken for ST segment changes.*
5	**Are the QT intervals and T waves normal?**	*The T wave shape is in keeping with the QRS complexes and the QT interval is appropriate for the rate.*
Clinical Steps		
6	**Is the heart generating a palpable pulse of appropriate rate and providing adequate perfusion?**	*No.*
7	**Is the rhythm unstable and at risk of deterioration?**	*Yes, could deteriorate to cardiac arrest rhythm.*
8	**Does the presenting rhythm support or change your working diagnosis?**	*Complete heart block supports a bradyarrhythmia hypotensive cause of collapse.*
9	**Are any clinical interventions required?**	*Yes. Brian is in a peri-arrest state and requires urgent interventions and transport to hospital. His ABCs need to be managed with high-flow oxygen. Atropine should be considered for his bradycardia (keeping in mind that it may not be effective as the cause is an AV block). Fluid therapy can also be considered; however, as Brian has heart failure there is a risk of creating a fluid overload. But with his current state, fluid therapy may be the only way to prevent a further BP drop during transport.*

References

1. Joint Royal College Ambulance Liaison Committee and Association of Ambulance Chief Executives, *JRCALC Clinical Guidelines 2019*. Bridgwater: Class Professional Publishing, 2019.

2. Resuscitation Council (UK), 'Peri-arrest arrhythmias', in *Resuscitation Guidelines 2015*. London: Resuscitation Council (UK), 2015.

3. F. Kusumoto et al., '2018 ACC/AHA/HRS guideline on the evaluation and management of patients with bradycardia and cardiac conduction delay: a report of the American College of Cardiology/American Heart Association Task Force on Clinical Practice Guidelines and the Heart Rhythm Society', *Circulation*, vol. 140, no. 8, 2019, pp. 383–482.

4. B. Olshankshy and R. Gopinathannair, 'Bradycardia', in *BMJ Best Practice* [Online]. London: BMJ Publishing Group, 2018.

5. P. A. Younge, 'Bradycardia', in *Royal College of Emergency Medicine Learning* [Online]. London: RCEM, 2017.

6. M. R. Ginks et al., 'Cardiac arrhythmias', in J. Firth, C. Conlon and T. Cox, eds., *Oxford Textbook of Medicine*, 6th edn. Oxford: Oxford University Press, 2020.

7. G. R. Nimmo and T. Walsh, 'Critical illness', in *Davidson's Principles and Practices of Medicine*. Edinburgh: Churchill Livingstone, 2014.

8. T. Standl et al., 'The nomenclature, definition and distinction of types of shock', *Continuing Medical Education*, vol. 115, no. 45, 2018, pp. 757–768.

9. F. G. Bonanno, 'Clinical pathology of the shock syndromes', *Journal of Emergency Trauma and Shock*, vol. 4, no. 2, 2011, pp. 233–243.

10. C. Vahdatpour, D. Collins and S. Goldberg, 'Cardiogenic shock', *Journal of the American Heart Association*, vol. 8, no. 8, 2019, pp. 1–12.

11. Joint Formulary Committee, 'Beta-adrenoceptor blocking drugs', *BMJ Group and Pharmaceutical Press* [Online]. Available: https://bnf.nice.org.uk/treatment-summary/beta-adrenoceptor-blocking-drugs.html.

12. Joint Formulary Committee, 'Calcium-channel blockers', *BMJ Group and Pharmaceutical Press* [Online]. Available: https://bnf.nice.org.uk/treatment-summary/calcium-channel-blockers.html.

13. Joint Formulary Committee, 'Cardiac glycosides', *BMJ Group and Pharmaceutical Press* [Online]. Available: https://bnf.nice.org.uk/treatment-summary/cardiac-glycosides.html.

14. Joint Formulary Committee, 'Analgesics', *BMJ Group and Pharmaceutical Press* [Online]. Available: https://bnf.nice.org.uk/treatment-summary/analgesics.html.

15. Joint Formulary Committee, 'Sodium chloride', *BMJ Group and Pharmaceutical Press* [Online]. Available: https://bnf.nice.org.uk/drug/sodium-chloride.html.

16. J. Brugada et al., 'ESC guidelines for the management of patients with supraventricular tachycardia: The task force for the management of patients with supraventricular tachycardia of the European Society of Cardiology (ESC)', *European Heart Journal,* vol. 41, no. 5, 2019, pp. 655–720.

17. T. Garcia, *12-Lead ECG: The Art of Interpretation*, 2nd edn. Burlington: Jones and Bartlett Learning, 2013.

18. R. Shadman and R. W. Rho, 'Assessment of tachycardia', in *BMJ Best Practice* [Online]. London: BMJ Publishing Group, 2018.

19. D. E. Newby, N. R. Grubb and A. Bradbury, 'Cardiovascular disease', in *Davidson's Principles and Practices of Medicine*, 22nd edn. Edinburgh: Churchill Livingstone, 2014.

20. A. Henning and C. Krawiec, 'Sinus tachycardia', *StatPearls* [Online], 2020.

21. D. Katritsis et al., 'European Heart Rhythm Association (EHRA) consensus document on the management of supraventricular arrhythmias, endorsed by Heart Rhythm Society (HRS), Asia-Pacific Heart Rhythm Society (APHRS), and Sociedad Latinoamericana de Estimulación Cardiaca y Elect', *EP Europace*, vol. 19, no. 3, 2016, pp. 465–511.

22. S. M. Stevens, S. C. Woller and G. V. Fontaine, 'Pulmonary embolism', in *BMJ Best Practice* [Online]. London: BMJ Publishing Group, 2018.

23. C. N. Sawchuk and J. P. Veitengruber, 'Panic disorders', in *BMJ Best Practice* [Online]. London: BMJ Publishing Group, 2019.

24. S. Konstantinides et al., '2019 ESC guidelines for the diagnosis and management of acute pulmonary embolism developed in collaboration with the European Respiratory Society (ERS)', *European Heart Journal*, vol. 41, no. 4, 2019, pp. 543–603.

25. R. Page et al., '2015 ACC/AHA/HRS guideline for the management of adult patients with supraventricular tachycardia', *Journal of the American College of Cardiology*, vol. 67, no. 13, 2016, pp. 27–115.

26. S. Goodacre and R. Irons, 'Atrial arrhythmias', *BMJ*, vol. 324, no. 594, 2002.

27. S. M. Fox, J. P. Naughton and W. L. Haskell, 'Physical activity and the prevention of coronary heart disease', *Annals of Clinical Research*, vol. 3, no. 6, 1971, pp. 404–432.

28. P. Reavley, 'Palpitations', in *Royal College of Emergency Medicine Learning* [Online]. London: RCEM, 2017.

29. Joint Formulary Committee, 'Arrhythmias', in *British National Formulary* [Online]. London: BMJ Group and Pharmaceutical Press, 2019.

30. B. Alzand and H. Crijns' Diagnostic criteria of broad QRS complex tachycardia: decades of evolution', *Europace*, vol. 13, 2011, pp. 465–472.

31. A. R. Houghton and D. Gray, 'Electrocardiography', in J. Firth, C. Conlon and T. Cox, eds., *Oxford Textbook of Medicine*, 6th edn. Oxford: Oxford University Press, 2020.

32. S. Meek, 'Supraventricular tachycardias', in *Royal College of Emergency Medicine Learning* [Online]. London: RCEM, 2019.

33. E. Docherty and F. P. Morris, 'Broad complex tachycardias', in *Royal College of Emergency Medicine Learning* [Online]. London: RCEM, 2017.

34. S. M. Al-Khatib et al., '2017 AHA/ACC/HRS guideline for management of patients with ventricular arrhythmias and the prevention of sudden cardiac death', *Circulation*, vol. 138, 2018, pp. 272–391.

35. J. Soar, C. D. Deakin, J. P. Nolan et al. 'Adult advanced life support guidelines', *Resuscitation Council UK* [online], 2021. Available: https://www.resus.org.uk/library/2021-resuscitation-guidelines/adult-advanced-life-support-guidelines.

36. Resuscitation Council (UK), 'Prehospital resuscitation', in *Resuscitation Guidelines* 2015. London: Resuscitation Council (UK), 2015.

37. P. Rautaharju, B. Surawicz and L. Gettes, 'AHA/ACCF/HRS recommendations for the standardization and interpretation of the electrocardiogram', *Journal of the American College of Cardiology*, vol. 53, no. 11, 2009, pp. 982–991.

38. A. J. Camm and N. Bunce, 'Cardiovascular disease', in P. Kumar and M. Clark, eds., *Clinical Medicine*, 7th edn. Edinburgh: Saunders Elsevier, 2009, pp. 717–720.

39. A. Vink et al., 'Determination and interpretation of the QT interval', *Circulation*, vol. 138, no. 21, 2018, pp. 2345–2358.

40. S. Meek and F. Morris, 'ABC of clinical electrocardiography: introduction. II—Basic terminology', *BMJ,* vol. 324, 2002, pp. 470–473.

41. National Institute for Health and Care Excellence, 'Transient loss of consciousness ("blackouts") in over 16s', *NICE Clinical Guideline 109*. London: NICE, 2010.

42. M. Beattie and M. Champion, *Essential Revision Notes in Paediatrics for the MRCPCH*, 3rd edn. Knutsford: PasTest, 2013.

43. M. Brignole et al., '2018 ESC guidelines for the diagnosis and management of syncope', *European Heart Journal*, vol. 39, 2018, pp. 1883–1948.

44. National Institute for Health and Care Excellence, 'Atrial fibrillation: management', *NICE Clinical Guideline 180*. London: NICE, 2014.

45. NHS, 'Atrial fibrillation' [Online], 2018. Available: www.nhs.uk/conditions/atrial-fibrillation.

46. P. Kirchhof et al., '2016 ESC guidelines for the management of atrial fibrillation developed in collaboration with EACTS', *European Heart Journal*, vol. 37, no. 38, 2016, pp. 2893–2962.

47. R. Kurapati, J. Heaton and D. R. Lowery, 'Atrial kick', *StatPearls* [Online], 2020.

48. V. Namana et al., 'Clinical significance of atrial kick', *Quarterly Journal of Medicine*, vol. 111, no. 8, 2018, pp. 569–570.

49. C. Mann, 'Atrial fibrillation', in *Royal College of Emergency Medicine Learning* [Online]. London: RCEM, 2019.

50. S. Levy et al., 'International consensus on nomenclature and classification of atrial fibrillation', *Journal of Cardiovascular Electrophysiology*, vol. 14, no. 4, 2003, pp. 443–445.

51. G. Hindricks et al., '2020 ESC guidelines for the diagnosis and management of atrial fibrillation developed in collaboration with the European Association for Cardio-Thoracic Surgery (EACTS)', *European Heart Journal*, vol. 29, ehaa612, 2020, pp.1–126.

52. N. J. Adderley et al., 'Prevalence and treatment of atrial fibrillation in UK general practice from 2000 to 2016', *Heart*, vol. 105, 2019, pp. 27–33.

53. J. Granada et al., 'Incidence and predictors of atrial flutter in the general population', *Journal of the American College of Cardiology*, vol. 36, no. 7, 2000, pp. 2242–2246.

54. S. Petkar, J. Pathiraja and A. Aziz, 'Atrioventricular block', in *BMJ Best Practice* [Online]. London: BMJ Publishing Group, 2019.

55. H. Hreybe and S. Saba, 'Location of acute myocardial infarction and associated arrhythmias and outcome', *Clinical Cardiology*, vol. 32, no. 5, 2009, pp. 274–277.

56. R. S. DePaula et al., 'Cardiac arrhythmias and atrioventricular block in a cohort of asymptomatic individuals without heart disease', *Cardiology*, vol. 108, no. 2, 2007, pp. 111–116.

57. S. Kinoshita, G. Konishi and Y. Kinoshita, 'Mechanism of ventricular extrasystoles with fixed coupling', in *Journal of Electrocardiology*, vol. 23, no. 3, 1990, pp. 249–254.

12-Lead ECG Problems

As we know from Section 2, arrhythmias can be identified from a lead II rhythm strip. However, the majority of ECGs reviewed in clinical practice will be 12-lead ECGs. The basics of interpreting a 12-lead ECG are covered in Section 1. In Section 3 we will look at the ECG changes that can only be identified on a 12-lead ECG and some of the underlying conditions that have led to these changes.

It is important to remember that the purpose of the 12-lead ECG is to 'look' at different anatomical areas of the heart. The majority of problems we will identify from a 12-lead ECG are location-based problems, either affecting only a certain anatomical area of the heart (for example, myocardial infarction) or affecting the heart in ways that mean the resulting ECG changes are only visible in certain ECG lead views (for example, axis deviation).

It often occurs that the underlying condition causing a location-based problem also causes, or is linked to the cause of, an arrhythmia. This can make the interpretation of an ECG more challenging, as multiple problems present themselves on the ECG. We will look at some examples of these more complex ECGs at the end of this section and in the scenario section at the end of the book.

Cardiac Muscle Damage

Cardiac muscle damage may occur suddenly if the blood supply to an area of muscle is cut off due to myocardial infarction (MI); cardiac muscle may also become damaged over time through heart failure and hypertrophy. We may even see signs of historic cardiac muscle damage on the ECG, such as when a patient has had a previous MI.

Any part of the heart can become damaged and it is important that we identify the area of the heart muscle that has been affected. To do this, we must assess all of the leads of the 12-lead ECG and look for changes based on the anatomical location of each lead view (page 22).

It is important to remember that cardiac muscle damage can often also lead to damage of the electrical conduction system within the heart. Therefore, we may see rate or rhythm disturbances along with the cardiac muscle damage on the ECG. Ectopic beats are also often present due to the increased strain on, and irritation of, the cardiac muscle. Arrhythmias are the most common complication of MI, with over 90% of patients suffering MI displaying some form of arrhythmia.[1]

Acute Coronary Syndrome and Myocardial Ischaemia

The term Acute Coronary Syndrome (ACS) is an umbrella term for unstable angina, ST Segment Elevation Myocardial Infarction (STEMI) and Non-ST Segment Elevation Myocardial Infarction (NSTEMI). All of these conditions are associated with a sudden and reduced blood flow to the cardiac muscle.[2, 3]

In the UK, around 275,000 women and 640,000 men will have an MI at some point during their lives. Around 175,000 MIs will occur annually. One in ten women and one in six men will die from coronary heart disease.[4] There are around 700,000 presentations of acute chest pain to emergency departments each year in England and Wales, and chest pain accounts for around 25% of emergency medical admissions.[5, 6]

Clinical Presentation of Acute Coronary Syndrome

In the out-of-hospital environment, ACS is identified through a combination of clinical presentation and analysis of the patient's 12-lead ECG. The classical, cardinal symptom of ACS is severe central or left-sided chest pain, described as tight, crushing or heavy in nature. The pain may also radiate to the patient's neck, jaw, back, arms or upper abdomen.[2, 7] Associated symptoms include nausea, vomiting, clamminess, shortness of breath, dizziness, anxiety and a sense of impending doom. It should be noted, however, that this 'classic' presentation of ACS can lend clinicians a dangerous and false sense of security when presented with an absence of the most well-known symptoms. Further to this, patients each have their own unique perception of pain and way of expressing themselves; their description of chest pain should be carefully analysed. Although chest pain is present in the majority of ACS patients, up to one third of ACS patients can present atypically, with an absence of the classic symptoms. They instead present with any number and combination of diffuse and less specific symptoms such as shortness of breath or collapse.[7] ACS may even present without any pain or discomfort whatsoever; termed a 'silent MI', these are notoriously difficult to diagnose, even with the aid of a 12-lead ECG. The silent MI is frequently diagnosed retrospectively when a patient presents with symptoms of the resulting heart failure and cardiac muscle damage. Women, older people and diabetic patients are more likely to present atypically or with a silent MI;[3] combine this with the fact that older patients, women and those with co-morbidities are less likely to receive an out-of-hospital ECG in the UK,[7, 8] and we are reminded that it is essential to have a low threshold for carrying out a 12-lead ECG on patients who may be presenting with an atypical MI. Research by the Myocardial Ischaemia National Audit Project in the UK has demonstrated favourable survival rates for patients suffering either STEMI or NSTEMI where out-of-hospital 12-lead ECGs were undertaken.[8]

It is important to note that even though the presence, or absence, of certain symptoms can suggest an increased or decreased likelihood of ACS occurring, none are specific enough to allow the diagnosis or exclusion of ACS, even in combination with a 12-lead ECG. This is especially the case in the out-of-hospital environment where near-patient blood testing is not usually available.[5, 7, 9]

> **!**
> - Clinicians should have a low threshold for suspecting ACS. It is not possible, or safe, to exclude ACS based on the presence or absence of specific symptoms alone.
> - A patient presenting with ACS signs and symptoms and an ECG which does not meet STEMI criteria should be managed following guidelines for ACS.[7, 9]

Clinical Signs and Symptoms of Acute Coronary Syndrome [1, 2, 3, 5, 7, 9, 10, 11, 12, 13, 14, 15]

- Chest pain or discomfort:
    - Often severe and of sudden onset.
    - Central or left side of the chest, though may be diffuse and not localised within the chest.
    - Described as tight, crushing, constricting or heavy in nature.
    - Often not affected by position or movement.
    - Possible radiation to the neck, jaw, arms or epigastric region of the abdomen.
    - Lasting longer than 15 minutes.
- Associated signs and symptoms:
    - Shortness of breath.
    - Dizziness.

- ‣ Nausea and vomiting.
- ‣ Pallor and clamminess.
- ‣ Anxiety, agitation or a sense of impending doom.
- ‣ Collapse.
- ‣ Palpitations.
- ‣ Tachycardia.
- ‣ Weakness or fatigue.
- ‣ Audible S3 or S4 heart sound.
- ‣ Atypical symptoms:
  - ‣ Non-'classic' chest pain.
  - ‣ Isolated upper epigastric pain.
- ‣ The damage to the heart muscle can be significant enough to cause a reduced cardiac output. The severity of the circulatory shock (page 14) and the associated symptoms is dictated by the degree of cardiac muscle damage. Symptoms associated with reduced cardiac output include:
  - ‣ Pale, cold and clammy skin.
  - ‣ Hypotension and weak or absent peripheral pulses.
  - ‣ Delayed capillary refill.
  - ‣ Tachypnoea.
  - ‣ Dizziness or near loss of consciousness.
  - ‣ Loss of consciousness or reduced level of consciousness.
  - ‣ Anxiety and confusion.

> **Remember!** Up to one third of patients having an MI will present atypically, without the classic chest pain associated with MI. Women, older patients and those with diabetes are at increased risk of having atypical or absent symptoms. Clinicians should have a low threshold for carrying out a 12-lead ECG.

Cardiac Risk Factors

When obtaining a history from a patient, it is important to consider what risk factors they may have that increase their risk of acute cardiac events.

The following all increase a patient's cardiac risk:[2, 5, 16]
- Smoking.
- Hypertension.
- Diabetes.
- Obesity.
- Sedentary lifestyle (physical inactivity).
- High cholesterol.
- Family history of cardiac events or coronary artery disease.
- Cocaine use.
- Sex: Greater risk to men than women.
- Age: Risk increases with age.
- Existing coronary artery disease.
- Renal insufficiency.

Pathophysiology of Acute Coronary Syndrome

To understand the differences between the conditions which together encompass ACS, we must first understand the pathophysiology which they share.

Ischaemia occurs when cardiac muscle cells are deprived of oxygen; cells cannot metabolise normally via aerobic respiration, and instead they start to metabolise via anaerobic respiration, which is metabolism without oxygen and therefore not sustainable. Anaerobic respiration produces lactic acid and other harmful metabolites which cause an increasing level of acidosis within the cardiac muscle tissue which will then lead to cardiac muscle cell damage. Acidosis, alongside the lack of oxygen and nutrient supply to the cardiac muscle cells, will lead to infarction (cardiac muscle necrosis – cell death) if blood flow is not restored.

Ischaemia can develop both when demand for oxygen exceeds the supply (demand ischaemia) and when the supply is decreased and falls below the demand (supply ischaemia).[5]

Angina Pectoris

Angina pectoris is an example of demand ischaemia. This is caused by long-term narrowing of the coronary arteries due to coronary artery disease (CAD), reducing blood flow to the cardiac muscle. When demand for oxygen within the cardiac muscle cells increases through exercise or other means, the narrowed and diseased coronary arteries are unable to meet the increased demand and myocardial ischaemia occurs. Cell death does not usually occur unless there is complete arterial obstruction preventing blood flow to the cardiac muscle. The cardiac muscle cells still receive some blood supply and the transient ischaemia resolves when the demand for oxygen decreases, usually through rest and stopping exertion.

Key Concept: Cardiac ischaemia is a restriction of blood supply to cardiac muscle tissue which if prolonged will result in cardiac muscle cell death (infarction).

Types of Angina[7, 17, 18, 19, 20]

Stable angina has a trigger, usually exercise, exertion or stress, and should resolve within a few minutes of resting, taking medication (glyceryl trinitrate – GTN) or both. Being called to a patient due to previously diagnosed angina often generates enough concern in itself to warrant further assessment in hospital, as many patients are able to manage episodes of stable angina without seeking medical assistance. Patients with stable angina are also at risk of transitioning into unstable angina and at increased risk of MI. Unlike unstable angina, stable angina is not considered part of the ACS triad.

Unstable angina may start without a trigger, even starting at rest, and symptoms will continue despite rest and medication. Unstable angina is defined as myocardial ischaemia occurring with minimal exertion or at rest, without biochemical evidence of myocardial damage. Differentiation between NSTEMI and unstable angina relies on the results of cardiac biomarkers which cannot normally be obtained in the out-of-hospital environment. The initial presentation and range of ECG changes are the same for both conditions. Patients should be treated for the worst-case scenario, NSTEMI, with standard ACS management.

Prinzmetal angina differs from other types of angina in that it is not caused by narrowed arteries; instead, vasoconstrictive spasms of the coronary arteries result in reduced blood flow to cardiac muscle and lead to the symptoms of angina. It can cause marked ST segment elevation which resolves rapidly with GTN treatment (though GTN treatment should not be used diagnostically to differentiate conditions).

Myocardial Infarction

Myocardial infarction (MI) is defined pathologically as myocardial cell death due to prolonged ischaemia; this is normally caused by coronary artery occlusion. Cell death does not occur immediately and begins around 20 minutes after the onset of ischaemia. Complete necrosis of all myocardial cells affected by the MI takes at least 2–4 hours or longer, depending on the degree of collateral circulation, if the occlusion is intermittent, the treatment received and the specific demand for oxygen of the affected cells.[21]

Coronary artery occlusion can occur due to acute thrombus formation within the coronary artery itself, due to coronary embolism or due to coronary artery dissection.

Acute thrombus formation occurs when an atherosclerotic coronary artery plaque is disrupted either by rupture (mechanical disruption) or erosion (inflammatory disruption). This disruption triggers thrombosis (clot formation) by platelet activation and aggregation.[5]

Coronary embolism occurs when a blood clot, calcium or piece of tissue or infection travels through the circulation from another part of the body and becomes lodged within the coronary circulation.

Coronary artery dissection can also cause MI, where a tear develops in a coronary artery and prevents blood supply beyond the area of dissection. This classically presents in women in their 20s or 30s or during pregnancy.[22]

When a blood clot forms and occludes a coronary artery, the blood supply to an area of cardiac muscle cells is completely lost. This causes supply ischaemia, which will progress to cardiac muscle cell death unless the patient receives some form of reperfusion therapy to restore blood flow and oxygenation to the affected area. Unlike ischaemia, cell death is irreversible and permanently damages an area of the cardiac muscle. The area affected by the coronary artery occlusion may be large enough to cause heart failure or cardiac arrest.

In myocardial infarction, speed is paramount; the phrase 'time is muscle' is widely used, and for good reason. The sooner reperfusion is achieved, the smaller the area of cardiac muscle cell death and the better the chances of survival, recovery and sustained quality of life.

The area of cardiac muscle deprived of blood flow due to coronary artery occlusion is known as the zone of ischaemia;[3] the location of the occlusion within the coronary artery will impact the size of the zone of ischaemia and the severity of the MI. Heart failure can occur if 25% of the myocardium is affected, and cardiogenic shock occurs when greater than 40% of the left ventricular myocardium is affected.[2]

Myocardial infarction is divided into two subcategories based on 12-lead ECG findings:[19]

- ST segment elevation myocardial infarction (STEMI) is identified when a patient presents with both ACS symptoms and ST segment elevation which meets STEMI criteria. STEMI is usually the result of acute thrombus formation where the clot remains at the site of formation within the coronary artery, creating a large zone of ischaemia.[5] The ST segment elevation on the ECG is caused by the electrical activity of cardiac conduction interacting with necrotic cells.
- Non-ST segment elevation myocardial infarction (NSTEMI) is identified when a patient has ACS symptoms but there is an absence of ST segment elevation on the 12-lead ECG. Despite the absence of ST segment elevation, there can still be signs of ischaemia on the ECG; these are discussed below. NSTEMI is usually the result of coronary embolism, where thrombus formation has occurred and fragmented into smaller emboli, causing many micro-infarctions in the distal cardiac muscle tissue, without causing complete occlusion in the coronary artery at the site of the initial clot formation.[5]

ECG Changes in Acute Coronary Syndrome

Before we proceed with ECG identification of ACS, we need to understand two key principles: How to identify and interpret the J point on the ECG, and how to relate contiguous ECG leads to their anatomical locations.

The J Point

The J point is the junction between the end of the QRS complex and the start of the ST segment, and is used to measure the extent of any ST segment depression or elevation that may be present in any given ECG lead.

When measuring the J point and ST segment changes, it is best to compare them to the TP segment since in patients with a stable baseline it provides the most accurate resting baseline (as it is the isoelectric interval between heartbeats).[23]

When assessing the J point (Figure 3.1) we must consider both its position and its shape. The **position** can be:

- Elevated: Possible STEMI.
- Depressed: Possible ischaemia.
- Isoelectric: Normal.

The **shape** can be:

- Normal.
- Notched: Suggestive of possible non-ischaemic cause of ST segment elevation.
- Slurred: Possible early repolarisation (page 110).

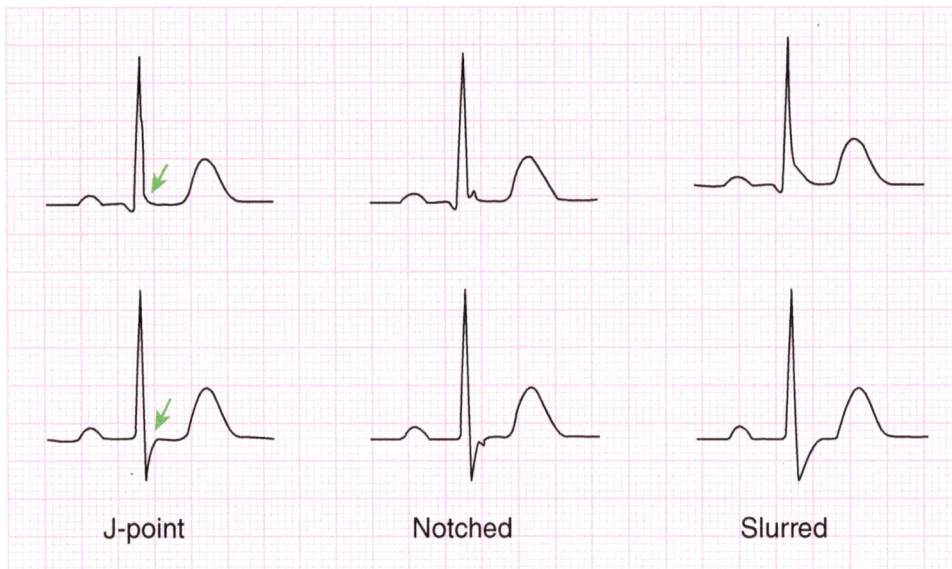

Figure 3.1 The J point.

Contiguous Leads

Contiguous leads are those which are anatomically adjacent in their views of the heart (Figure 3.2). Just because two leads are printed next to each other on an ECG print-out does not necessarily mean they are focusing on the same area of the heart. Equally, there are leads which are not printed together but are considered anatomically adjacent and therefore are contiguous.[21, 22]

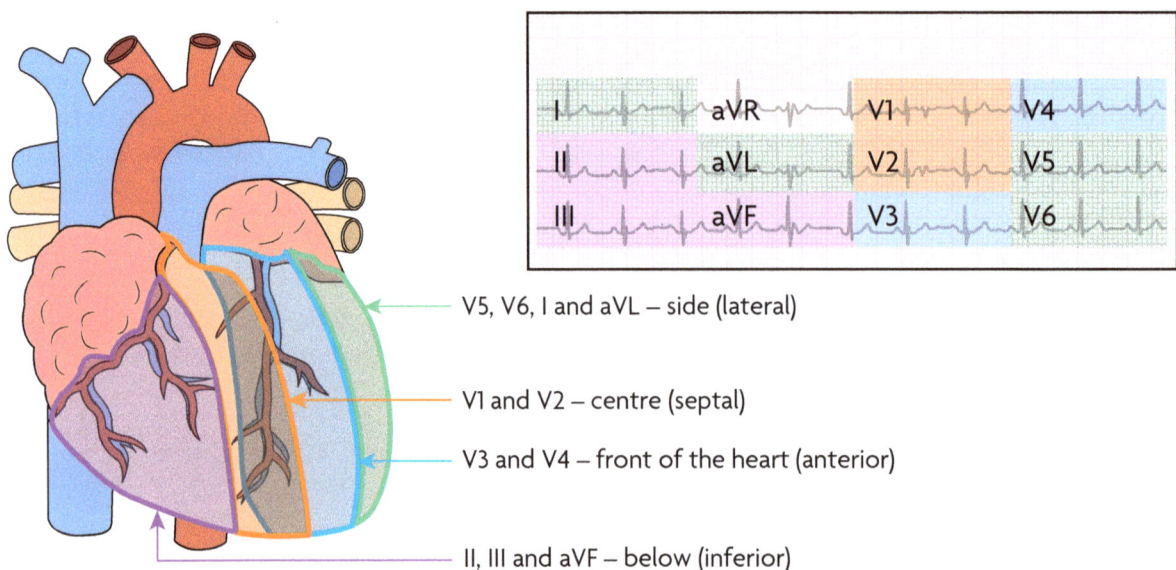

V5, V6, I and aVL – side (lateral)

V1 and V2 – centre (septal)

V3 and V4 – front of the heart (anterior)

II, III and aVF – below (inferior)

Figure 3.2 Anatomical viewpoints of the standard 12-lead ECG.

ECG Identification[7, 23]

When a patient presents with clinical signs and symptoms of ACS, they will often fall into one of three possible groups of findings on the ECG:

- The ECG has no significant changes and no signs of ischaemia. Note: Ischaemia may still be occurring despite the absence of ECG changes. **A 12-lead ECG should not be used to exclude ACS.**
- The ECG has signs of myocardial ischaemia, such as:
  - ST segment depression: Horizontal or downward-sloping ST segment depression, > 0.5 mm in two or more contiguous leads.
  - T wave changes: Inverted, biphasic or hyperacute.
  - ST segment elevation that does not meet STEMI criteria.
- The ECG meets STEMI criteria (see page 102).

- A patient presenting with ACS signs and symptoms and an ECG which does not meet STEMI criteria should be managed following guidelines for ACS.
- It is not possible to differentiate between unstable angina and NSTEMI in the out-of-hospital environment.
- A 'normal' ECG in a patient with ACS signs or symptoms does not exclude a cardiac cause and does not rule out significant myocardial damage or injury.

It is not possible, or safe, to exclude ACS based on the presence or absence of specific symptoms alone.[5, 7, 9]

Myocardial Ischaemia

There are multiple changes that can be identified on a 12-lead ECG that are suggestive of myocardial ischaemia. The main two are ST segment depression and inverted or biphasic T waves. Around half of patients found to have ST segment depression and a third of patients with T wave inversion will be found to have myocardial infarction.[5]

ST Segment Depression

Measured from the J point, ST segment depression can be described as horizontal, upward-sloping or downward-sloping (Figure 3.3).

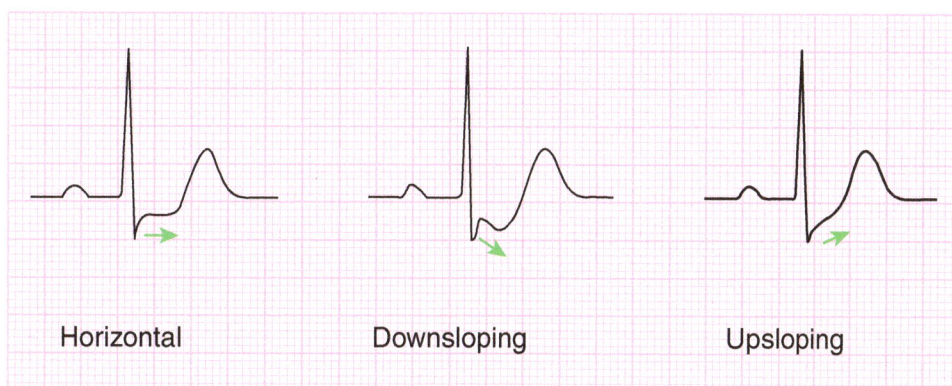

Horizontal   Downsloping   Upsloping

Figure 3.3 Different presentations of ST segment depression.

Horizontal or downward-sloping ST segment depression, measured at the J point, greater than 0.5 mm in two or more contiguous leads, is widely accepted as being indicative of myocardial ischaemia.[23] The greater the degree of ST segment depression, the more specific and indicative of myocardial ischaemia it is.

ST segment depression is also the main reciprocal change found in STEMI. When ST segment depression is localised to a specific anatomical area, ST segment elevation should be sought in the reciprocal leads; this may mean conducting a right-sided or posterior ECG (page 264).

ECG 3.1 – ST Depression

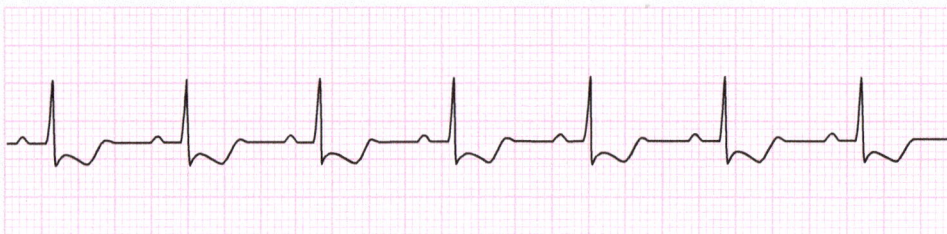

Remember, ST depression can occur in any ECG lead view.

De Winter's Sign[24]

One exception to upward-sloping ST segment depression is De Winter's sign, which presents with hyper-acute T waves persisting for hours with deep, upward-sloping ST segment depression in the precordial leads. It is a sign of proximal LAD occlusion. The presence of De Winter's sign is treated as a STEMI equivalent (despite not meeting criteria).

ECG 3.2 – De Winter's Sign

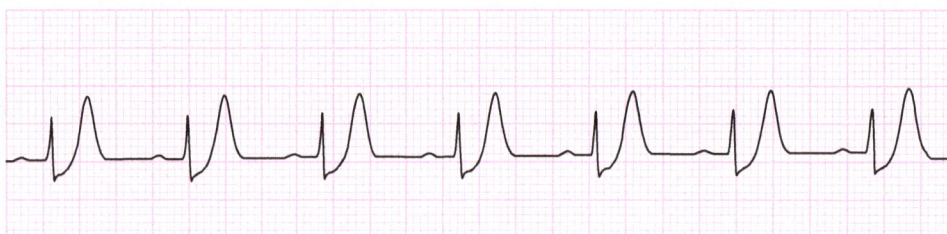

T Wave Changes

Remember, the T wave represents the repolarisation of the ventricles (page 7), meaning that myocardial cell death and ischaemia can both cause changes to T waves as well as to the ST segment.

T Wave Inversion (T wave Concordance)

We need to consider the relationship between the T wave and the QRS complex in regard to their direction. If the T wave is pointing in the same direction as the QRS complex it is referred to as being concordant. If the T wave is pointing in the opposite direction from the QRS complex this is referred to as being discordant or inverted. In most leads viewed on the ECG the QRS complex and T wave are upright, meaning that in most cases T wave inversion is seen as a T wave with a negative deflection below the isoelectric line.

Symmetrically inverted T waves can indicate myocardial ischaemia. To do so they must be at least 1 mm deep and be present in two or more contiguous leads with prominent R waves or an R/S ratio >1.16;[21] T wave inversion is a normal variant in lead aVR and can be a normal variant in leads III, V1, V2 and aVL.[25]

Non-ischaemic causes of T wave inversion include bundle branch blocks (page 124), ventricular hypertrophy (page 119) and hypokalaemia (page 145). Hypertrophic cardiomyopathy can also cause T wave inversion in the precordial leads (V1–V6).

ECG 3.3 – Inverted T Waves

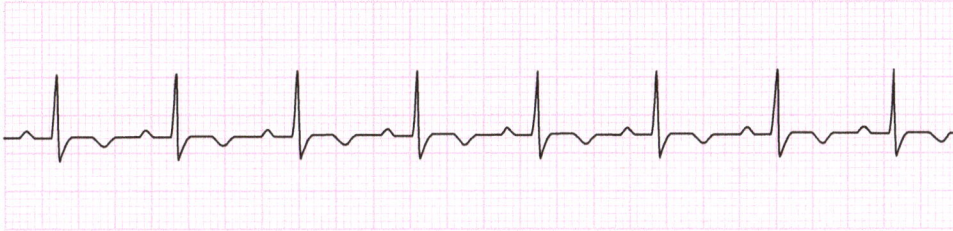

Remember, Inverted T waves can occur in any ECG lead view.

Biphasic T Waves

Biphasic T waves present with both a positive and a negative deflection. This can occur in either combination of positive deflection followed by negative deflection, or negative deflection followed by positive deflection. Biphasic T waves can be caused by both ischaemia and hypokalaemia (page 145).

A biphasic T wave is classified as either positive or negative based on its terminal portion, so if the last (terminal) part of the T wave is positive, it would be considered a positive T wave.

Wellen's Syndrome

Wellen's syndrome is an exception where isolated T wave inversion is a significant and acute sign likely requiring urgent recognition and transport to hospital. Wellen's syndrome is best seen in Leads V1–V6, though it can appear in other leads such as I and aVL. It is an evolving process that starts with biphasic T waves, where the first deflection is positive and followed by a second, negative deflection as seen in ECG 3.4a. It can then progress to deep, symmetrical and inverted T waves (ECG 3.4b). In both cases there is usually no significant ST segment depression or elevation. Wellen's syndrome is caused by significant stenosis (narrowing) of the left anterior descending coronary artery. Patients presenting with Wellen's syndrome have up to a 75% risk of developing significant anterior myocardial infarction within weeks.[26]

ECG 3.4a (left) and ECG 3.4b (right) – Wellen's Syndrome

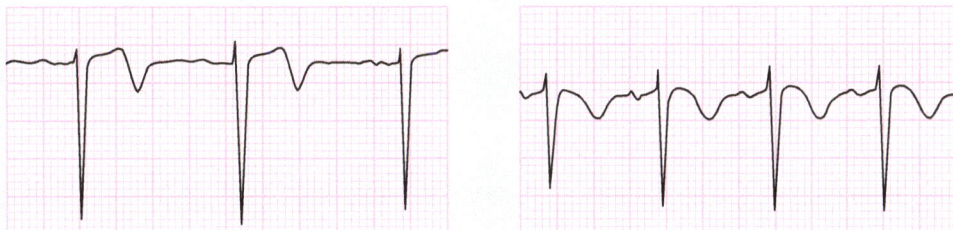

The Digoxin Effect[25, 27]

The digoxin effect is a classic pattern of ECG changes that can occur in patients on therapeutic levels of digitalis (digoxin). These changes include flattened or inverted T waves, shortening of the QT interval, prolongation of the PR interval and, most notably, 'scooped' ST segment depression. This classic 'scooped' ST segment depression is usually most prominent in the inferior and lateral ECG leads and can be confused with signs of ischaemia.

ST Segment Elevation Myocardial Infarction

ST Segment Elevation Myocardial Infarction (STEMI) is identified when ST segment elevation is present in at least two contiguous leads (measured from the J point). The degree of ST segment elevation required to diagnose a STEMI will depend on which of the ECG leads are showing the elevation.

> The ECG criteria for identification of STEMI depends on local guidelines but the widely accepted and used criteria for STEMI is:[7, 23]
> - Two or more contiguous leads with >1 mm of ST segment elevation, measured from the J point, except in leads V2 and V3 where age and sex need to be considered:
>   - Men > 40 years old: > 2 mm of ST segment elevation is required.
>   - Men < 40 years old: > 2.5 mm of ST segment elevation is required.
>   - Women of any age: > 1.5 mm of ST segment elevation is required.

The initial ECG obtained for patients who are suffering a STEMI is not always conclusive, emphasising the importance of the need for repeated ECGs as diagnostic changes may not become visible for several hours. Repeat ECGs increase the sensitivity of identifying STEMI to 95%.[18]
Of patients who suffer a STEMI:

- 50% have diagnostic changes on their initial ECG.
- 40% have an abnormal initial ECG that is not diagnostic.
- 10% have a normal initial ECG.

It is important that repeated ECGs are performed when attending a patient with ACS symptoms. It may be the case that the patient has presented too early for ST segment elevation to have developed from the time when the first ECG was taken.[7]

> !
> - A patient presenting with ACS signs and symptoms and an ECG which does not meet STEMI criteria should be managed following guidelines for the treatment of ACS.
> - A 12-lead ECG should not be used to exclude ACS.
> - A 'normal' ECG in a patient with ACS signs or symptoms does not exclude a cardiac cause and does not rule out significant myocardial damage or injury.[7, 5]

When we identify ST segment elevation we should take note of which ECG leads are involved. We can locate the anatomical area of the heart affected by the infarction and also judge the size of the affected area as indicated by the number of ECG leads involved. The presence of reciprocal changes will help to further confirm the diagnosis of STEMI. A reciprocal change is described as ST segment depression in the ECG leads with opposite anatomical views to those showing ST segment elevation. As described on page 22, each ECG lead views the heart from a different anatomical direction. If ST segment elevation is present, it appears as ST segment depression in the reciprocal lead, as can be seen in ECGs 3.5 and 3.6.

Reciprocal changes may not always be present. The leads showing ST segment elevation may not have reciprocal leads on the standard 12-lead ECG; the magnitude of the ST segment elevation may be not sufficiently manifest as ST segment depression in the reciprocal lead. Other ECG abnormalities such as bundle branch blocks (page 124) may mask or mimic reciprocal changes.[28]

> **Remember!** If previously undiagnosed left bundle branch block is found on the ECG when a patient is presenting with ACS symptoms, it is treated as a STEMI. !

ECG 3.5 – Inferior STEMI

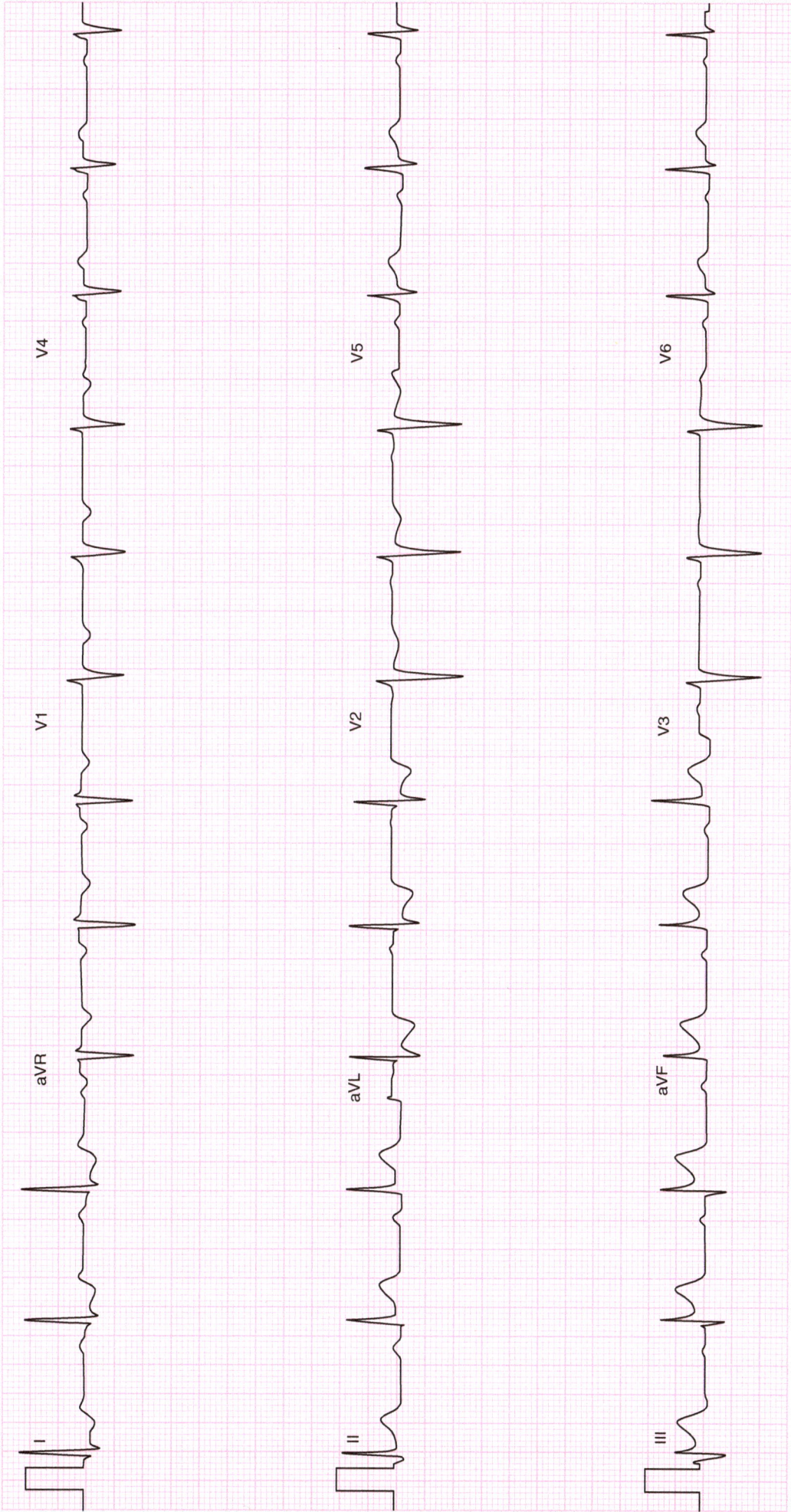

ST segment elevation can be seen in leads II, III and aVF, making this an inferior STEMI. There are also reciprocal changes visible in the high lateral leads I and aVL with ST segment depression and inverted T waves.

103

ECG 3.6 – Anterior STEMI

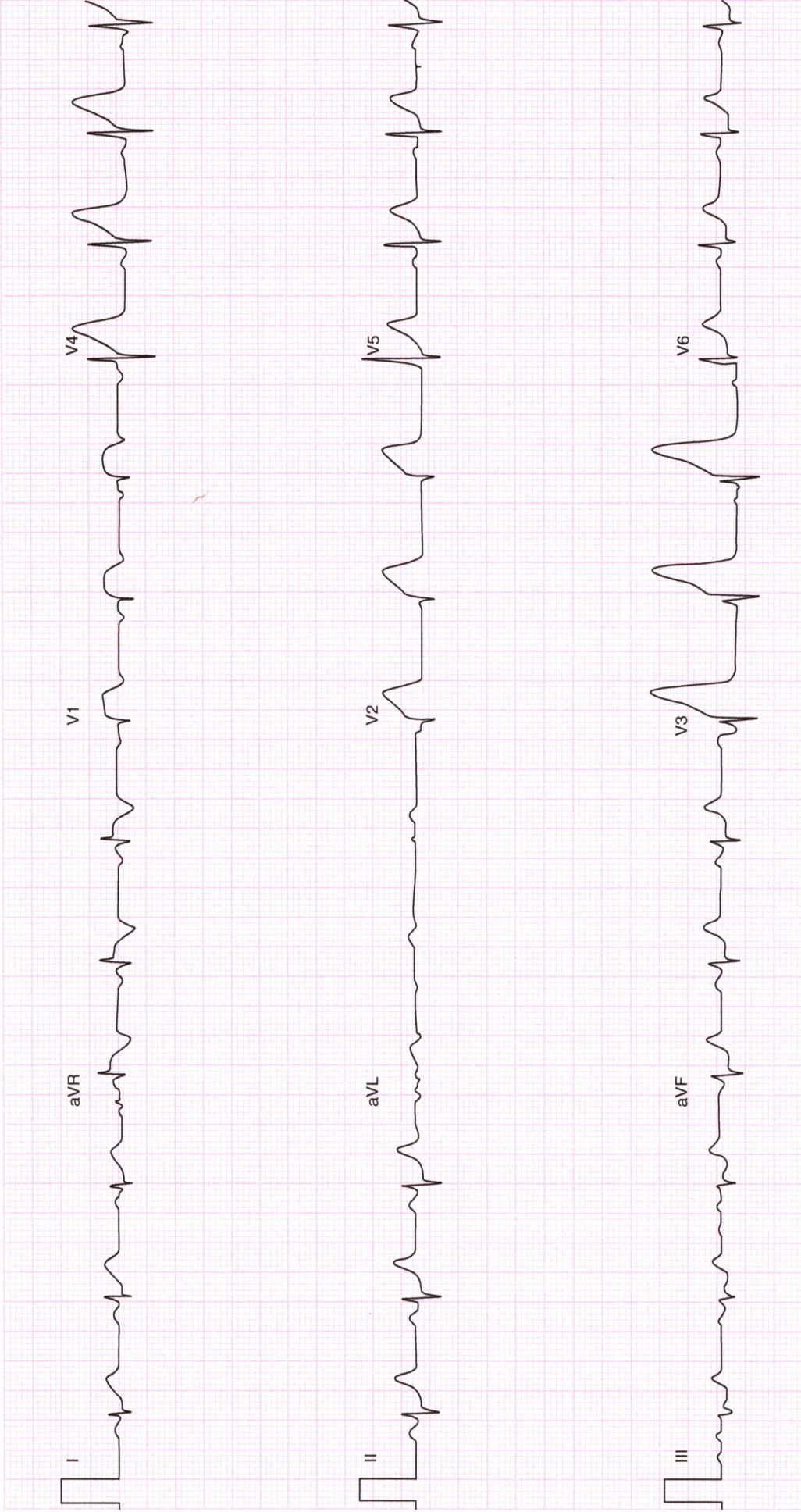

ST segment elevation is present in leads V1–V4, making this an anterior STEMI. There is also ST segment elevation in lead aVR; when combined with the presence of elevation in lead V1 this is suggestive of left anterior descending coronary artery occlusion. There are reciprocal changes in the form of widespread ST segment depression in lateral and inferior leads.

ECG 3.7 – Lateral STEMI

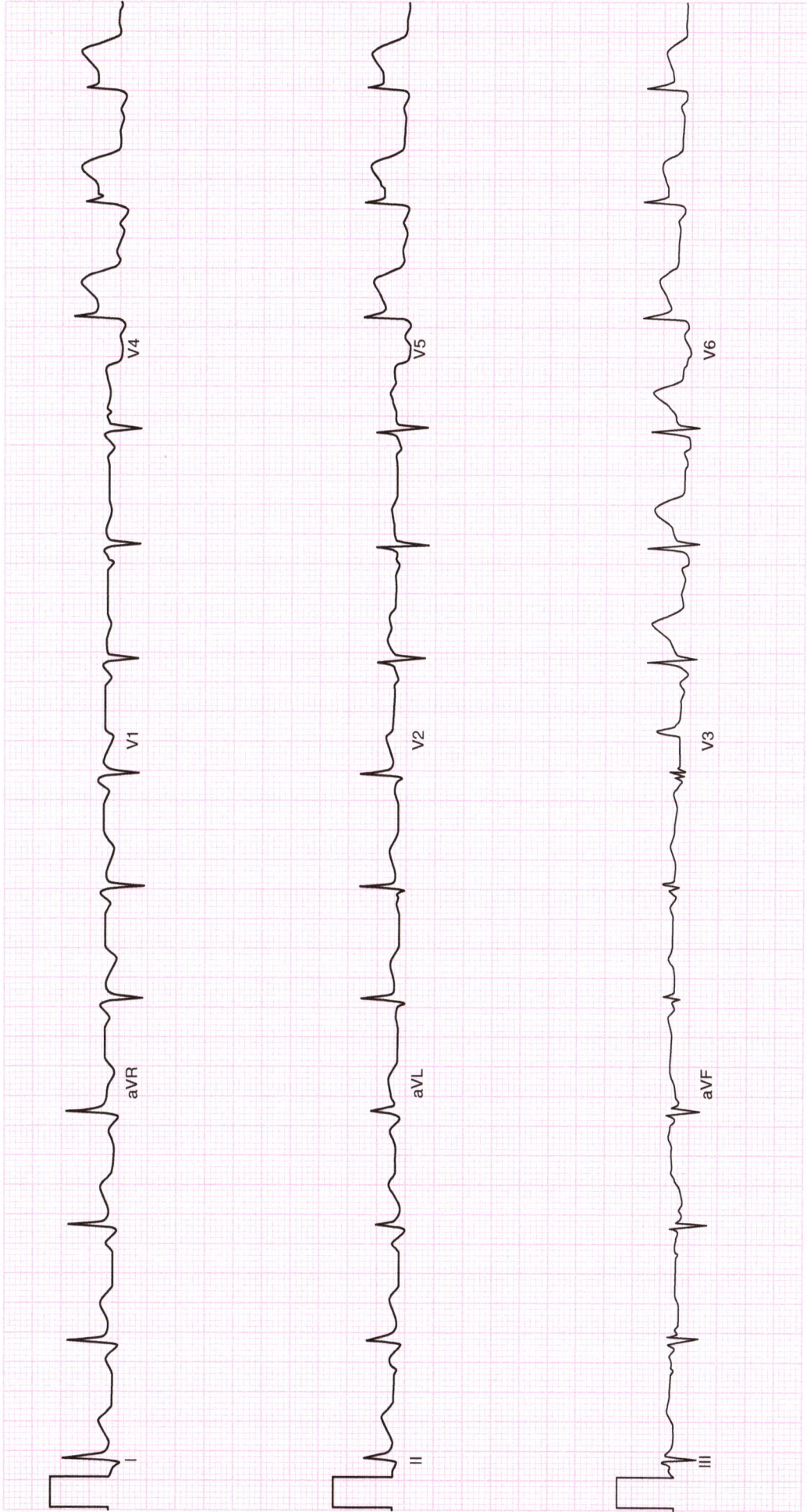

ST segment elevation is present in leads I, aVL, V3–V6, making this a lateral STEMI. The ST segment elevation is most prominent in leads V4–V6, though the more subtle elevation in leads I and aVL is still clearly visible.

The Progression of STEMI[1, 23, 26, 28]

The ECG changes that occur with STEMI are an evolving process that develops from the point at which coronary artery occlusion occurs. From this point the ECG will evolve and move through the phases outlined below and shown in Figure 3.4. Different sources will group these ECG changes in different ways, based on time or specific changes, which can be confusing. The key principle to note is that a myocardial infarction will appear differently on an ECG depending on the time since coronary artery occlusion has occurred, and that ST segment elevation is only visible for a limited period in the infarction process.

In the first few minutes following coronary artery occlusion, hyperacute T waves will develop. The T waves become pointed and are usually at least 50% as tall as their preceding R wave. The hyperacute T waves are named as such because they are only visible in the first minutes of myocardial infarction before resolving. Thus, they are rarely captured on a 12-lead ECG as they have usually resolved before the patient has sought medical attention, or before the ambulance arrives.

ST segment elevation usually begins to develop within the first hour of coronary artery occlusion and continues to elevate for several hours before beginning to normalise over several more.

As the ST segment begins to normalise and return to the baseline, pathological Q waves and T wave inversion begin to develop and R wave definition may be lost.

Pathological Q waves are an indication that cardiac tissue has died and can develop within hours of infarction, but may also take several days to appear. Pathological Q waves often remain on the ECG permanently as an indication that previous myocardial infarction has occurred. On occasions where pathological Q waves do resolve and normalise, it will happen months or years after the initial event.

For a Q wave to be classified as pathological it must be more than 0.04 seconds in duration, greater than one third the amplitude of the associated R wave or greater than 2 mm in amplitude.

Pathological Q waves can provide useful diagnostic information about a patient's current clinical presentation. They may be the only clue that a myocardial infarction has occurred recently and explain why the patient's clinical presentation is in keeping with post-myocardial infarction conditions such as heart failure and cardiomyopathy (page 122).

- **Minutes**:
  - ▸ Hyperacute T waves occur.
- **Minutes to hours**:
  - ▸ Hyperacute T waves resolve.
  - ▸ ST segment elevation begins and continues to elevate for several hours.
- **Hours to days**:
  - ▸ ST segment elevation starts to resolve.
  - ▸ T wave inversion and pathological Q waves develop.
  - ▸ R wave definition may be lost.
- **Days to months**:
  - ▸ T wave inversion resolves.
  - ▸ Pathological Q waves remain.

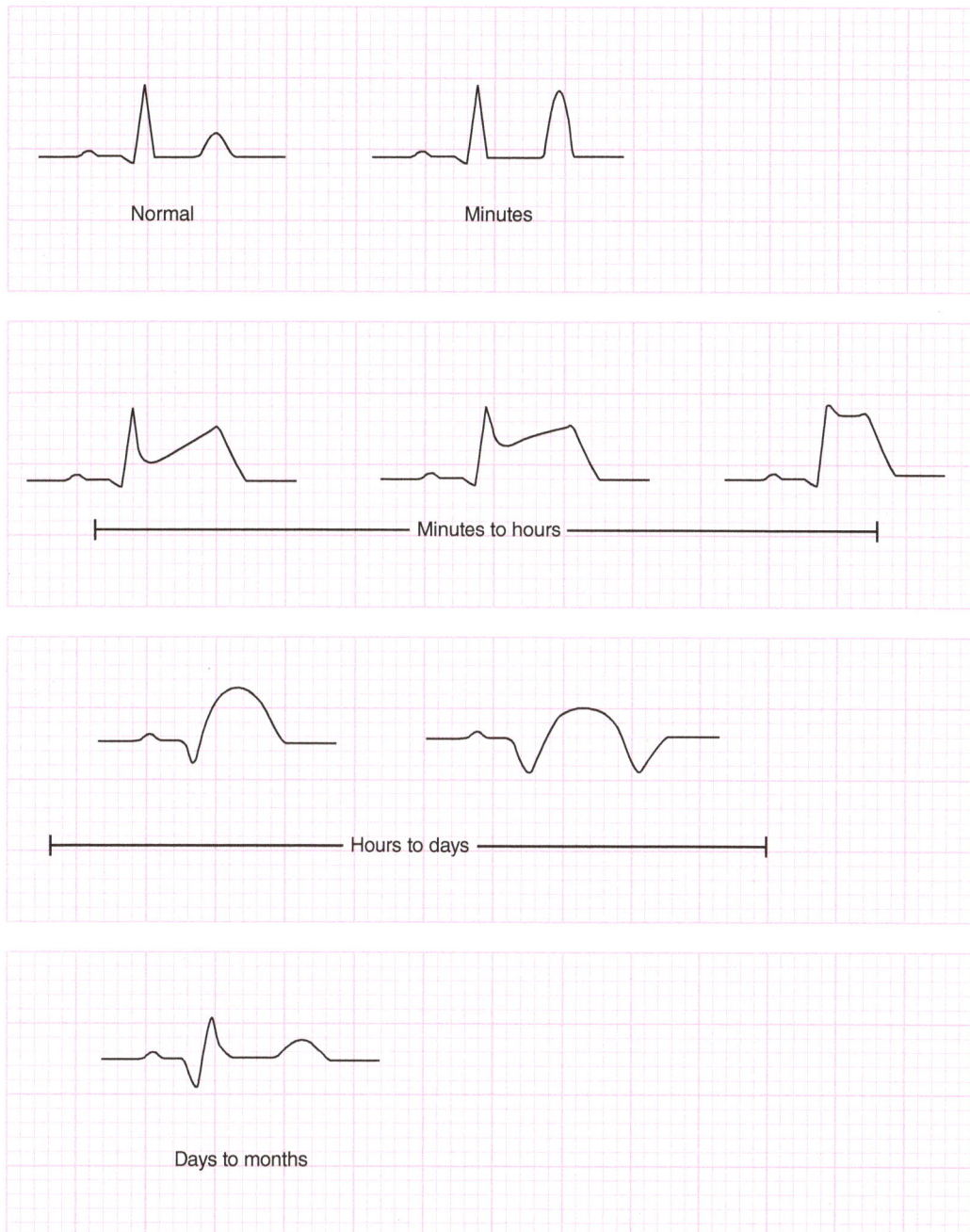

Figure 3.4 Progression of STEMI.

The Physiological Cause of ST Segment Elevation and Depression[29, 30]

Ischaemia affects the electrical properties of myocardial cells. In cases of severe and acute ischaemia, the resting membrane potential is lowered, and the action potential duration is shortened. These changes create a voltage gradient between the ischaemic and healthy myocardial cells. This voltage gradient means that an electrical current flows between the ischaemic and healthy regions of myocardial tissue. These electrical current flows are seen on the ECG as ST segment changes. The changes seen depend on the location and extent of the area of ischaemia (Figure 3.5).

If the area of ischaemia is transmural or epicardial, the electrical vector of the ST segment is moved towards the outer layer of the heart, creating ST segment elevation in the ECG leads 'facing' the area of injury, and, if the area of ischaemia is transmural, ST segment depression is present in the reciprocal leads. T wave inversion is also caused by these voltage gradient changes affecting ventricular repolarisation.

If the area of ischaemia is subendocardial, then the electrical vector of the ST segment is moved towards the inner layer of the heart, creating ST segment depression in the ECG leads 'facing' the area of injury.

Transmural or full thickness ischaemia describes when the full thickness of the myocardial tissue becomes ischaemic.

Partial thickness ischaemia can be either subendocardial ischaemia, where the inner layer of myocardial tissue is ischaemic, or epicardial, where the outer layer of myocardial tissue is ischaemic.

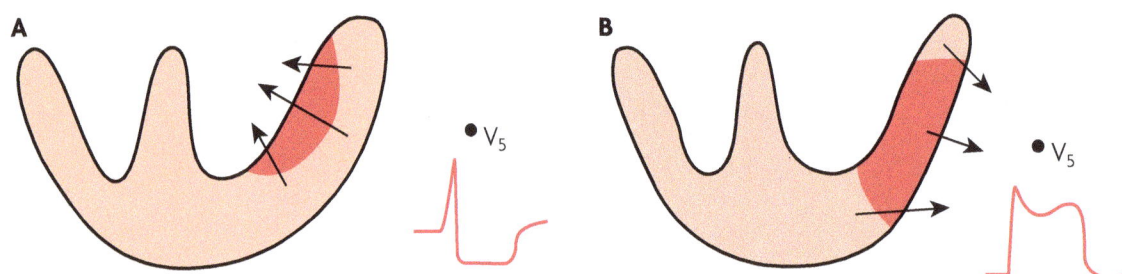

Figure 3.5 Examples of subendocardial (A) and transmural (B) areas of ischaemic injury with ECG vectors.

Management of ACS and STEMI[5, 7, 19, 31, 32]
- Time-critical transfer with hospital pre-alert call to appropriate receiving unit:
  - STEMI should be transported directly to a heart attack centre with PPCI capability following local pathways.
  - ACS should be transported to a cardiac centre if local pathways allow, otherwise to the nearest appropriate emergency department.
- Monitor en route and be prepared for sudden deterioration or cardiac arrest.
- Gain IV access.
- Administer ACS drugs, following local protocols:
  - Aspirin.
  - Clopidogrel.
  - Glyceryl trinitrate.
  - Morphine.
  - Consider oxygen therapy only if signs of poor perfusion are present, following current oxygen administration guidelines.
- Consider whether right ventricular involvement is present and if this impacts pre-load-reducing ACS drugs (page 116).

Acute Complications of STEMI[29, 32, 33, 34]

Patients with STEMI are at risk of complications and deterioration. In the out-of-hospital setting it is often not possible to identify a specific STEMI complication. Instead, the recognition of the deterioration and management of any resulting ABCDE problems is key.

- Complications of STEMI include:
  - Arrhythmias, including:
    - Heart blocks.
    - Ectopic beats.
    - AF.
    - VF and VT – cardiac arrest.
  - Cardiogenic shock, due to:
    - Left ventricular dysfunction (responsible for around 70% of cases of cardiogenic shock in MI).
    - Right ventricular dysfunction.
  - Mechanical complications:
    - Ventricular septal rupture
      - Most common in anterior or posterior MI.
      - May present with signs of acute heart failure including hypotension and pulmonary oedema.
    - Ventricular septal defect
      - Occurs in 1–2% of STEMI patients.
      - Associated with high mortality at 12 months.
    - Mitral regurgitation
      - The most common mechanical complication of MI.
      - Associated with worse outcomes in MI.
      - May present with signs of acute heart failure including hypotension and pulmonary oedema.
    - Acute cardiac wall rupture
      - A potential cause of sudden death in MI.
      - More common in elderly patients.
      - Leads to cardiac tamponade and sudden deterioration, with potential for classic tamponade signs of hypotension, distended neck veins and muffled heart sounds.

Pericarditis[1, 2, 15, 35, 36, 37]

Pericarditis is an inflammation of the pericardium. Up to 90% of cases are either preceded by a viral infection or are idiopathic, although other causes include pericarditis following cardiac surgery, or myocardial infarction (commonly occurring 1–3 days after infarction, but may also occur weeks or months after infarction; known as Dressler's syndrome and occurs in 5%–10% of patients who have survived MI).

Pericarditis can cause widespread concave ST segment elevation and PR segment depression with reciprocal changes seen in lead aVR. Sinus tachycardia is also often present due to infection, pain or both. Some form of ECG change occurs in around 90% of patients with pericarditis.

The cardinal symptom of pericarditis is central or left-sided sharp chest pain, which is worse when lying flat, breathing deeply or innovating the muscles of the chest wall. The pain can range from mild to severe and may be eased or relieved when leaning forward. It may also radiate to the epigastric region, neck, back or shoulders.

The differentiation between pericarditis and ACS in the out-of-hospital environment is challenging due to the similarity in symptoms and potential ECG changes.

ST Segment Elevation in Lead aVR[23, 31, 38]

ST segment elevation in lead aVR coupled with ST segment depression >1 mm in the inferior or lateral leads is associated with left main coronary artery obstruction or multivessel ischaemia. These findings are especially suggestive in patients who are also haemodynamically unstable.

The same can be applied to lead V1, but with less diagnostic accuracy.

ST segment elevation in aVR combined with RBBB or >2.5 mm of ST segment elevation in lead V1 has been found to be predicative of obstruction of the left anterior descending artery.

Late Complications of Heart Attack Patients[2]

The long-term prognosis of a patient following MI is influenced by multiple contributing factors: The severity of the myocardial infarction, how quickly medical help was summoned and how rapidly treatment and reperfusion therapy were carried out. The severity of any underlying coronary artery disease, the health of the cardiac muscle prior to infarct and other co-morbidities also contribute to prognosis. A patient who has suffered an MI in recent weeks is at increased risk of associated conditions and further cardiac events, including:

- **Heart failure**, which may develop due to reduced left ventricular function.
- The formation of myocardial scar tissue in ways that allow a re-entrant circuit to occur, causing **ventricular tachycardia** (page 49) or narrow complex tachycardia (page 39).
- Thromboembolism, which may develop at the site of the previous infarct and cause a further **MI**, **stroke** or occlusion in other blood vessels causing localised ischaemia to the tissues and organs they supply.
- **Pericarditis**, which can be caused by full thickness MI several weeks after the infarct.

Early Repolarisation[39, 40, 41]

Commonly known as 'high take off', early repolarisation has long been considered a normal variant that is not linked to cardiac disease or injury. The term 'benign early repolarisation' is often used, but should be avoided as early repolarisation is not always benign. A recent study has shown a link between early repolarisation in the inferior ECG leads and an increased risk of death due to cardiac causes in middle-aged men.[39] Early repolarisation is most commonly seen in younger men, with up to 90% of young men found to have 1–3 mm of ST segment elevation in at least one precordial lead. Age decreases the likelihood of early repolarisation in men and simultaneously increases cardiac risk factors. Compared to men, women showed only around 20% prevalence, which did not increase with age.[40]

In clinical practice, 'high take off' can be a dangerous conclusion to make when assessing an ECG. If the patient's clinical presentation were enough to prompt an ECG to be obtained in the first place, then any J point deviation should be considered a serious finding and approached by adopting a low threshold for transport to further care. If the patient is presenting with ACS symptoms then a diagnosis of early repolarisation is not appropriate as ST segment changes will act only to aid differentiation between STEMI and ACS (NSTEMI and unstable angina).

ECG 3.8 – Early Repolarisation

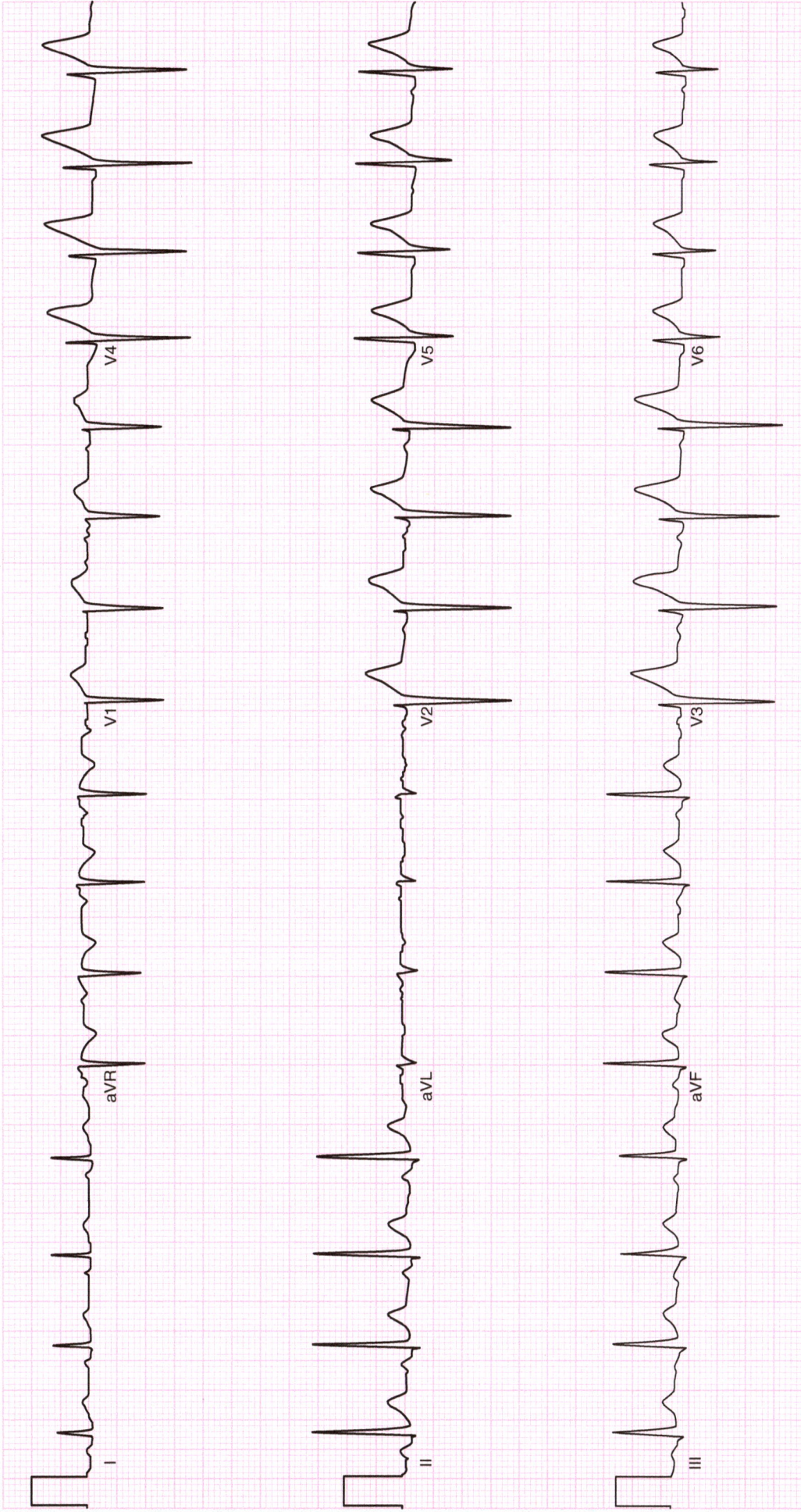

The J point in leads V2–V6 is elevated, in this case due to early repolarisation.

Brugada Syndrome

There is a high incidence of sudden death associated with Brugada syndrome in otherwise healthy individuals. Patients showing Brugada sign on their ECG may present asymptomatically with no associated cardiac symptoms. However, they may also present with syncope or in the event of sudden death.

ECG Identification of Brugada Sign[42, 43]

- At least 2 mm of J point ST segment elevation in ECG leads V1–V3 with a coved ST segment leading into an inverted T wave.

To diagnose Brugada syndrome, the ECG showing Brugada sign must be associated with syncope, a family history of sudden cardiac death or witnessed VF or VT. In the out-of-hospital environment, the identification of the ECG changes alone is enough to warrant transfer to further care.

Key Points: ACS and STEMI

- Patients presenting with signs and symptoms of ACS should be treated for ACS; it is not possible, or safe, to exclude ACS in the out-of-hospital environment based on ECG findings or the presence or absence of specific signs or symptoms.
- STEMI is not the only ECG change associated with ACS; pathological Q waves, ST segment depression and T wave changes can also indicate the presence of ACS.
- ACS is time critical; treatment and transport should not be delayed. Delays can lead to more extensive cardiac damage and worse outcomes for patients.
- Patients presenting with STEMI are at increased risk of rapid deterioration and cardiac arrest. Monitor them closely and be ready to manage rapid deterioration.

Supplemental ECG Leads (Posterior and Right-Sided ECGs)

It is important at this point to reemphasise that the heart is a three-dimensional physical organ which we are viewing as a two-dimensional graph of electrical activity.

The standard 12-lead ECG does not view every aspect of the heart. It is possible for a myocardial infarction to occur and affect an area which is not shown, or is only partially shown, in the standard 12-lead ECG.

If a patient presents with signs and symptoms of ACS and there is no STEMI identified on the initial standard 12-lead ECG, it is appropriate to carry out further ECG traces having repositioned the electrodes to view the right side and posterior aspects of the heart.

Even if a patient does meet STEMI criteria on their initial 12-lead ECG, there are times when further ECG views are indicated to assess the extent of the ST segment elevation and the associated cardiac damage. There are some findings on a standard 12-lead ECG which give clear indication that right-sided or posterior ECGs are required and that right coronary artery occlusion may have occurred. Right-sided and posterior ECG leads should be obtained routinely in any patient with inferior STEMI or with ST depression in anteroseptal leads (V1–V4).[5]

ECG 3.9 – Brugada Syndrome

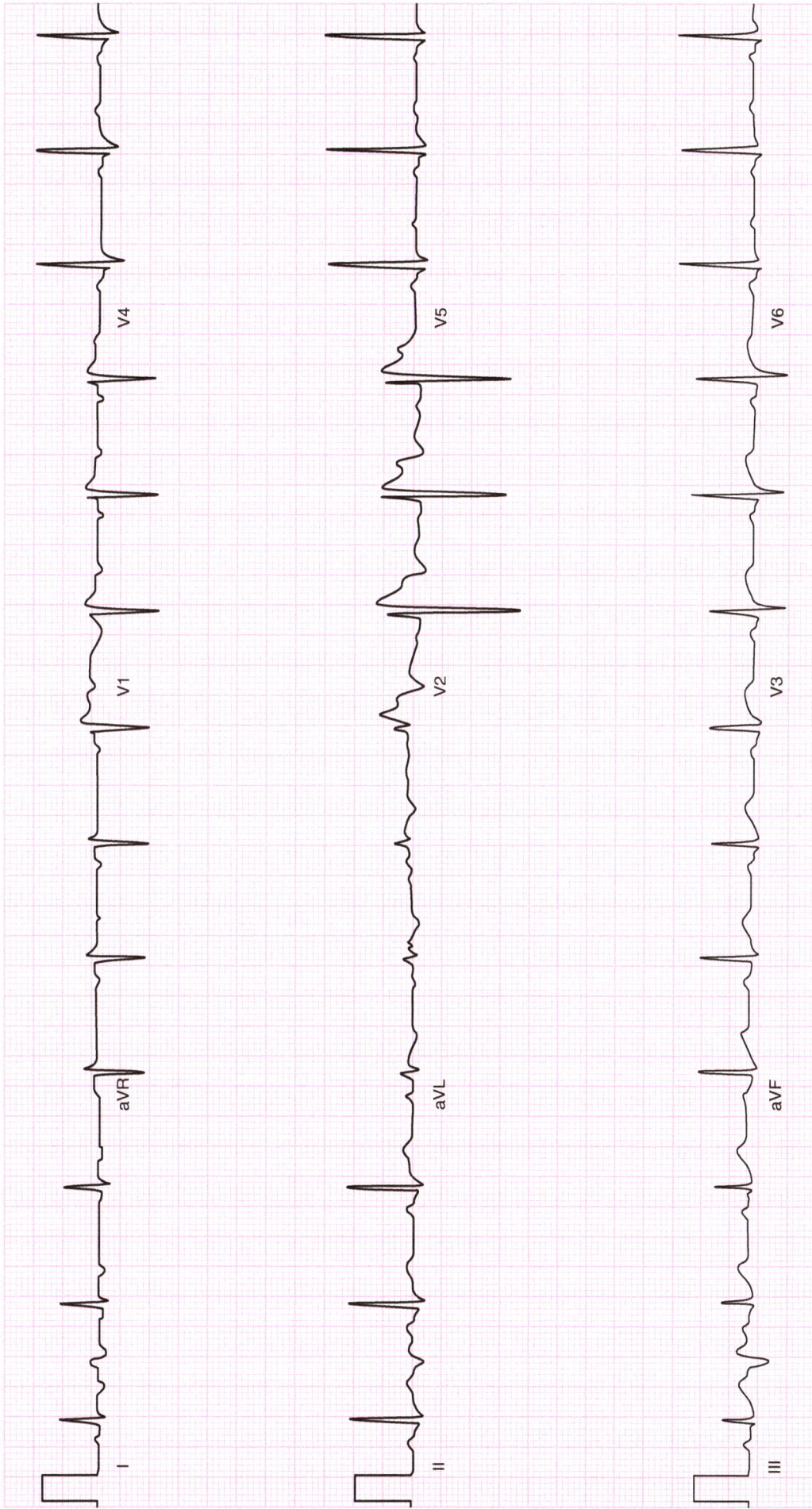

Leads V1 and V2 display the signs of Brugada syndrome – the ST segment elevation with a downward-sloping, coved ST segment leading into inverted T waves.

A right-sided ECG is obtained by swapping the precordial leads to the right side of the patient's chest. They then become right-sided precordial leads, with an 'R' added to their names to indicate that they are from the right side of the chest (V4 becomes V4R and so on); these right-sided leads represent the free wall of the right ventricle.[21] All six precordial leads can be swapped to a right-sided view, but in the out-of-hospital environment it is common to find that only V4, or V3 and V4, are used. V4R is the single most useful lead of choice in right ventricular involvement.[28, 30, 44]

A posterior ECG is also obtained by repositioning some precordial leads to a different anatomical location. Leads V4, V5 and V6 may be removed and placed on the left side of the patient's back so that V4 becomes V7, V5 becomes V8 and V6 becomes V9.[21]

> **!**
>
> Right-sided and posterior ECG leads should be obtained in all patients with inferior STEMI or with ST depression in anteroseptal leads.

When printing a right-sided or posterior ECG trace, it should immediately be annotated with pen to indicate which leads have been repositioned and the views they now represent. At the time you may be confident that you will remember which ECG print-out is which, but it is highly likely that you will struggle to differentiate the different ECGs on arrival at the receiving hospital.

Right-sided ECG and STEMI

Around 40% of inferior STEMIs will have Right Ventricular Involvement (RVI). As a right-sided ECG represents the free wall of the right ventricle, ST segment elevation in lead V4R is highly specific of RVI.

Isolated V4R ST segment elevation is uncommon.[44]

> **ECG Identification of Right Ventricular Involvement MI**[3, 23, 28, 31, 44]   ⎍
>
> **Standard 12-Lead ECG**
> - Any of these signs in the presence of an inferior STEMI would suggest right ventricular involvement. Any inferior STEMI should prompt you to carry out a right-sided ECG:
>   - ST segment elevation in leads II and III where the ST segment elevation in lead III is greater than the ST segment elevation in lead II is suggestive of right coronary artery occlusion. This is because lead III is more 'rightward facing' than lead II.
>   - > 1 mm ST segment elevation in lead V1 or aVR.
>   - ST segment depression in lead V2 accompanied by either ST segment elevation or an isoelectric ST segment in lead V1 is highly suggestive of right coronary artery occlusion.
>
> **Right-Sided ECG**
> - ST segment elevation > 0.5 mm in ECG lead V3R and V4R is strongly suggestive of right coronary artery occlusion affecting the right ventricle.
> - ST segment elevation of 1 mm or more in any right-sided ECG lead V3R–V6R in the presence of inferior STEMI is suggestive of right coronary artery occlusion.

ECG 3.10 – Inferior and V4R Elevation STEMI

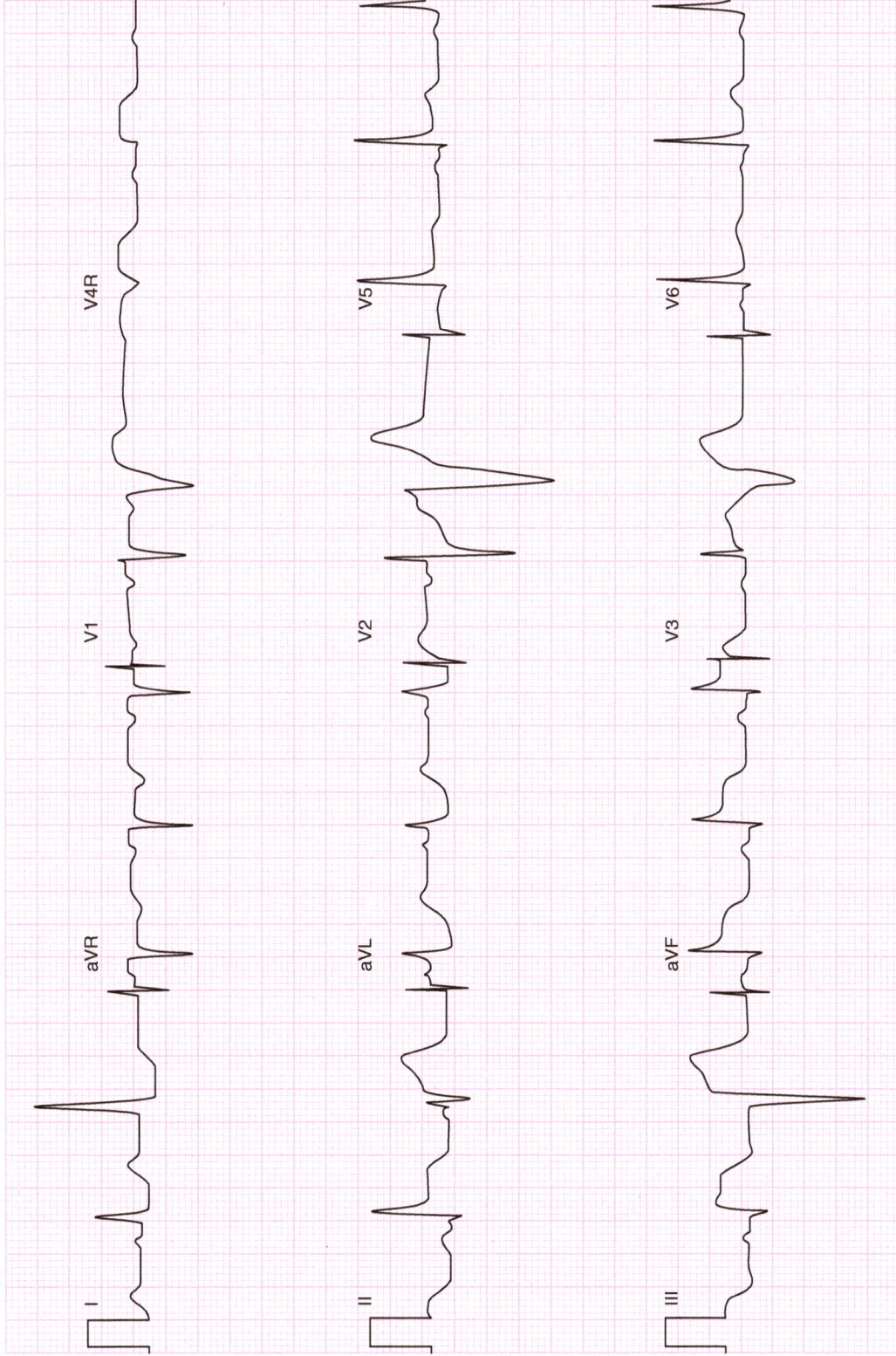

We can see the inferior STEMI in leads II, III and aVF, but we can also see some ST segment elevation in leads V3 and V5 and most importantly in this case in lead V4R. This tells us that there is a high probability that there is right ventricular involvement. The ST depression in leads V1–V2 also suggests possible posterior involvement, which is discussed next.

Clinical Signs and Symptoms of Right Ventricular Involvement MI[5, 22, 31]

A patient suffering an MI with RVI will have the same potential signs, symptoms and considerations that are associated with a 'normal' MI (page 94), with the following additional potential findings:

- An estimated 10–15% of patients will present with the 'RVI triad':
  - Hypotension.
  - Jugular venous distension.
  - Clear lung fields (absences of pulmonary oedema).
- Patients with RVI have an increased risk of:
  - Ventricular arrhythmias and heart blocks (due to RCA occlusion).
  - Reduced cardiac output.
  - Circulatory shock.

Management of Right Ventricular Involvement MI[3, 5, 7, 31]

Management of RVI MI is the same as with 'normal' MI, with the following considerations:

- The right coronary artery supplies the majority of the cardiac muscle of the right ventricle. Infarction that damages and weakens the right ventricle makes it pre-load sensitive. A drop in pre-load can lead to a significant drop in cardiac output from the right side of the heart into the pulmonary artery. This in turn leads to a significant reduction in the volume of blood reaching the left ventricle and thus being returned to the body.
- Standard ACS management includes the administration of glyceryl trinitrate (GTN) and morphine; both drugs have pre-load-reducing effects. If a patient with RVI is given these medications, the resulting drop in pre-load combined with the reduced effectiveness of the right ventricle's contractions can lead to a drop in cardiac output that is significant enough to cause cardiac arrest.
- The 2019 JRCALC Clinical Guidelines list RVI MI as a caution for the administration of GTN. You must rely on your clinical judgement during each patient care episode when deciding if administration of GTN is appropriate.
- A patient presenting with RVI has an increased chance of being in a hypotensive state. Hypotension should be managed with fluid therapy to attempt to increase and maintain pre-load to the heart (as per clinical practice guidelines for medical hypotension).

Posterior ECG

The posterior and basal walls of the left ventricle are not visible on a standard 12-lead ECG; they are seen via the posterior lead positions of leads V7, V8 and V9. Fifteen to twenty per cent of STEMIs involve the posterior of the heart and are most often seen alongside inferior or lateral ST segment elevation. Isolated posterior STEMI is less common and may be missed; it should be considered and watched for when assessing any patient presenting with ACS. Posterior involvement in STEMI is suggestive of a wider area of myocardial muscle being affected and therefore further increases the risk of rapid deterioration during transport to the cardiac centre.[44]

Reciprocal changes of posterior ST segment elevation may be seen in leads V1–V3. If these are identified, a posterior ECG should be carried out to establish if ST segment elevation is present.

ECG Identification of Posterior Involvement MI[3, 5, 23, 28, 31]
Standard 12-Lead ECG
- Any of these signs should prompt you to carry out a posterior ECG:
  - \> 0.5 mm horizontal ST segment depression in leads V1–V3.
  - Inferior STEMI.

Posterior ECG
- ST segment elevation > 0.5 mm in any of ECG leads V7–V9.

ECG 3.11a – Inferior STEMI with Signs of Posterior Involvement

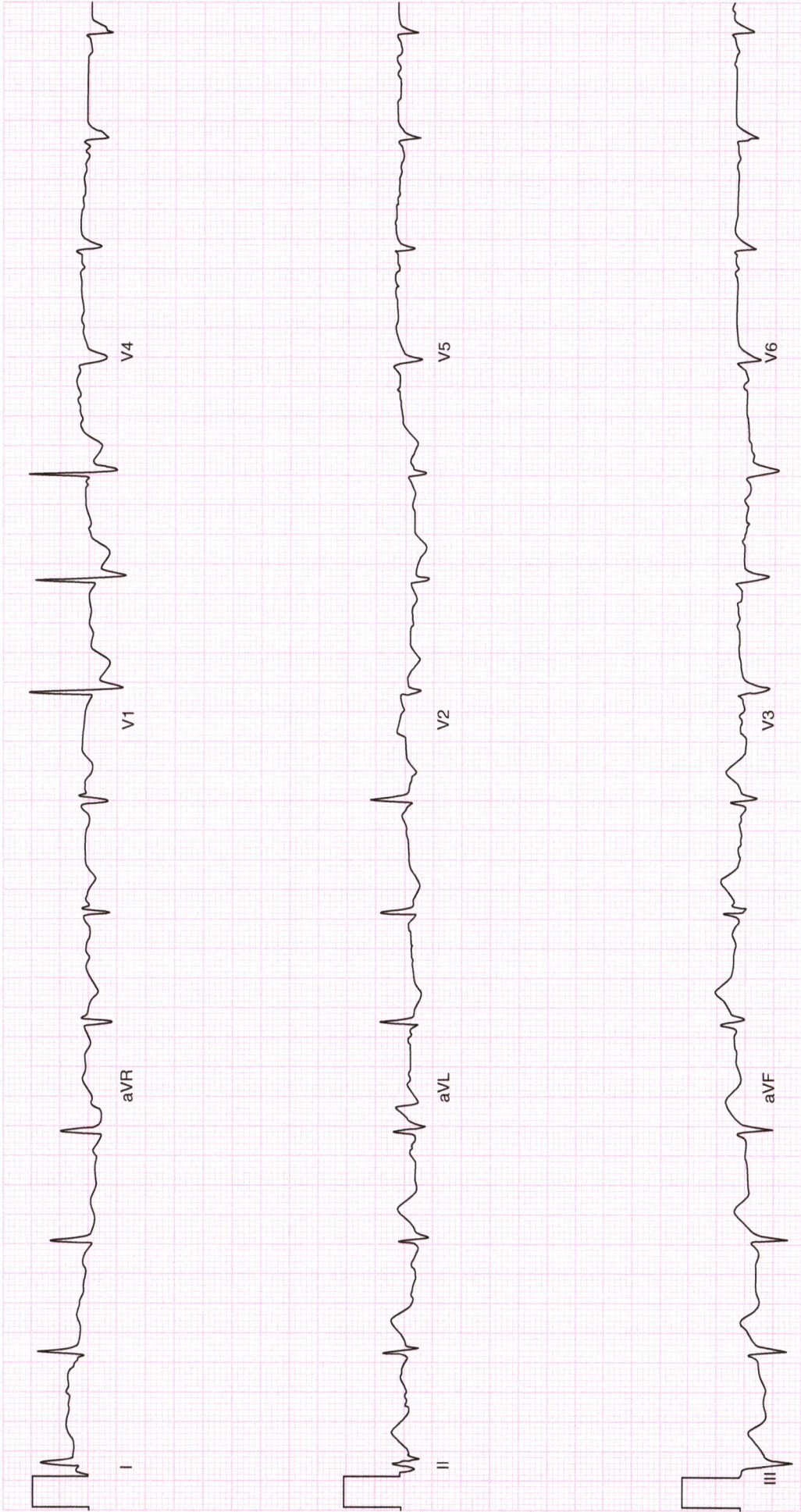

This ECG shows some slight inferior ST segment elevation in leads III and aVF. However, it also shows ST segment depression and T wave inversion in leads V1–V2. This indicates the necessity for a posterior ECG, as can be seen in ECG 3.11b.

ECG 3.11b – Posterior STEMI

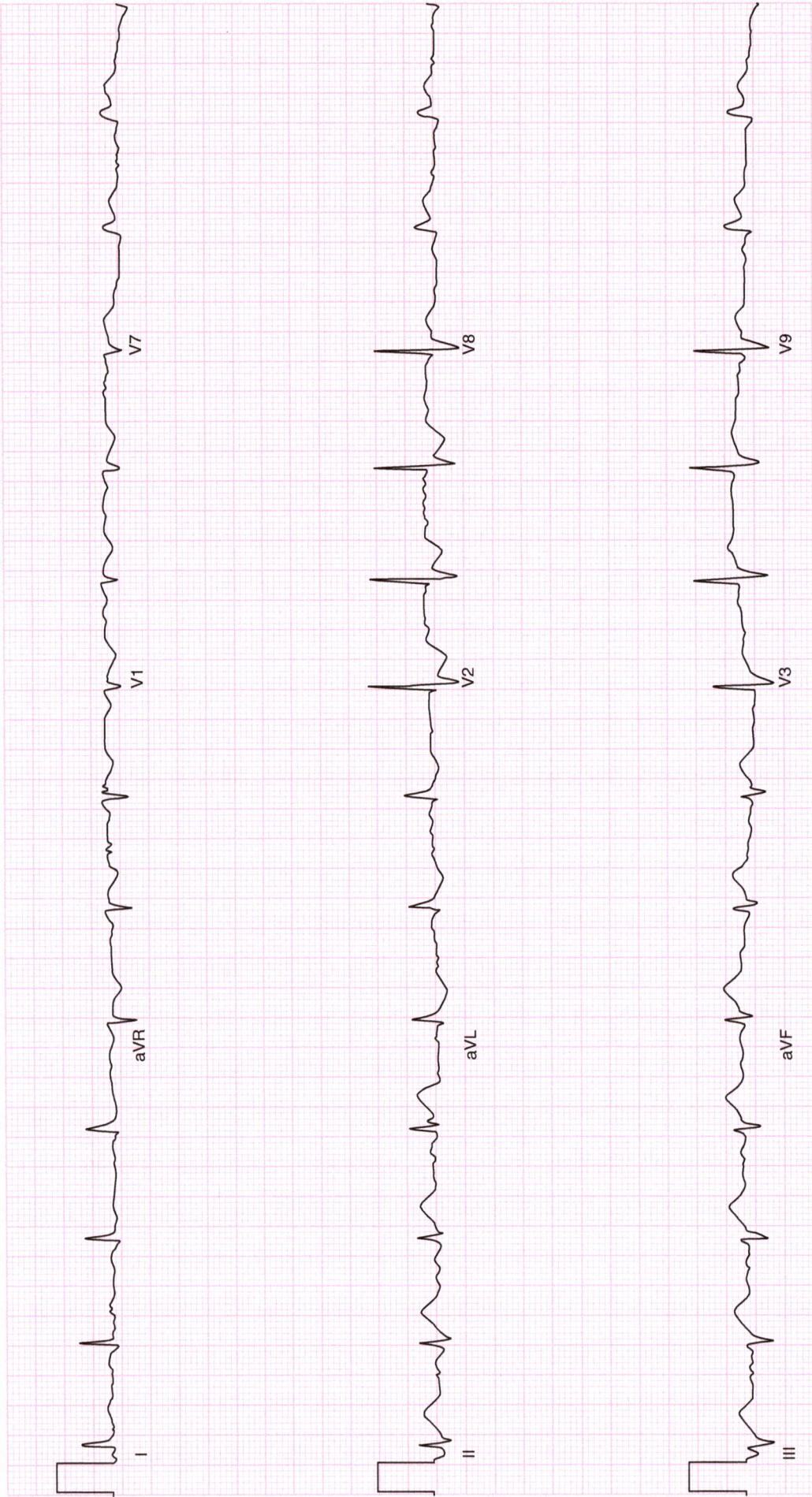

This posterior ECG shows ST segment elevation in leads V7–V9, making this a posterior STEMI. The ST segment changes in leads III and aVF would not be enough to activate most cath lab pathways; this emphasises the importance of adopting a low threshold for obtaining additional ECG lead views.

Management of Posterior Involvement MI[7, 21]

The principles of managing a posterior STEMI do not differ from standard STEMI management.

Posterior ST segment elevation alongside ST segment elevation on the standard 12-lead ECG strongly suggest that a larger area of the myocardium is affected by the infarction and therefore the patient is at increased risk of rapid deterioration and cardiac arrest.

As we know from Section 1, the posterior descending artery originates from the right coronary artery in around 80% of the population. This produces a considerable likelihood that if posterior ST segment elevation is present, then the infarction is also affecting the right side of the heart. It is difficult to differentiate, though the presence of inferior ST segment elevation further increases the likelihood of right coronary artery occlusion. Unless there is right-sided ST segment elevation present in V4R, standard ACS treatment should be followed.

Key Points: Supplemental ECG Leads

- Right-sided and posterior ECG leads should be obtained in all patients with inferior STEMI or with ST depression in anteroseptal leads.
- Patients with STEMI that is affecting the right ventricle are likely to be pre-load sensitive and at risk of severe hypotension and deterioration, especially if GTN is administered.
- Patients with RCA occlusion are at increased risk of developing heart blocks and other arrhythmias.

Left Ventricular Hypertrophy

Hypertrophy is when an area of muscle becomes enlarged and less elastic. This can occur in the left ventricle due to prolonged periods of pumping against increased resistance (increased afterload, see page 15), or sustained periods of overfilling of the left ventricle.

Left Ventricular Hypertrophy (LVH) is a chronic, gradual and abnormal increase in left ventricular size (mass) which is most often caused by chronic hypertension and is a form of hypertrophic cardiomyopathy. The increased thickness and overall size of the left ventricular myocardium reduce the contractile strength of the left ventricle as it becomes more rigid and less elastic; this also leads to a reduction in the size of the left ventricular cavity, thus reducing its capacity to hold blood. The loss of elasticity also reduces the amount the ventricles can stretch with pre-load prior to contraction. These factors reduce stroke volume and cardiac output (page 13).

ECG Identification of Left Ventricular Hypertrophy[18, 25, 28]

ECG changes in left ventricular hypertrophy relate to the increased size of the left ventricular heart muscle and the leftward rotation of the heart due to its increased size.

Due to the increased size of the left side of the myocardium, an increase in amplitude of T and S waves can be expected. More heart muscle means more electrical activity. Signs of myocardial ischaemia may also be seen in the left-facing leads.

- Amplitude changes in QRS complexes:
  - Increased height of R waves in leads I, aVL, V4, V5 and V6 (the leads that look at the left side of the heart).
  - Increased depth of S waves in leads V1 and V2 (leads looking at the more rightward side of the heart).
- May also see:
  - Left axis deviation (page 22).
  - Downward-sloping ST segment depression and inverted T waves, similar to myocardial ischaemia, in left-facing leads.
  - ST segment elevation in the rightward-facing leads V1 and V2, which could mimic STEMI.
  - Increased QRS duration – the larger mass of the left ventricle will take longer to depolarise.
  - Increased QT interval – The larger mass of the left ventricle causes increased depolarisation and repolarisation times.

There are multiple diagnostic indexes and criteria that each set out to measure QRS amplitude to diagnose LVH. These indexes have varying degrees of accuracy and reliability as many things affect QRS amplitude other than ventricular mass. Body shape and size also affect QRS amplitude due to changes in the distance between the heart and the ECG electrodes. For these reasons, in the out-of-hospital setting it is advisable to use the above ECG signs of LVH as a guide alongside clinical history-taking and physical examination to recognise the possible presence of LVH in a patient.

Causes of Left Ventricular Hypertrophy

Causes of left ventricular hypertrophy include:
- Aortic stenosis.
- Hypertension.
- Aortic regurgitation.
- Cardiomyopathy.

Management of Left Ventricular Hypertrophy

There is no specific out-of-hospital treatment for LVH. You may find signs of LVH when assessing a patient who is suffering from an acute cardiac presentation such as ACS (page 93) or from heart failure (page 122). Finding ECG signs of LVH can help to build your overall clinical picture and provide suggestions as to the patient's overall health state.

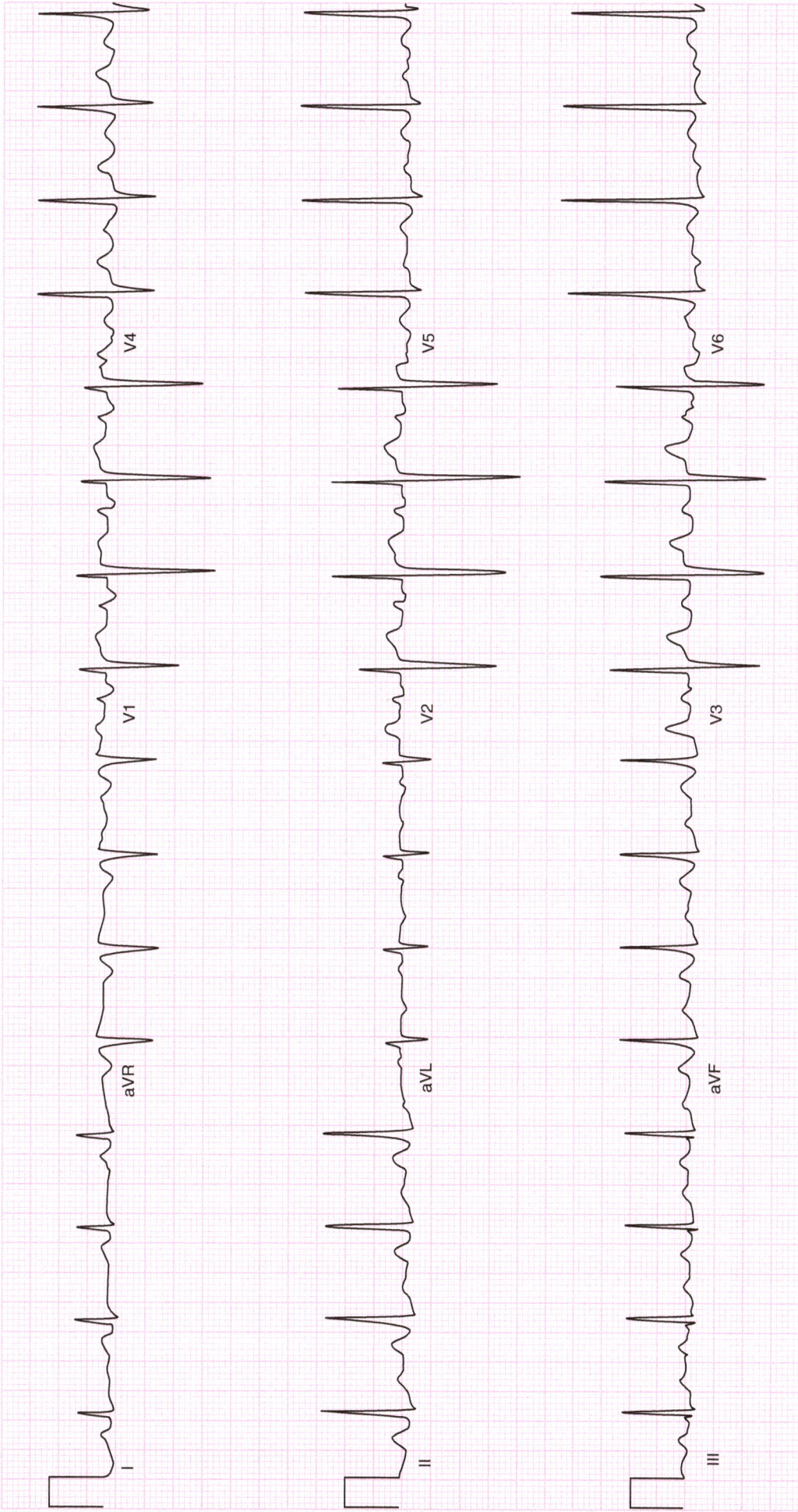

ECG 3.12 – Left Ventricular Hypertrophy

This ECG shows multiple features of LVH; we can see some ST segment elevation in leads V1–V2 and depression in the left-facing leads V4–V6. Most obviously, there is increased amplitude of R waves in leads V4–V6 and increased amplitude of S waves in leads V1–V2.

Cardiomyopathy and Heart Failure[7, 29, 45, 46, 47, 48, 49]

Cardiomyopathies are diseases of the heart muscle. They can be divided into three main groups: hypertrophic cardiomyopathy, dilated cardiomyopathy and restrictive cardiomyopathy.

Hypertrophic cardiomyopathy: Through increased work the heart muscle becomes thicker, larger, more rigid and less elastic. Causes include left ventricular hypertrophy and genetic inheritance.

Dilated cardiomyopathy: The left ventricular cavity stretches and becomes 'baggy' as the heart works to deal with increased volumes of blood; this causes the left ventricle to become enlarged. Primary causes of dilated cardiomyopathy include aortic valve regurgitation, mitral valve regurgitation and genetic inheritance. The most common secondary cause of dilated cardiomyopathy is chronic alcoholism.

Restrictive cardiomyopathy: Caused either by infiltration and build-up of abnormal materials into the myocardium or by fibrosis. It is similar to hypertrophic cardiomyopathy in that it results in myocardium becoming larger, thicker and less elastic.

Heart failure results from structural or functional problems with the heart muscle, leading to the heart not operating effectively as a pump. Cardiomyopathies are a common cause of heart failure. Heart failure is a long-term health condition, referred to as chronic heart failure. Acute heart failure occurs when either chronic heart failure worsens or there is sudden cardiac injury, such as an MI.

Right ventricular hypertrophy

Because the right ventricle is comparatively much smaller than the left ventricle, the signs of right ventricular hypertrophy (RVH) are not commonly seen unless the RVH is significant. This is compounded by the fact that if LVH or other cardiac conditions are present they may further mask the signs of RVH on the patient's ECG.

ECG changes that may indicate the presence of RVH include:
- Amplitude changes in QRS complexes:
  - Increased height of R waves in leads V1 and aVR.
  - Increased depth of S waves in left ventricular leads I, aVL, V4, V5 and V6.
- Right axis deviation (page 22).
- There may also appear to be incomplete right bundle branch block (page 129) in leads V1 and V2.

Causes of RVH include right-sided heart valve problems (pulmonary valve stenosis, tricuspid valve regurgitation), pulmonary hypertension, lung disease, ventricular or atrial septal defects and pulmonary embolism.[18, 29, 50, 51]

ECG 3.13 – Right Ventricular Hypertrophy

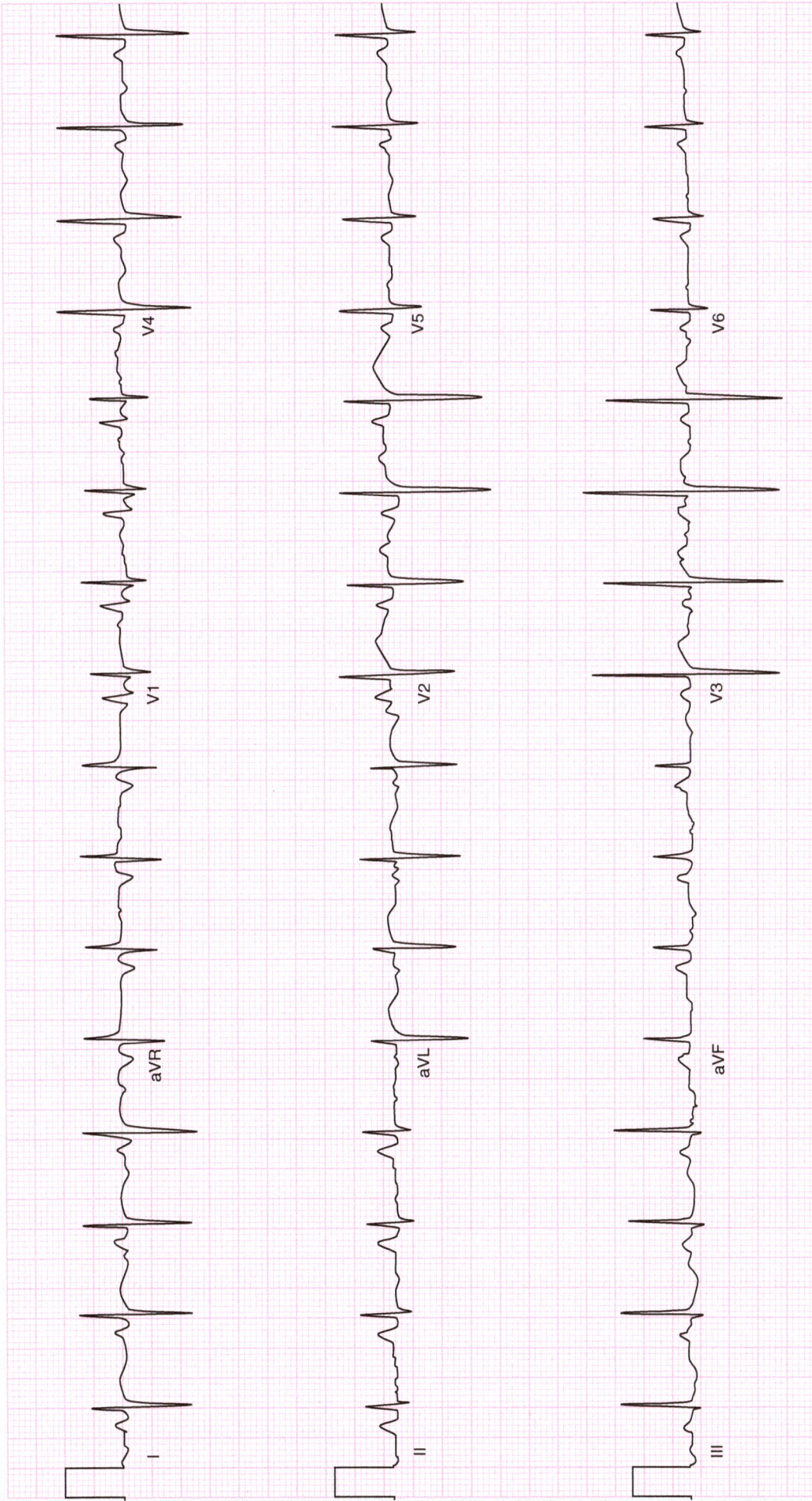

We can see the increased amplitude of R waves in leads V1 and aVR as well as the increased amplitude of S waves in the left-facing leads (I, aVL, V4–V6). There is also right axis deviation. These findings tell us that RVH is present.

Bundle Branch Blocks

There are two bundle branches: The left bundle branch and the right bundle branch. The bundle branches form part of the normal electrical conduction pathway. Each bundle branch provides an electrical 'motorway' to their respective ventricle. If a bundle branch ceases to function and becomes blocked to electrical impulses, the impulses will need to reach that ventricle using an alternative, slower pathway. In bundle branch blocks the alternative pathway is usually through the other ventricle and ventricular septum which increases the time it takes for the electrical impulse to reach its destination; this is why the QRS complex appears wider than the expected 0.12 seconds (3 small squares) when bundle branch blocks are present.

Bundle branch blocks are a form of heart block; they originate below the level of the AV node and are a form of vesicular block. They are identified by examining the 12-lead ECG and assessing the morphology of the QRS complexes in different leads. Remember that the shape of a QRS complex tells us about the route the electrical impulse has taken whilst travelling through the ventricles.

Left bundle branch block and right bundle branch block each have their own criteria for identification. The left bundle branch divides into two fascicules; if one of these fascicles becomes blocked it is known as a fascicular block.

Non-specific intraventricular conduction defect occurs if the QRS duration is greater than 0.12 seconds (3 small squares) and does not have a typical right or left bundle branch block pattern.[28]

Left Bundle Branch Block

Left Bundle Branch Block (LBBB) is often caused by myocardial ischaemia and associated ischaemia of the left bundle branch. This is why a patient presenting with clinical signs and symptoms of acute coronary syndrome (page 93) who is found to have new onset LBBB on their ECG should be treated as though they are having a STEMI (page 108).[23, 31, 52]

When a pathology causes the left bundle branch to become blocked (Figure 3.6), the electrical impulse travelling down from the bundle of His is prevented from continuing to the myocardium of the left ventricle via its normal pathway. This means that there is a delay in the left ventricular contraction as the electrical impulse finds an alternative slower route. The ECG will show a prolonged QRS complex of greater than 0.12 seconds (3 small squares) because the left ventricle contracts just after the right ventricle, instead of them both contracting at the same time as would be the case if normal conduction were present.

ECG Identification of Left Bundle Branch Block[18, 25, 28]

- Normally the right and left ventricle depolarise simultaneously; in LBBB the left ventricle depolarisation is delayed, which results in the following changes seen on the 12-lead ECG (Figure 3.7):
  - QRS complex prolongation of greater than 0.12 seconds (3 small squares).
  - Predominantly negative QRS complex in lead V1 with a dominant S wave.
  - Predominantly positive QRS complex in lateral leads V5, V6 and I.
- Other features of LBBB that may be present:
  - 'Notching' or 'M'-shaped R waves in the lateral leads.
  - Left axis deviation (page 22).
  - Discordant QRS waves and T waves (page 100); the T waves go in the opposite direction to their preceding QRS complex.

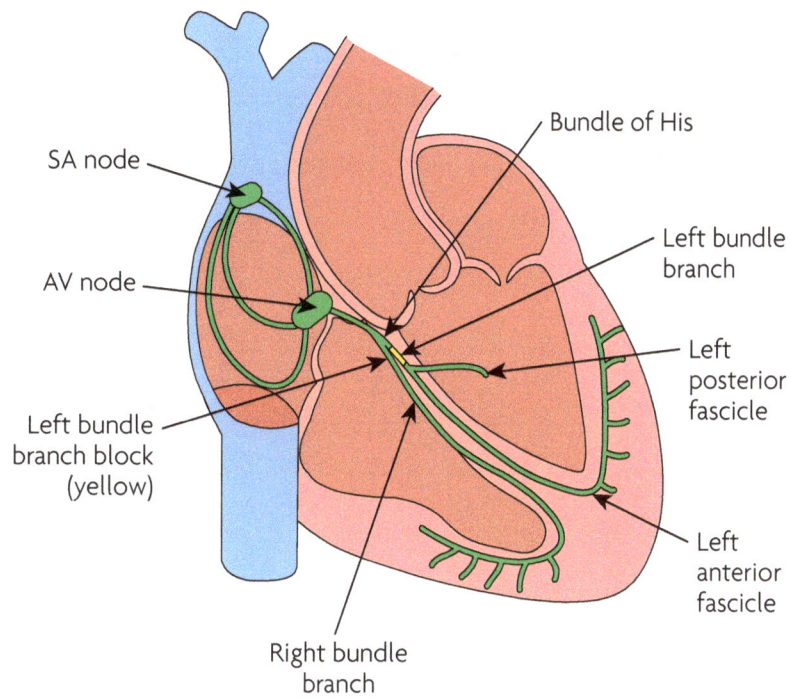

Figure 3.6 Left bundle branch block anatomy.

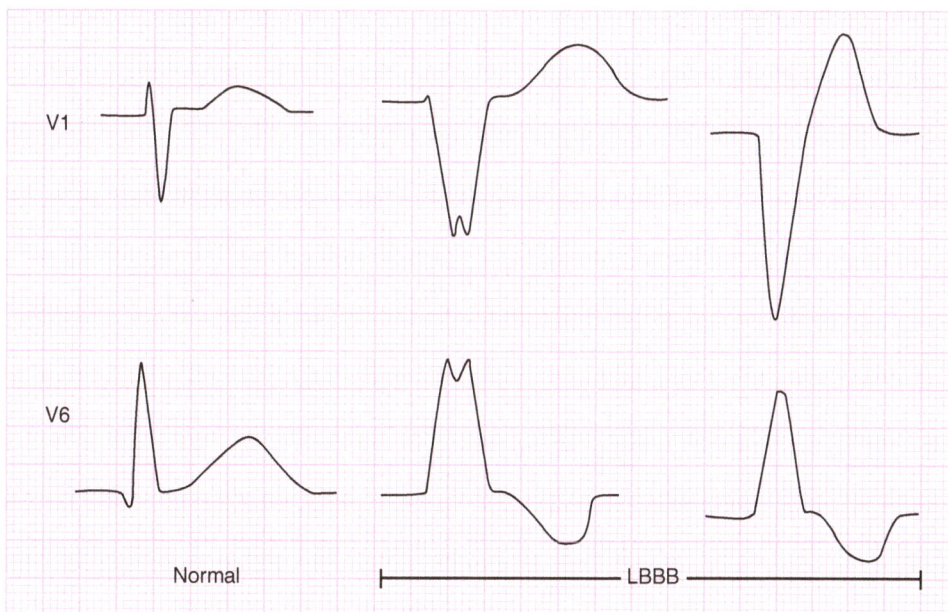

Figure 3.7 Left bundle branch block ECG views.

Causes of Left Bundle Branch Block[28, 29, 33]

- Acute causes:
  - Myocardial infarction.
  - Acute heart failure.
  - Pericarditis.
  - Myocarditis.
- Coronary artery disease.
- Hypertension.
- Aortic valve disease (for example, aortic stenosis).
- Primary fibrosis and degeneration of the cardiac conduction system.
- Cardiomyopathy.

ECG 3.14 – Left Bundle Branch Block

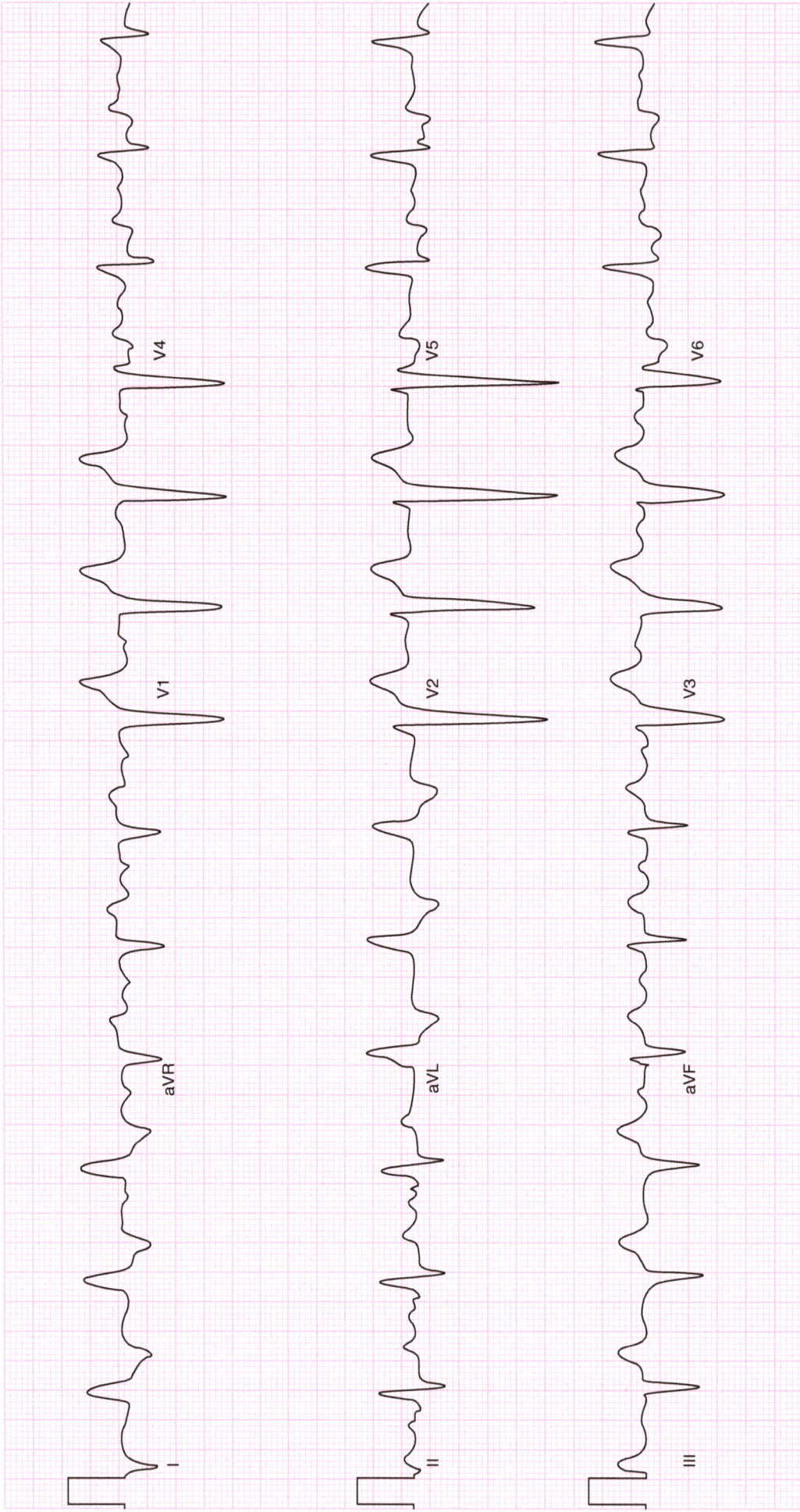

This ECG meets all of the criteria for LBBB. The QRS complexes are prolonged greater than 0.12 seconds (3 small squares). The QRS complexes in lead V1 are predominantly negative; note the deep, wide S waves. The lateral leads I, V5 and V6 are predominantly positive.

Concordance and Discordance[25, 28]

In the context of ECG interpretation, concordance is when two waves in the same P-QRS-T complex both occur in the same direction, either both with positive or both with negative deflections.

Discordance is when two waves are in opposite directions to each other, one being positive and the other being negative.

For example, in Test ECG 1.1 of sinus rhythm, the QRS complex and T waves are concordant; they both are positive, pointing upwards.

In LBBB, the QRS complex and T waves should be discordant; the QRS complex is negative and the T wave is positive, or vice versa. This can be seen in ECG 3.14. Lead V1 has a predominantly negative QRS complex and positive T wave, making them discordant, which is appropriate in LBBB.

If in LBBB the QRS complex and T wave are inappropriately concordant, it may be due to myocardial ischaemia and the ECG may meet Sgarbossa criteria (page 128).

Incomplete Left Bundle Branch Block[33]

Incomplete LBBB occurs when an ECG meets the criteria for LBBB except for the duration of the QRS which remains less than 0.12 seconds (3 small squares) and as such does not meet the full criteria for LBBB. There is no clinically significant difference between the incomplete LBBB and LBBB in the out-of-hospital setting; the same possible causes and differentials should be considered.

Clinical Presentation and Management of Left Bundle Branch Block[7, 31, 53]

A patient with LBBB will fit into one of four groupings based on their clinical presentation and previous cardiac history (Table 3.1):

- **Group 1**: Patients with new onset LBBB on their ECG and signs and symptoms of ACS (page 94). LBBB naturally has ST segment elevation and as such can mask signs of STEMI. Patients should be treated for STEMI (page 108) following local guidelines.
- **Group 2**: Patients with new LBBB on their ECG and *no* signs or symptoms suggestive of ACS. The treatment needs to be based on their clinical presentation and history. Transport to hospital will likely be indicated due to the restrictions of being unable to further interpret the ECG or to investigate the cause of LBBB. The LBBB may be a sign of a recent cardiac event which has now resolved or cannot be identified in the out-of-hospital environment.
- **Group 3**: Patients with previously diagnosed LBBB on their ECG and signs and symptoms of ACS. Treat for ACS (page 108). Consider Sgarbossa criteria to evaluate likelihood of underlying STEMI. If Sgarbossa positive, then consider contacting the STEMI pathway to see if the patient can be accepted directly at the cardiac centre. This decision will be based on local pathways and guidelines, in combination with relative travel times and the patient's clinical presentation.
- **Group 4**: Patients with previously diagnosed LBBB and no signs or symptoms suggestive of ACS. Consider the presenting clinical signs and symptoms and if these would warrant hospital conveyance. The likelihood of needing to convey to hospital is increased, as the LBBB may mask other ECG changes, particularly if the patient's clinical presentation is potentially cardiac in origin.

Table 3.1 Clinical presentation and management of LBBB presentations

	Signs or Symptoms of ACS	No Suggestion of ACS
New LBBB	Treat for STEMI (page 108).	Likely conveyance to hospital on presenting clinical symptoms and to investigate cause of LBBB.
Previously Diagnosed LBBB	Treat for ACS (page 108). Consider Sgarbossa criteria – if positive, consider contacting STEMI pathway to ask if patient can be brought directly to the cardiac centre.	Treatment and transport based on clinical presentations and findings, excluding ECG. Low threshold for conveyance if clinicians believe LBBB may be masking another ECG abnormality or if patient presents with symptoms that are potentially cardiac in origin.

Modified Sgarbossa Criteria[7, 31, 41, 52, 53]

Current guidelines emphasise that algorithms such as the Sgarbossa criteria do not provide diagnostic certainty in regard to identifying the presence or absence of underlying STEMI in patients with LBBB. However, it is important to be aware of these criteria as they can provide some degree of suggestion that can be considered as part of the patient's wider clinical picture. The absence of Sgarbossa criteria does not rule out MI. The presence of Sgarbossa criteria in LBBB is suggestive of, but does not confirm, underlying STEMI.

In the context of LBBB, the presence of any one of the following three criteria is suggestive of ongoing myocardial infarction:
- One or more leads with 1 mm or more of concordant ST segment elevation.
- One or more leads in V1–V3 with 1 mm or more of concordant ST segment depression.
- One or more leads anywhere with greater than 1 mm of ST segment elevation and proportionally excessive discordant ST segment elevation (defined by greater than 25% of the depth of the preceding S wave).

> **Remember:** The presence of negative Sgarbossa criteria does not rule out ACS. **!**

Key Points: Left Bundle Branch Block
- LBBB is most often caused by myocardial infarction.
- If undiagnosed LBBB is found, assume ACS until proven otherwise.
- Sgarbossa criteria can be used to help assess the likelihood of LBBB being caused by ongoing myocardial infarction.

Right Bundle Branch Block

When a pathology causes the right bundle branch to become blocked (Figure 3.8), the electrical impulses travelling down from the bundle of His are prevented from continuing down to the myocardium of the right ventricle. This means that there is a delay in right ventricular contraction as the electrical impulse finds an alternative, slower route. The ECG will show a prolonged QRS complex of greater than 0.12 seconds (3 small squares), because the right ventricle contracts *after* the left ventricle, instead of them both contracting at the same time as would be the case if normal conduction were present.

ECG Identification of Right Bundle Branch Block[18, 25, 28]

- Normally the right and left ventricle depolarise simultaneously; in RBBB, the right ventricle depolarisation is delayed, which results in the following changes seen on the 12-lead ECG (Figure 3.9):
  - QRS complex prolongation of greater than 0.12 seconds (3 small squares).
  - Predominantly positive QRS complex in lead V1 with rSR, pattern.
  - Slurred S wave in lateral leads V5, V6, I and aVL.
    - The slurred S waves are a vital aid in identifying RBBB. The rSR pattern in V1 is not always clearly recognisable. When you have a wide and predominantly positive QRS complex in lead V1 that does not show an obvious rSR pattern, you should look for the slurred S waves in the lateral leads.
- Other possible ECG changes:
  - Inverted T waves in leads V1 and V2.
  - Downward-sloping ST segment in leads V1 and V2.

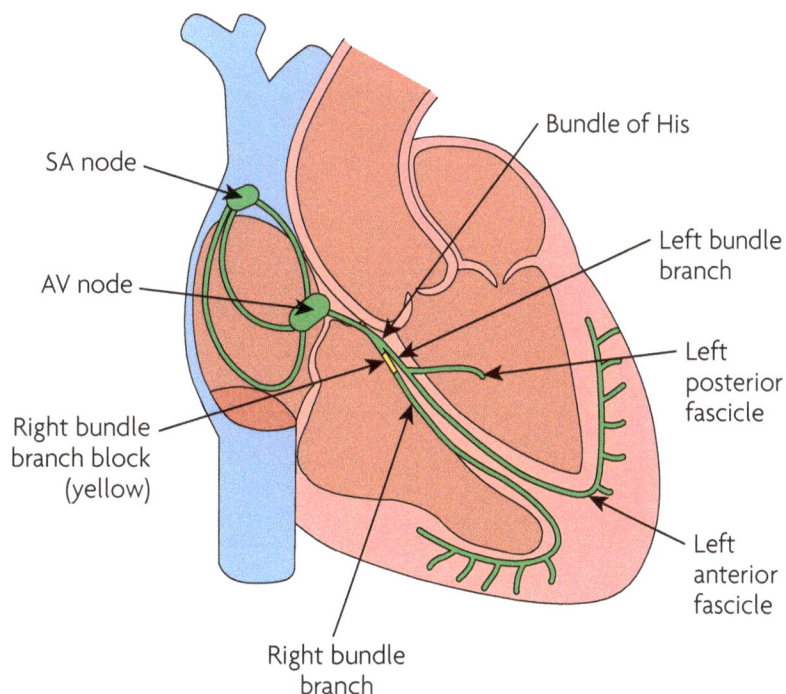

Figure 3.8 Right bundle branch block anatomy.

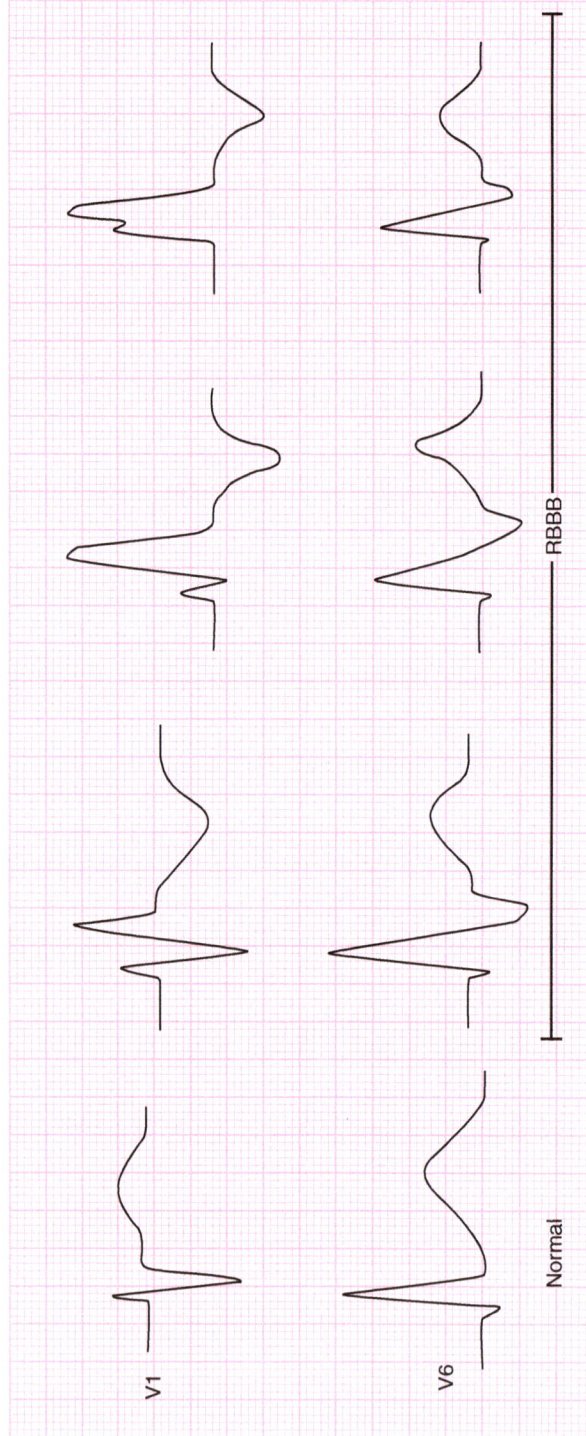

V1

V6

Normal

RBBB

Figure 3.9 Right bundle branch block ECG views.

ECG 3.15 – Right Bundle Branch Block

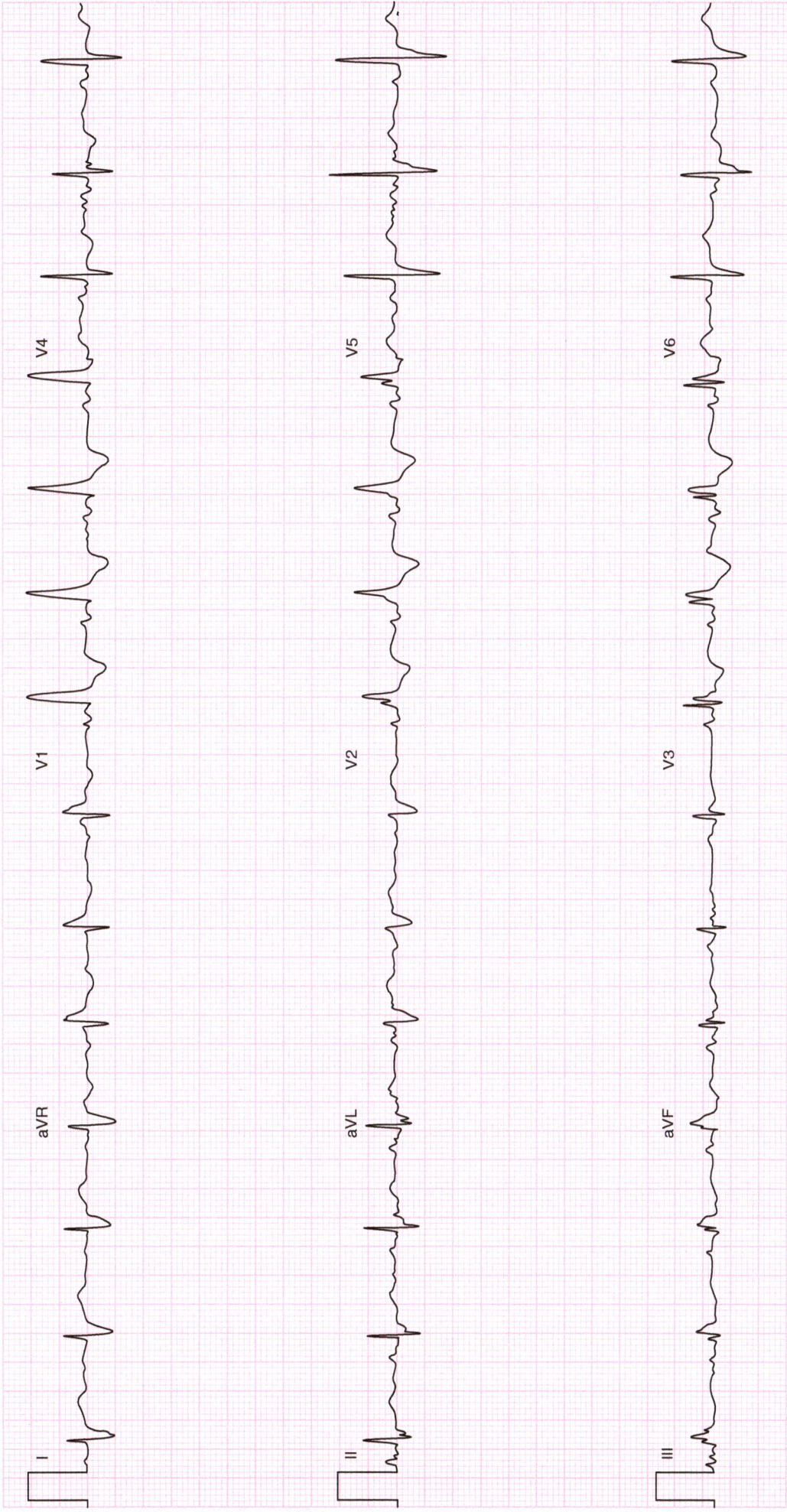

In this example of RBBB we can see the widened QRS complex in lead V1; though at first glance it does not have the 'classic' rSR pattern, it still meets the RBBB criteria. This lack of rSR emphasises that the slurred S waves we can see in leads I and V6 are reliable indicators of RBBB when combined with a widened QRS complex and positive QRS in lead V1. We can also see inverted T waves in leads V1–V2 which are also in keeping with RBBB.

rSR Complex

The staggered contraction of the ventricles is observed on the ECG in leads V1 and V2 in the form of a second R wave. The second R wave represents the contraction of the right ventricle, as this is the contraction that has been delayed due to the right bundle branch block. This leads to the terminology 'rSR' because the QRS complex is made up of two R waves separated with an S wave, instead of the usual QRS waves.

Clinical Presentation and Management of Right Bundle Branch Block[7, 28, 29, 33]

- The clinical presentation of a patient with RBBB varies dramatically. As can be seen from the below list of potential causes, there are a wide variety of conditions that can lead to RBBB.
- The patient may be showing clinical signs and symptoms of ACS (page 94).
- There may be a respiratory pathology leading to a presentation of shortness of breath or difficulty breathing.
- In many cases, the RBBB will be pre-existent and not relate directly to the patient's current clinical presentation. If the RBBB has not been previously identified and formally diagnosed then due consideration must be given to the likelihood that it is related to the current presentation.
- There is no specific management for RBBB itself. Instead, consideration should be given to management of the potential underlying cause, which is likely to be cardiac, cardiovascular or respiratory in origin.

Causes of Right Bundle Branch Block[28, 29, 33, 50]

- Myocardial infarction.
- Coronary artery disease.
- Right ventricular strain due to:
  - Acute:
    - Pulmonary embolism.
  - Chronic:
    - Cor pulmonale.
    - Chronic obstructive pulmonary disease.
    - Pulmonary hypertension.
    - Recurrent pulmonary embolism.
- Right ventricular failure.
- Congenital heart disease.
- Primary fibrosis and degeneration of the cardiac conduction system.
- Cardiomyopathy.
- RBBB is a normal variant in up to 5% of older adults and 1% of young adults.

qR Wave[25]

A pathological Q wave in lead V1 is a sign of either a new or previous anteroseptal myocardial infarction. Instead of the expected rSR complex in V1, RBBB in patients who also have a new or previous anteroseptal myocardial infarction may present with a qR complex. This still meets the criteria for RBBB, as the QRS complex is wide and predominantly positive; a slurring or change in the gradient of the R wave can also be seen. More information on pathological Q waves may be found on page 106.

Incomplete RBBB[33]

If RBBB morphology is showing on an ECG but the QRS complex duration is under 0.12 seconds (3 small squares), this is referred to as incomplete right bundle branch block. There is no clinically significant difference between the incomplete RBBB and RBBB in the out-of-hospital setting; the same possible causes and differentials should be considered.

Right Ventricular Strain Patterns

There are multiple ways in which right ventricular strain can manifest on an ECG. There are also multiple causes of right ventricular strain. This means that an ECG showing a possible right ventricular strain pattern cannot be used to diagnose the cause of the right ventricular strain. Instead, the finding of a right ventricular strain pattern on an ECG should be used to form part of a wider clinical picture alongside thorough history-taking and physical examination.

- Potential causes of right ventricular strain:
  - ▸ Lung disease, including chronic obstructive pulmonary disease.
  - ▸ Pulmonary hypertension.
  - ▸ Pulmonary embolism.
  - ▸ Mitral regurgitation or other right-sided heart problems.
- Potential manifestation of right ventricular strain on an ECG (right ventricular strain patterns):
  - ▸ RBBB.
  - ▸ Right axis deviation and other signs of right ventricular hypertrophy.
  - ▸ 'S1 Q3 T3' – a deep S wave in lead I, a deep Q wave and inverted T wave in lead III.

The acuity of the cause of the right ventricular strain will affect what ECG changes are potentially present. An acute cause such as pulmonary embolism is more likely to cause electrical changes such as RBBB, whereas a sub-acute or chronic cause of right ventricular strain, such as lung disease or pulmonary hypertension, is more likely to cause structural changes such as right ventricular hypertrophy.

There have been recent associations made with right ventricular strain patterns preceding cardiac arrest (asystolic or PEA) due to respiratory failure, with right ventricular strain preceding up to 47% of in-hospital cardiac arrests.[54]

S1 Q3 T3 in Pulmonary Embolism[33, 50, 54, 55, 56, 57]

S1 Q3 T3 is often wrongly thought of as 'the' sign of pulmonary embolism on an ECG. In reality this is a rare ECG finding. Sinus rhythm or sinus tachycardia are the most common ECG changes in pulmonary embolism, followed by other changes such as ST segment elevation or depression or signs of right ventricular strain. Ten to twenty-five per cent of patients with pulmonary embolism will have a normal ECG. If S1 Q3 T3 is found on an ECG, it serves as an indication of possible right ventricular strain, which could have been caused by pulmonary embolism, but also could be due to any other cause of right ventricular strain.

Key Points: Right Bundle Branch Block

- If undiagnosed RBBB is found, the clinician should assume that a respiratory or cardiac pathology has occurred or is occurring.
- Treatment should be guided by the the patient's overall clinical presentation, with the ECG acting only as a part of the information used to formulate a working diagnosis.
- Previously undiagnosed RBBB must be treated as pathological until proven otherwise.

ECG 3.16 – Right Ventricular Strain with S1 Q3 T3

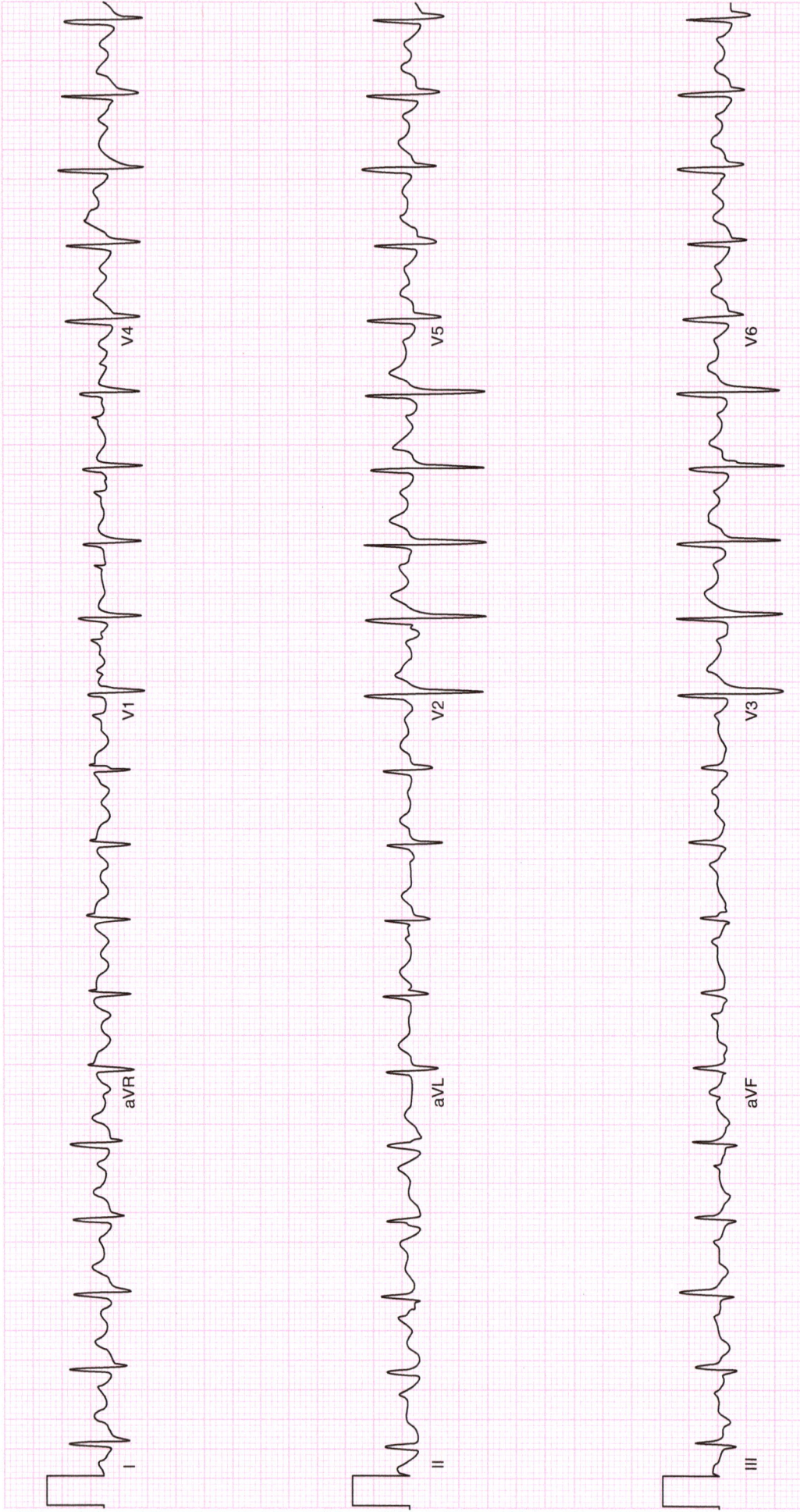

We can see in lead I that there is a prominent S wave. There are also Q waves and inverted T waves in lead III. This indicates that right ventricular strain may be present. Combined with the tachycardia of just under 150 beats per minute, we can consider the potential cause of the right ventricular strain to be acute.

Fascicular Blocks[18, 25, 33]

The left bundle branch subdivides into two fascicules, or sub-branches: The left anterior fascicle and the left posterior fascicle, as shown in Figure 3.10. The right bundle branch remains undivided and is, in itself, a single fascicule. A single fascicle within the left bundle branch can become blocked to electrical activity, leading to the development of a fascicular block.

Left Anterior Fascicular Block (LAFB) occurs when electrical impulses are unable to travel through the left anterior fascicule and instead reach the left ventricle only through the left posterior fascicle. This is identified with the following ECG changes:

- Left axis deviation (page 22).
- QRS duration on the longer side of the normal range, up to 0.11 seconds.
- Tall R wave with small Q wave in the high lateral leads I and aVL.
- Small R wave with deep S wave in the inferior leads II, III and aVF.

Left Posterior Fascicular Block (LPFB) occurs when electrical impulses are unable to travel through the left posterior fascicule and instead reach the left ventricle only through the left anterior fascicle. This is identified on the ECG with the following criteria:

- Right axis deviation (page 22).
- QRS duration on the longer side of the normal range, up to 0.11 seconds.
- Small R wave with deep S wave in the high lateral leads I and aVL.
- Tall R wave with small Q wave in the inferior leads II, II and aVF.

Bifascicular and trifascicular blocks

Bifascicular block occurs when RBBB is combined with either left anterior fascicular block or left posterior fascicular block. This causes RBBB ECG features to be seen, combined with either left or right axis deviation.

Trifascicular block occurs when bifascicular block is combined with an AV block (page 60). This is an accepted misnomer in cardiac terminology as the AV node is not a fascicle.

Bifascicular block combined with 1st or either of the 2nd degree AV blocks (page 62) is referred to as incomplete trifascicular block.

Bifascicular block combined with 3rd degree AV block (page 64) is referred to as complete trifascicular block.

Patients presenting with complete trifascicular block are managed in the same way as patients in 3rd degree heart block (page 61).

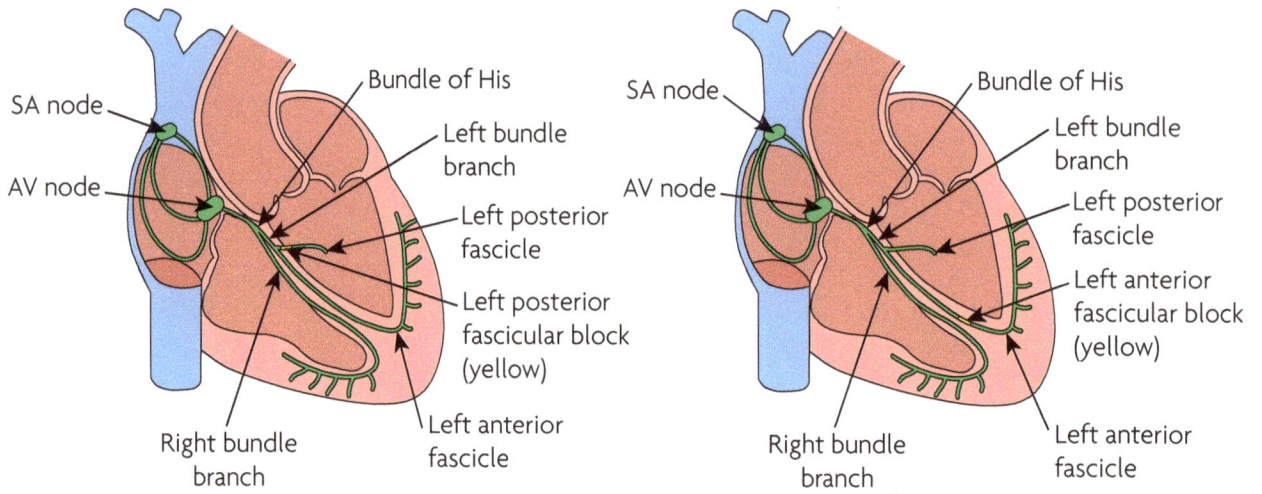

Figure 3.10 Left anterior and posterior fascicular block anatomy.

ECG 3.17 – Left Anterior Fascicular Block

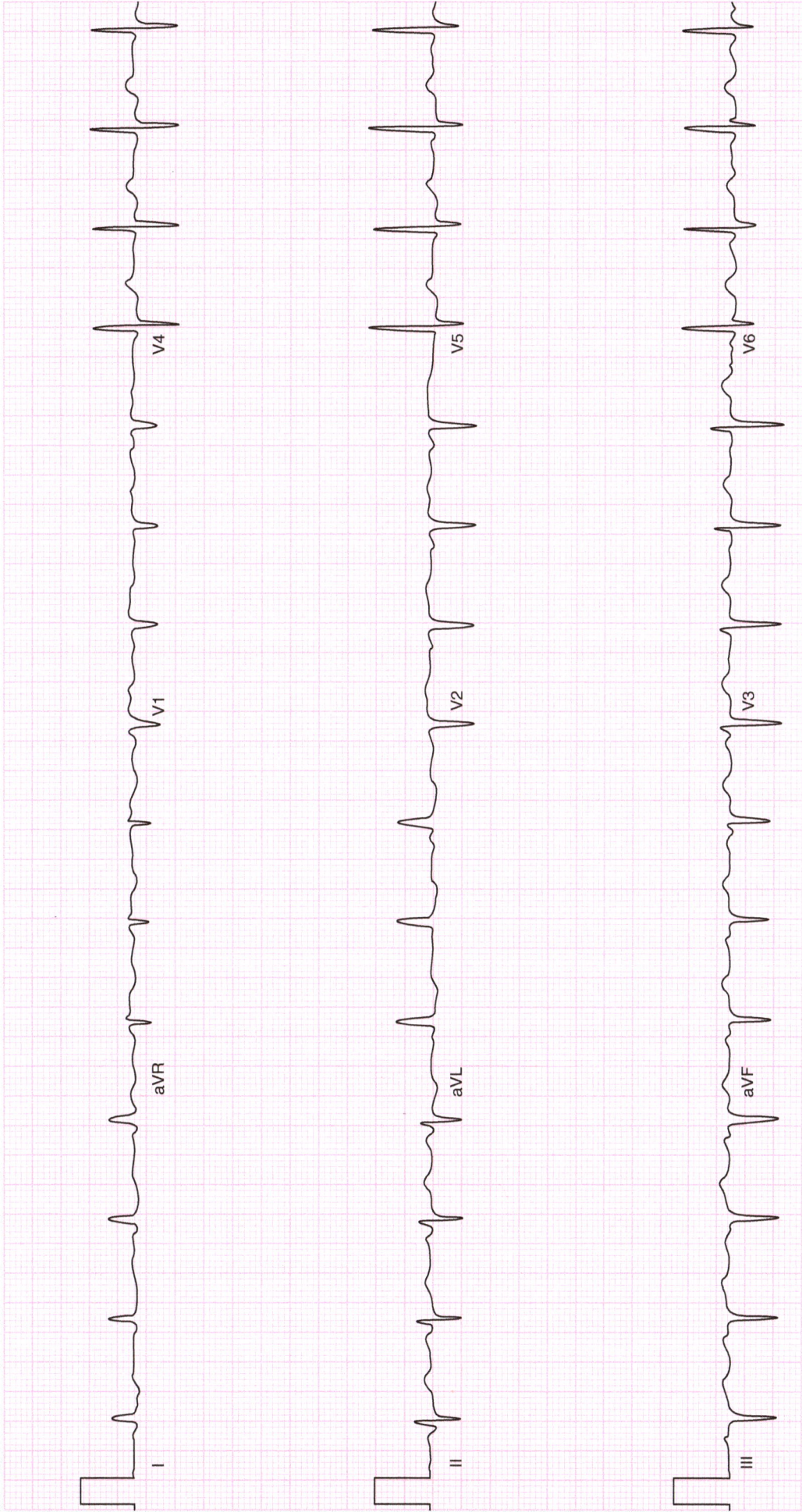

This ECG shows signs of LAFB; there is left axis deviation (lead I is positive and lead aVF is negative), the QRS duration is on the longer side of normal nearing 0.12 seconds (3 small squares) and there are tall R waves in leads I and aVL and deep S waves in the inferior leads II, III and aVF.

ECG 3.18 – Left Posterior Fascicular Block

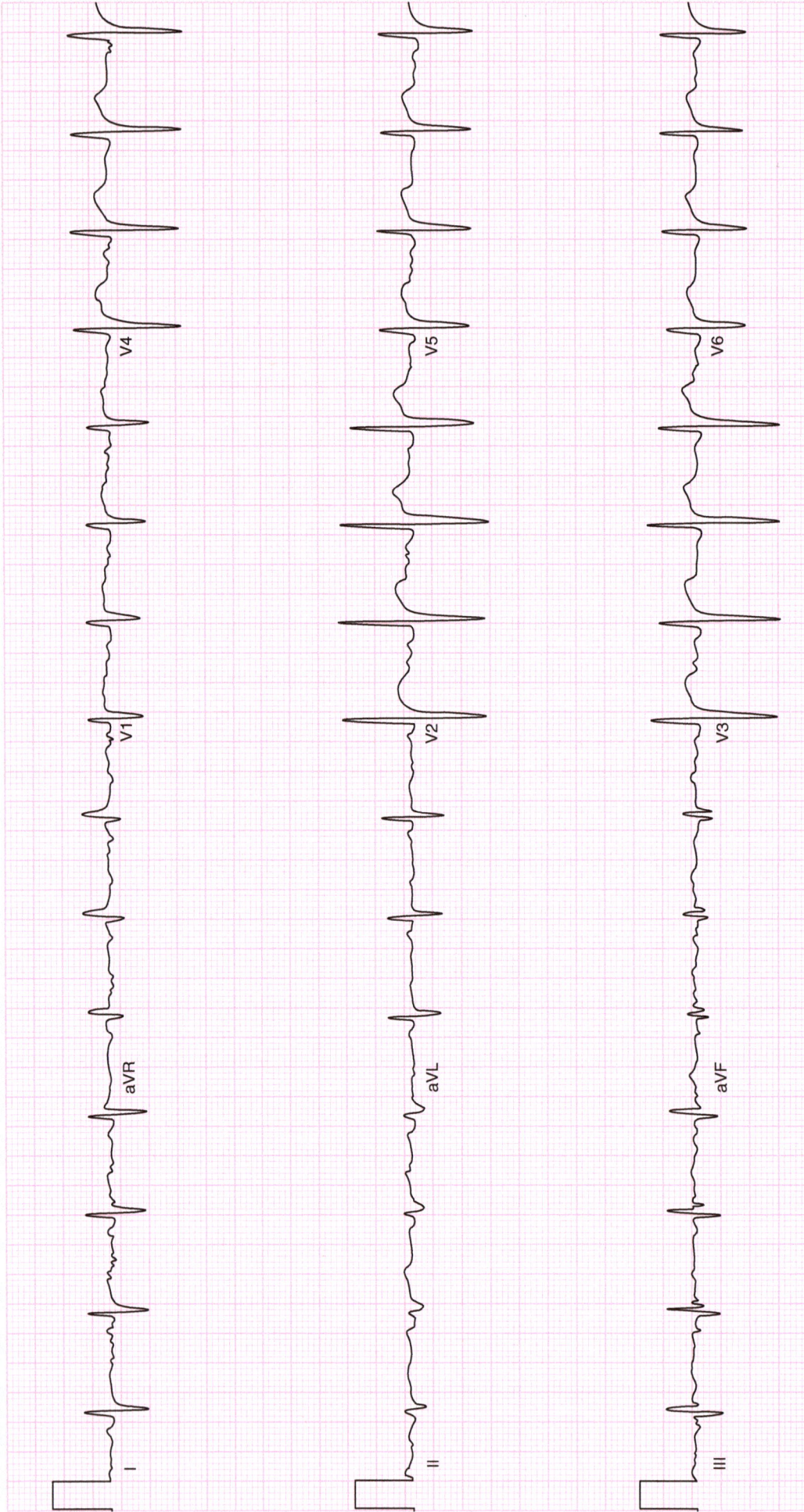

I

II

III

aVR

aVL

aVF

V1

V2

V3

V4

V5

V6

Here we can see an example of LPFB; there are right axis deviation, deep S waves in leads I and aVL, and tall R waves in lead III.

ECG 3.19 – Bifascicular Block

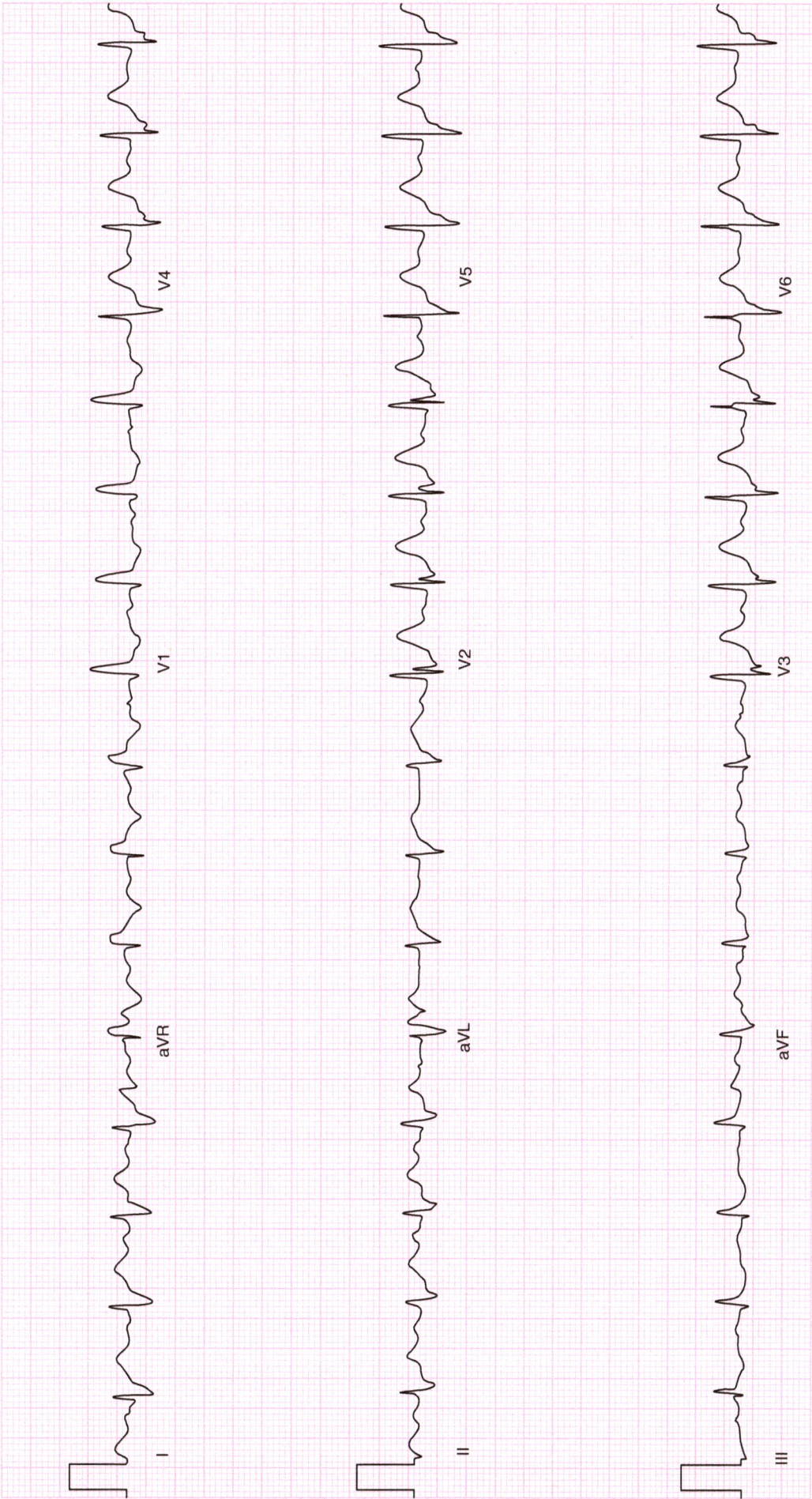

I
aVR
V1
V4

II
aVL
V2
V5

III
aVF
V3
V6

This ECG meets the criteria for both LPFB and RBBB, making it a bifascicular block.

ECG 3.20 – Trifascicular Block

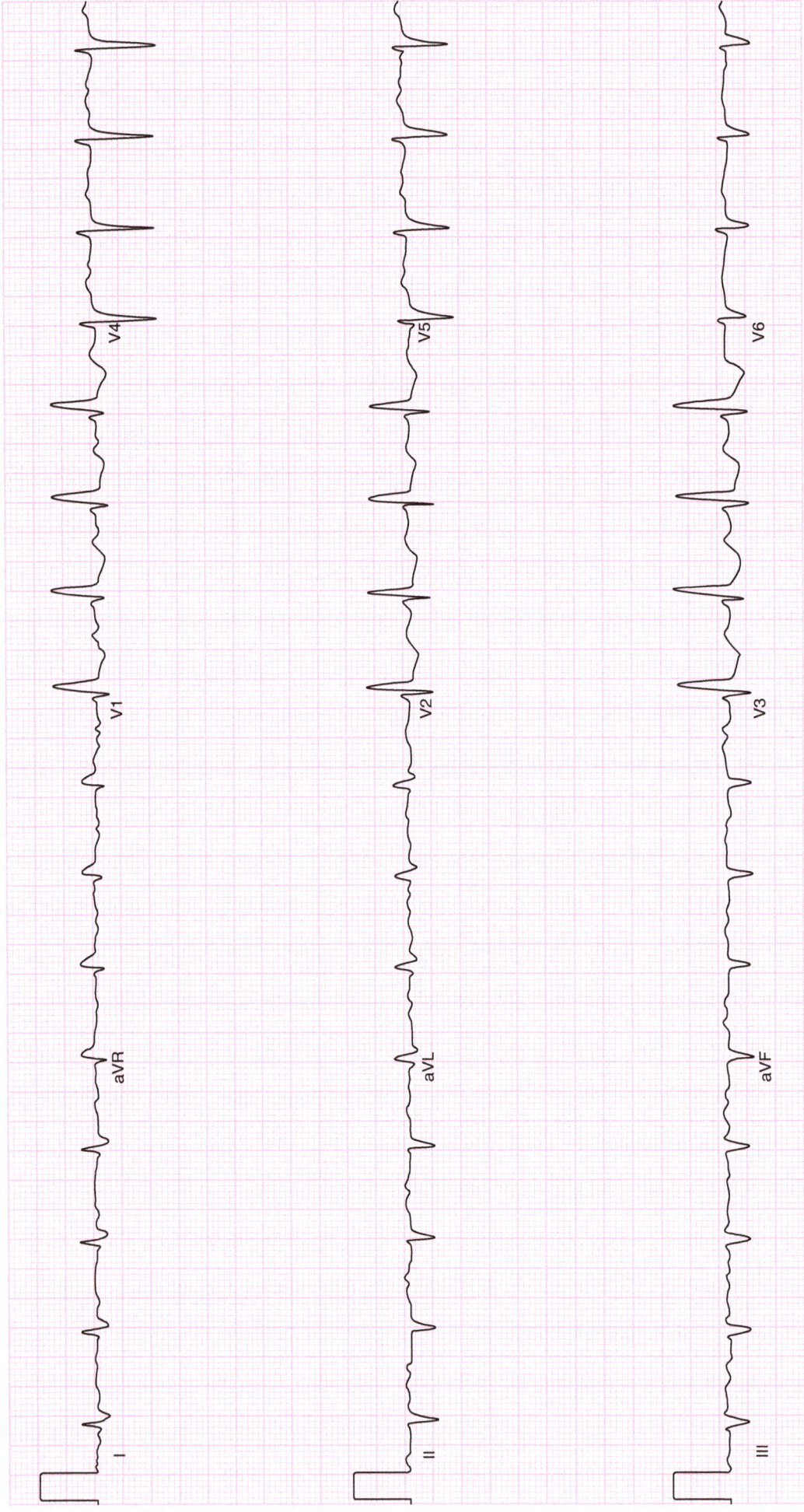

I

II

III

aVR

aVL

aVF

V1

V2

V3

V4

V5

V6

This ECG shows LAFB and RBBB (together making bifascicular block) and a 1st degree AV block; these, together, are identified as trifascicular block.

Paced Rhythms[29, 45, 33, 58, 59]

Pacemakers are surgically implanted devices that produce an electrical impulse which triggers a heartbeat. If a pacemaker is operating, there will be notable changes seen on the ECG. There are two main types of pacemaker: Those that pace only on demand and those that pace constantly. Demand pacemakers only pace the heart when they sense it is needed – when the heart does not beat for a predetermined amount of time. Some pacemakers pace the heart constantly at a fixed rate. This reduces the body's ability to react and alter cardiac output accordingly (page 13). Other pacemakers are rate responsive, sensing possible signs of exertion (increased respiratory rate, shortening QT interval) and altering the paced heart rate to an appropriate rate for the level of exertion. Pacemakers can introduce an electrical impulse to different parts of the heart depending on where the pacing wire has been placed.

On the ECG, all pacemaker rhythms will have a pacing spike visible before each heartbeat. If the pacing spike precedes the P wave then it is atrial pacing. If the pacing spike precedes the QRS complex, this indicates ventricular pacing.

In paced rhythms the QRS complex may appear to have a bundle branch block morphology, because the ventricle which has the pacing wire will depolarise before the other ventricle.

A pacing spike is a narrow, tall 'spike' of electrical activity on the ECG. The presence of pacing spikes can be difficult to identify in some 12-lead ECG views. The pacing spike only lasts around 0.02 seconds. An example can be seen in ECG 3.21, page 142.

The two main reasons for a patient having pacemaker therapy are for bradyarrhythmias or for heart failure (where both ventricles are usually paced). Patients can also have implantable cardiac devices for tachyarrhythmias, but there are usually implantable defibrillators designed to automatically cardiovert any tachyarrhythmia. Combined pacemaker–defibrillator devices are also available which serve both functions.

The Sgarbossa criteria can be used to assess for signs of underlying STEMI in ventricular-paced rhythms as well as in LBBB.

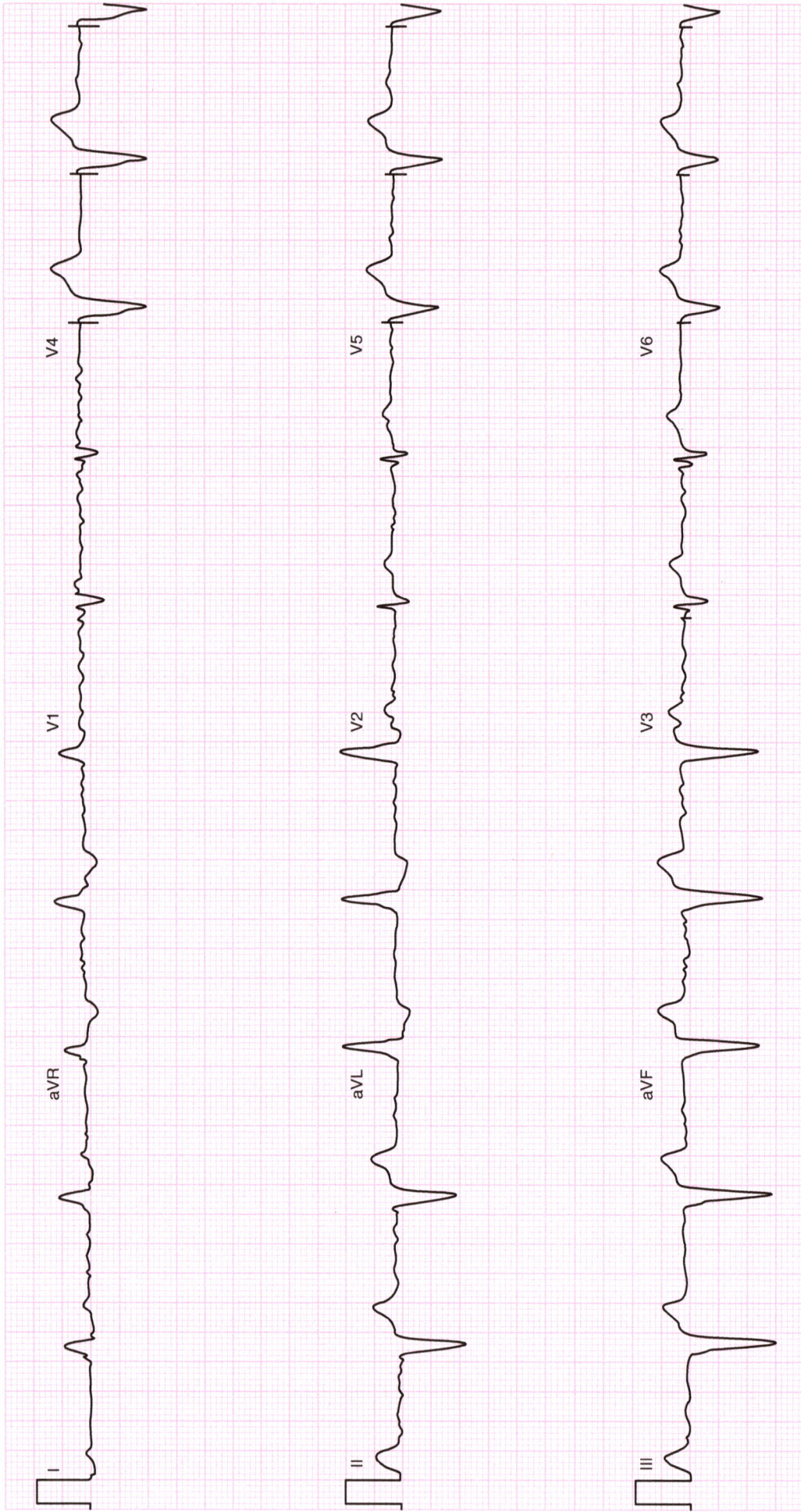

ECG 3.21 – Paced Rhythm

The pacing spikes on this ventricular pacing ECG are best seen in leads V4 and V5. The wide QRS complexes combined with the rate of 60 beats per minute and presence of pacing spikes tell us that this ECG shows ventricular pacing.

Other ECG Abnormalities

Electrolyte Imbalances

The correct balance of electrolytes, sodium, potassium and calcium is a vital part of the normal functioning of the electrical activity within the heart. An elevated or decreased serum level of potassium or calcium causes disruption to the electrical functioning of the heart. The disruption increases the more deranged the serum level becomes, until a fatal level is reached and cardiac arrest occurs.

Most paramedics in the UK do not have access to near-patient blood testing and are unable to determine a patient's electrolyte levels in the out-of-hospital setting. The ECG changes caused by an electrolyte imbalance can be difficult to identify, especially when the imbalance is only marginal. Often the patient's clinical presentation is the best clue to the presence of an electrolyte imbalance.

There are different causes for each electrolyte imbalance, but common themes include renal failure, kidney disease and fluid loss.

Hyperkalaemia

A high potassium in the extracellular space decreases myocardial excitability, causing depression of both the conducting and pace-making cardiac tissues. It is important to note that there is poor sensitivity and specificity of ECG changes in hyperkalaemia and that ECG changes only occur in under 50% of patients with hyperkalaemia.[60, 61] The most common cause of hyperkalaemia is associated with medications, especially if the patient also has heart failure, hypertension or chronic kidney disease. Hyperkalaemia is also common in diabetic ketoacidosis. There are also many other potential causes of hyperkalaemia.[62]

ECG Identification of Hyperkalaemia[25, 30, 63]

- Peaked T waves. Often the earliest sign of hyperkalaemia, but only present in up to 22% of cases.
- As potassium levels further increase and hyperkalaemia worsens:
  - Increased PR segment duration.
  - Widening and flattening of P waves; eventually P waves disappear completely.
  - ST segment changes that can appear as STEMI.
- Severe hyperkalaemia:
  - Atrial fibrillation (page 54) or bradycardia (page 35).
  - Wide and bizarre QRS complexes.
  - Development of heart blocks (page 60).

3

ECG 3.22 – Hyperkalaemia

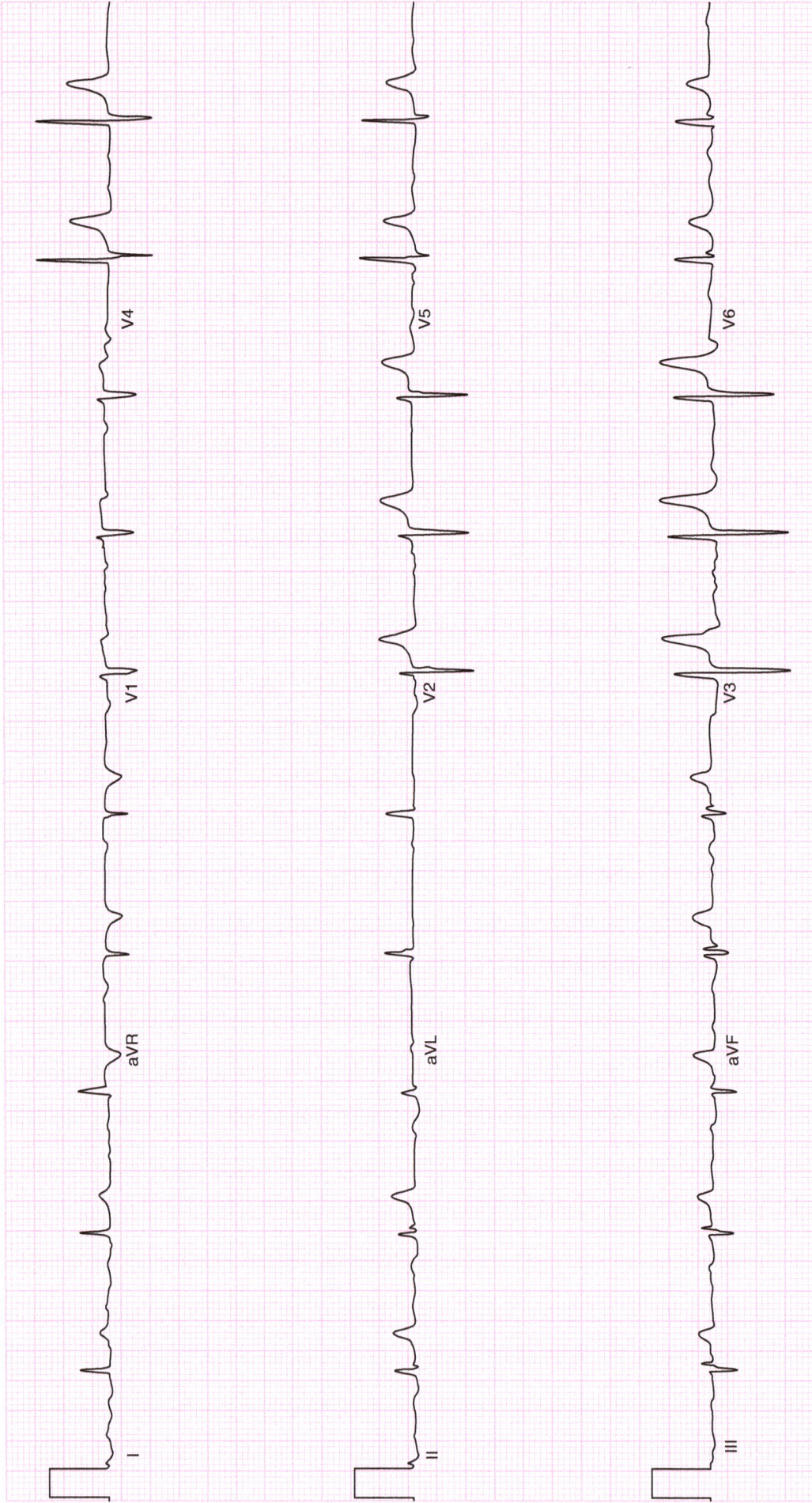

This ECG displays multiple signs of hyperkalaemia. Tall, peaked T waves are present, particularly in leads V2–V6. The PR segment duration is increased and P waves are flattened and in some places hardly visible.

Causes of Hyperkalaemia Include:[60, 64, 65]

- Ineffective elimination of potassium from the body:
  - Decreased kidney function, kidney disease and renal failure.
  - Medications, including:
    - ACE inhibitors.
    - Beta blockers.
    - Angiotensin receptor blockers.
    - Spironolactone.
    - NSAIDS.
    - Trimethoprim.
- Increased potassium release from cells:
  - Metabolic acidosis.
  - Insulin deficiency.
  - Diabetic ketoacidosis.
  - Rhabdomyolysis.
  - Exercise.
- Increased intake of potassium.
  - Excessive consumption of bananas.
  - Overdose of potassium supplement tablets or multivitamins containing potassium.

Hypokalaemia

A decreased level of potassium in the extracellular space increases myocardial excitability and can lead to the development of re-entrant tachycardias (page 42).

ECG Identification of Hypokalaemia[25, 30, 64]

- Increased PR interval.
- Increased width and height of P waves.
- ST segment depression.
- Inversion and flattening of T waves.
- Biphasic T waves.
- Presence of U waves (page 8).

Hypokalaemia can also cause other ECG arrhythmias to develop:

- Ectopic beats (page 68).
- Atrial fibrillation (page 54), atrial flutter (page 57) and other forms of SVT (page 32).
- VF and VT (page 49).

Causes of Hypokalaemia Include:[60, 65]

- Increased renal excretion; for example, loop diuretics and thiazides.
- Renal disease.
- Liver failure.
- Heart failure.
- Nephrotic syndrome.
- Cushing syndrome.
- Fluid loss from diarrhoea and vomiting.
- Excessive sweating.
- Other pharmacological:
  - Furosemide.
  - Beta-2 agonists.
  - Penicillin.

ECG 3.23 – Hypokalaemia

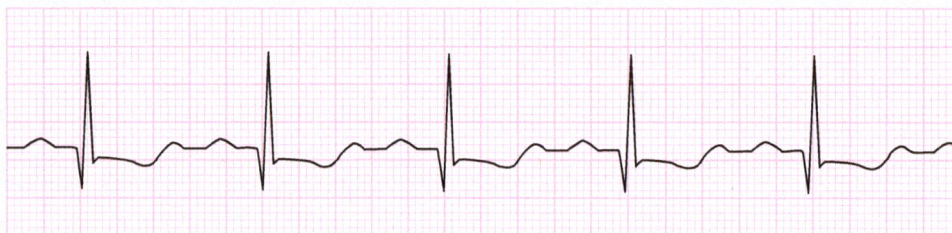

The increased width of the P waves, the ST segment depression, the flattened, inverted T waves and the presence of U waves (which could appear as biphasic T waves) are all suggestive of hypokalaemia.

Hypercalcaemia

An increased level of calcium can cause increased heart rate and contractility of the cardiac muscle. Severe hypercalcaemia can cause ventricular ectopics (page 69), bradycardia (page 35) and VF (page 28).

ECG Identification of Hypercalcaemia

- Short QT interval and short ST segment.
- Possible flattening of T waves.
- Severe cases may produce Osborn waves.

Hypocalcaemia

Atrial and ventricular arrhythmias can occur due to hypocalcaemia but are far less common than in other electrolyte imbalances.

ECG Identification of Hypocalcaemia[25, 64]

- Long QT interval and prolonged ST segment.

Hypothermia

Hypothermia is not an ECG diagnosis, but it can cause ECG changes. As body temperature is lowered and hypothermia sets in, several ECG changes and arrhythmias can develop. The heart rate slows and bradycardia develops. Atrial fibrillation (page 54) can also occur. When the body's core temperature drops too far, VF and asystole occur.

ECG Changes in Hypothermia[25]

- Osborne waves appear
  - Also known as J waves, Osborne waves occur as a positive deflection at the J point.
- The PR interval, QRS complex and QT interval durations increase.
- Depending on the degree and type of hypothermia, the patient may also be bradycardia.

ECG 3.24 – Hypothermia

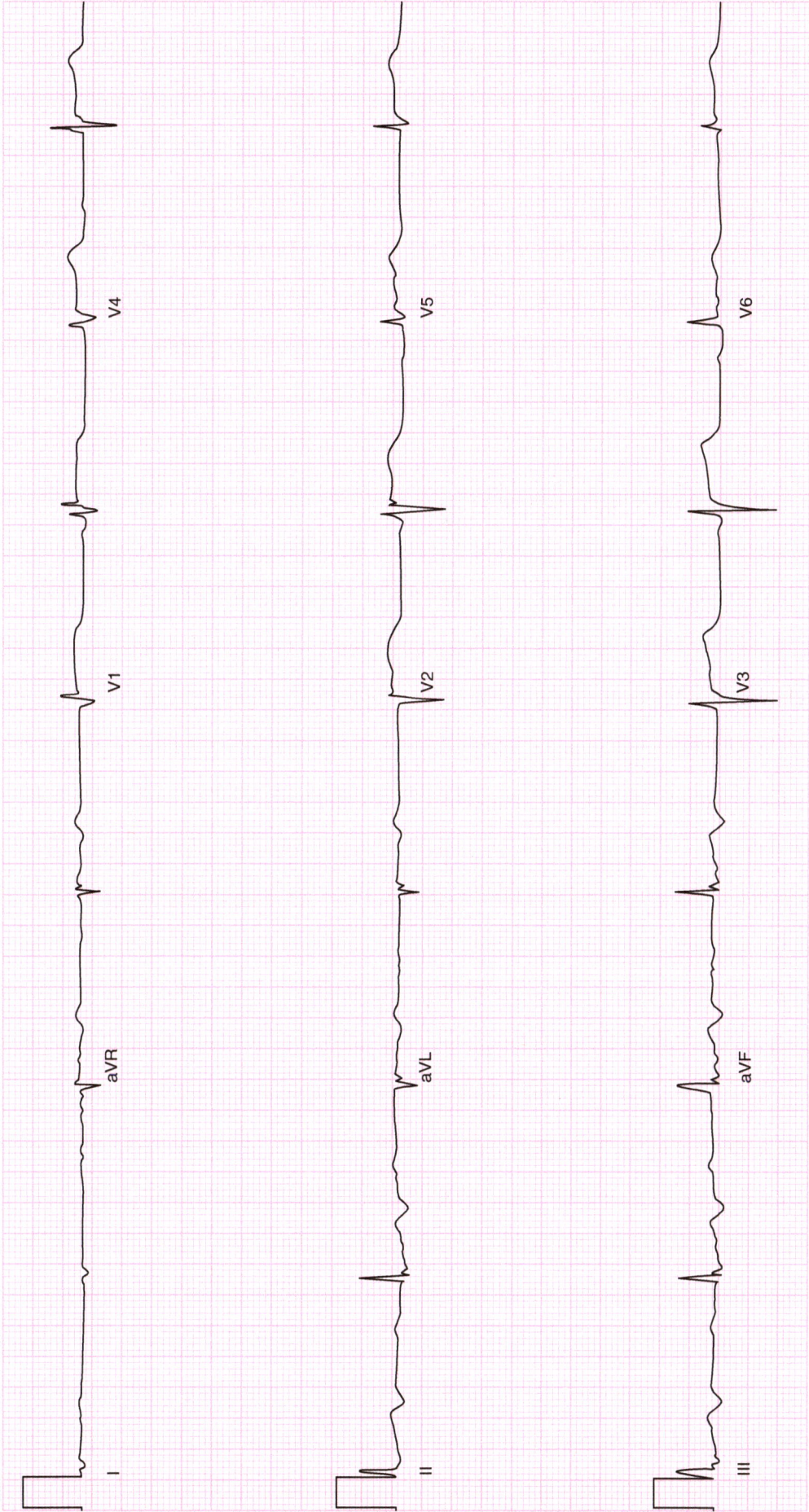

This bradycardic ECG displays Osborne waves and increased duration of the PR interval, QRS complexes and QT interval, all signs indicative of hypothermia.

Neurological ECG Changes

ECG changes can occur in patients with stroke or raised intracranial pressure (ICP). Causes of raised ICP include subarachnoid haemorrhage, traumatic brain injury and haemorrhagic stroke. Twenty-five per cent of patients with subarachnoid haemorrhage will demonstrate ECG changes.[41]

Usually, the clinical presentation of the patient will point towards a neurological pathology and ECG changes should not be sought as part of the assessment and diagnosis. Obtaining a 12-lead ECG in a patient with a clear neurological presentation causes unnecessary delay. Most emergent neurological conditions are time-critical and rapid transfer to hospital should not routinely be delayed by obtaining a 12-lead ECG as it is unlikely to have any additional diagnostic value and is associated with worse outcomes.[7]

If, however, a 12-lead ECG is obtained as part of the assessment of a patient presenting with an undifferentiated set of symptoms, the finding of any of the below changes could aid in identifying a potential neurological cause.

ECG Changes Due to Neurological Conditions Include:[7, 66, 67, 68]

- Widespread T wave inversion; often T waves are very deep and wide, known as 'neurological T waves'.
- Prolonged QT interval.
- Bradycardia.
- Ectopics.
- ST segment changes that may appear as ischaemia or STEMI.

ECG 3.25 – Neurological ECG Changes

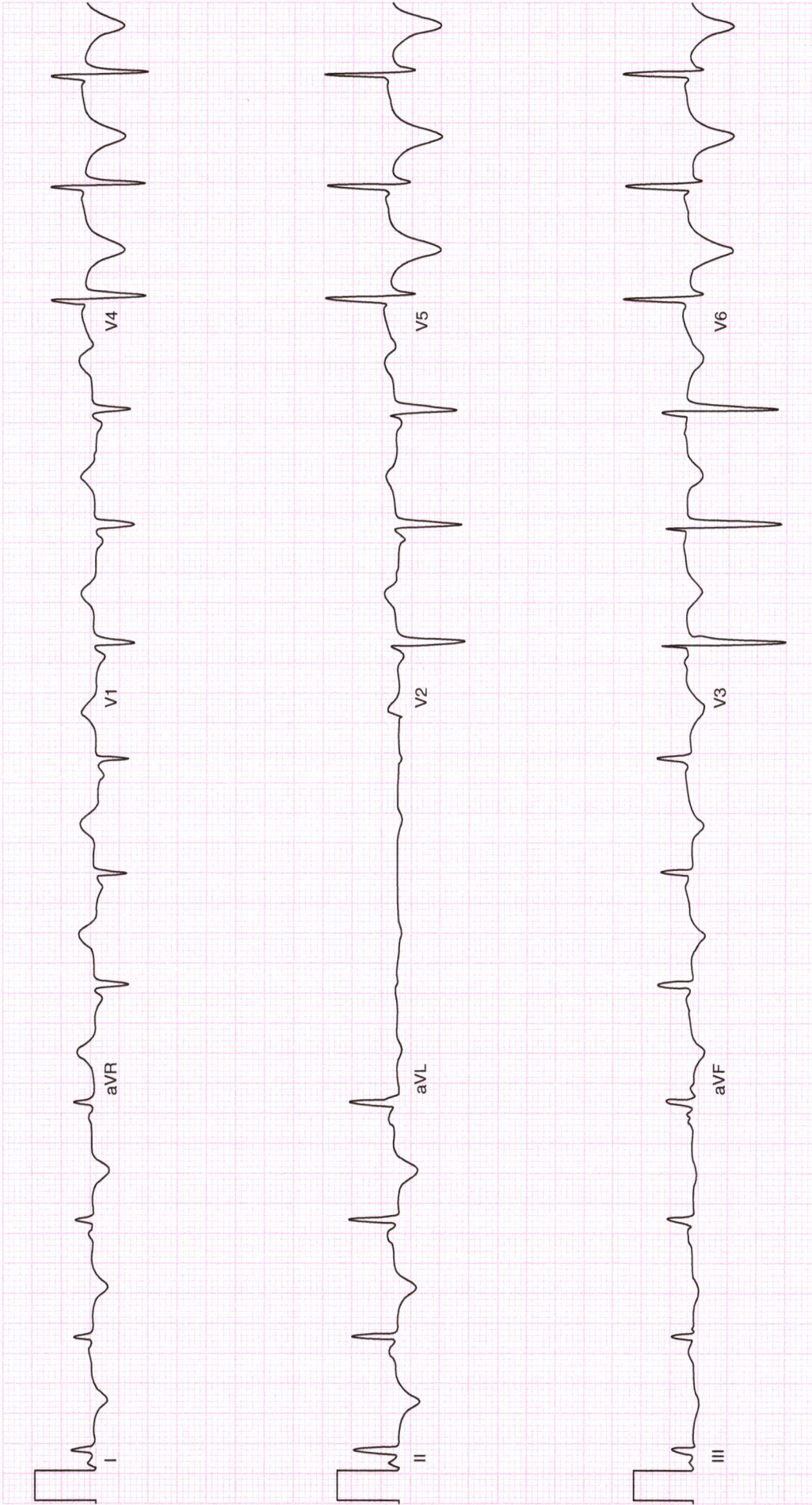

There are multiple changes on this ECG that suggest potential neurological pathology. Deep, wide and inverted 'neurological T waves' can be seen in most leads (note that even the T waves in lead aVR are inverted in that they are positive). The QT interval is also prolonged and there are ST segment changes in many leads.

Test ECG 3.1

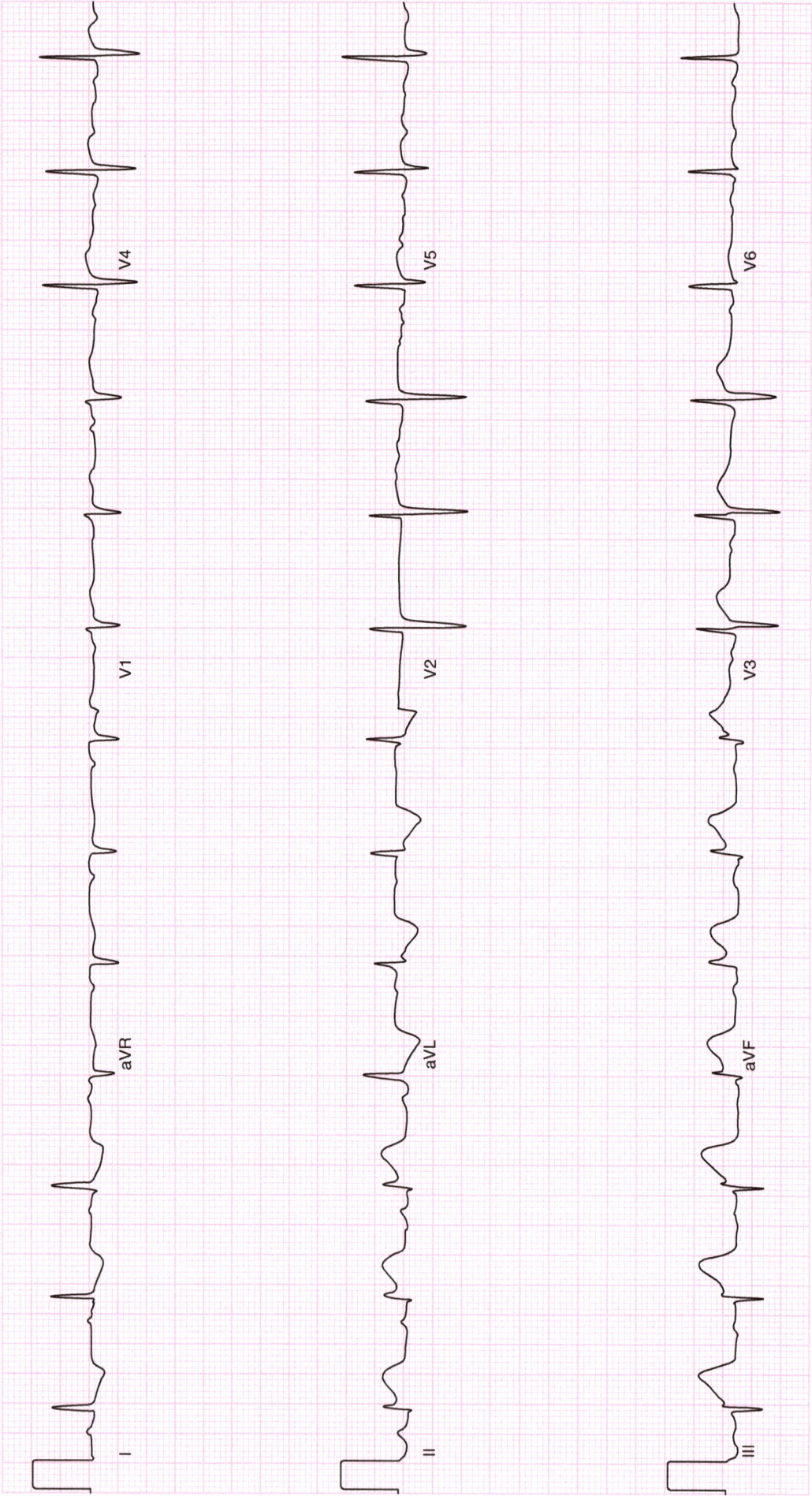

Test ECG 3.2

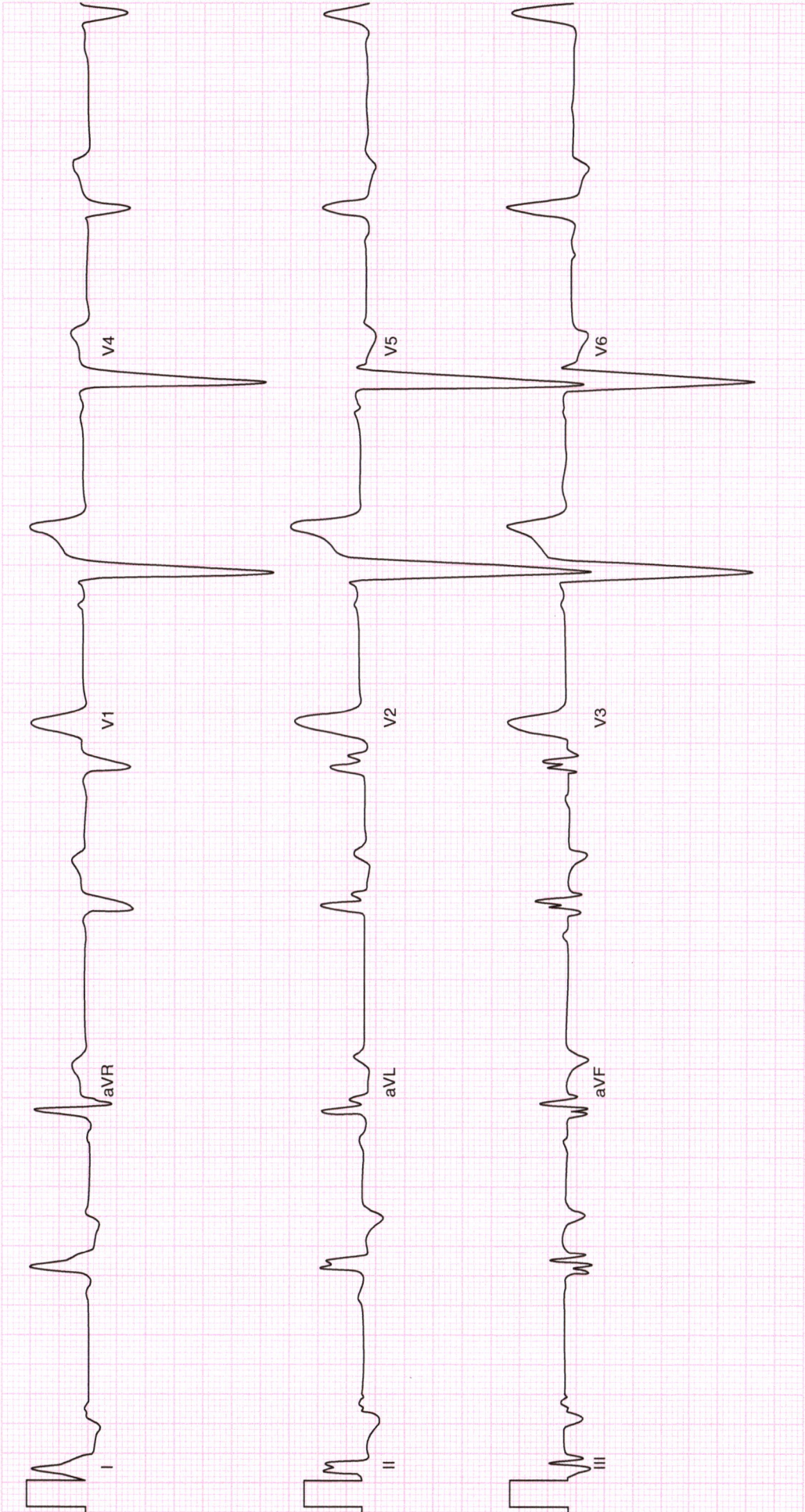

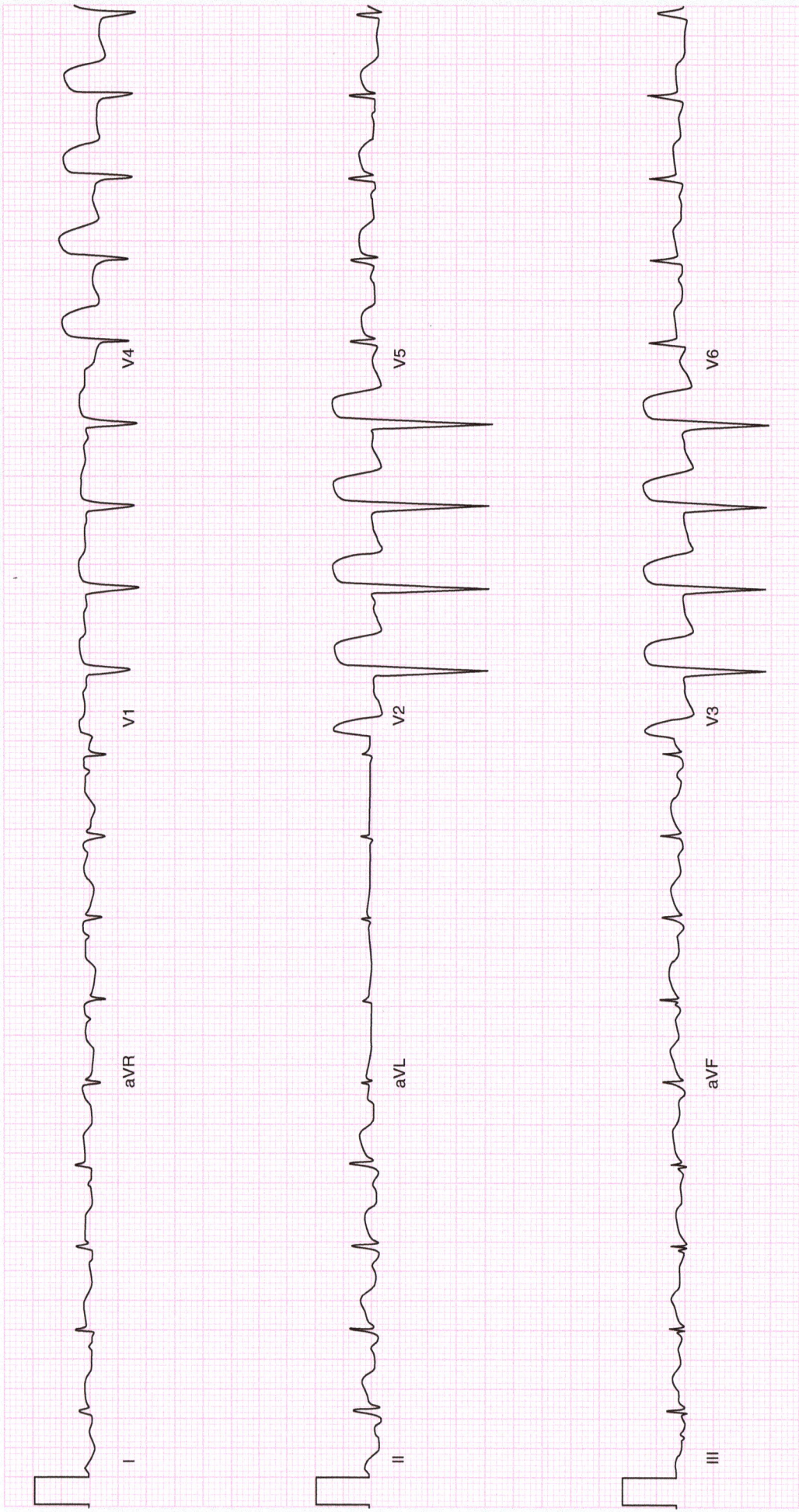

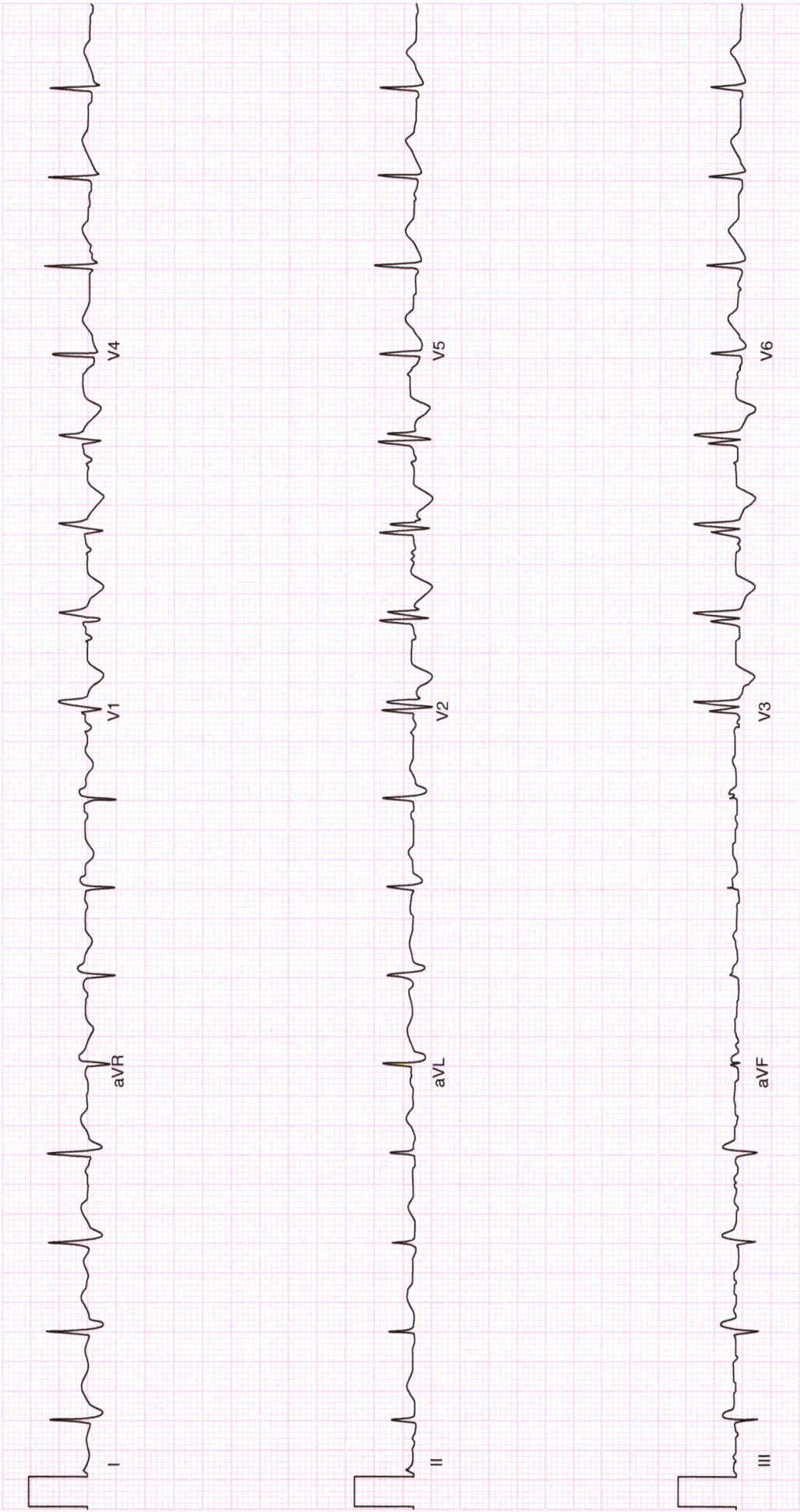

Test ECG 3.4

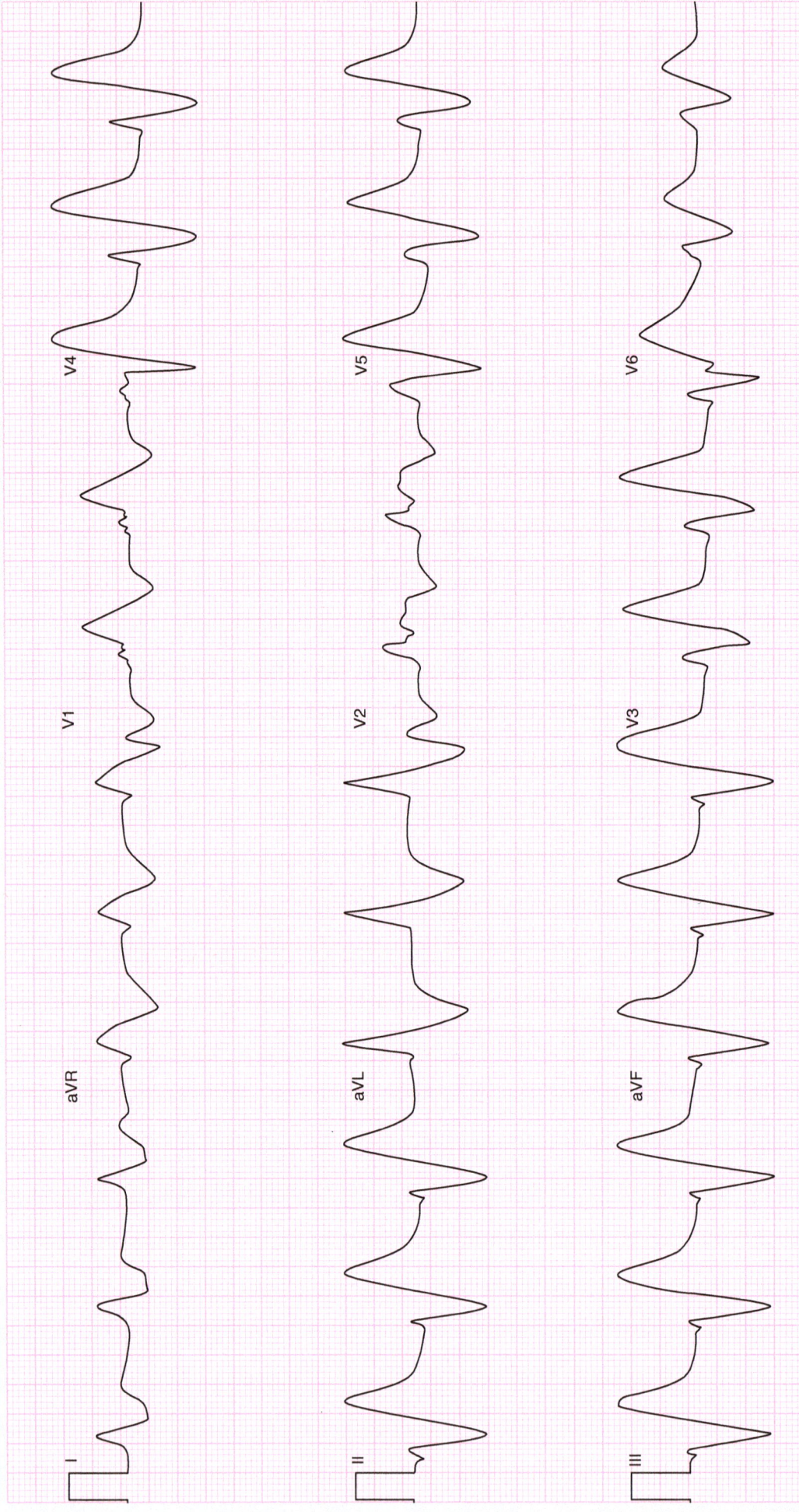

Test ECG 3.5

Test ECG 3.6

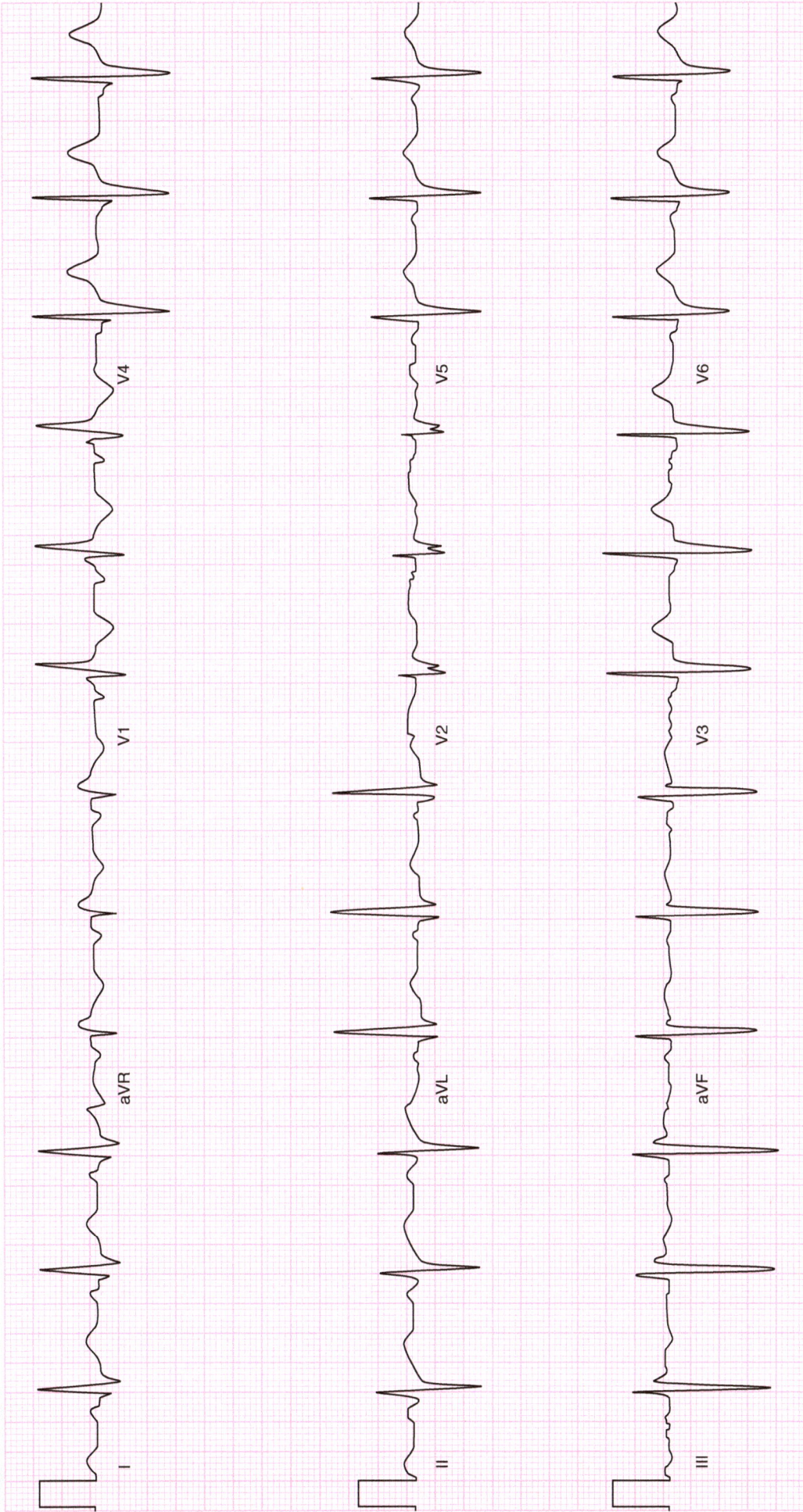

I   aVR   V1   V4

II   aVL   V2   V5

III   aVF   V3   V6

Test ECG 3.7

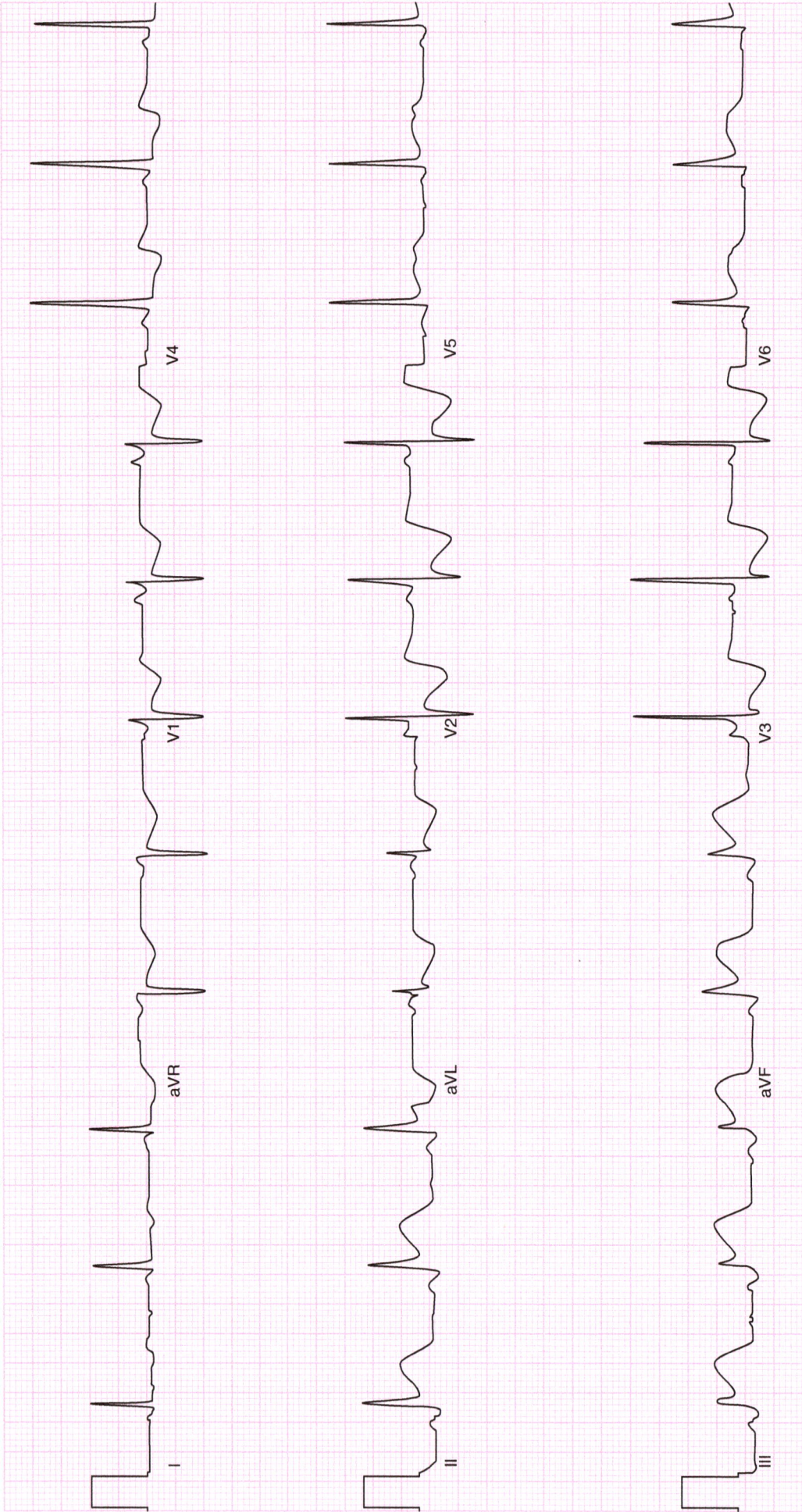

I
aVR
V1
V4

II
aVL
V2
V5

III
aVF
V3
V6

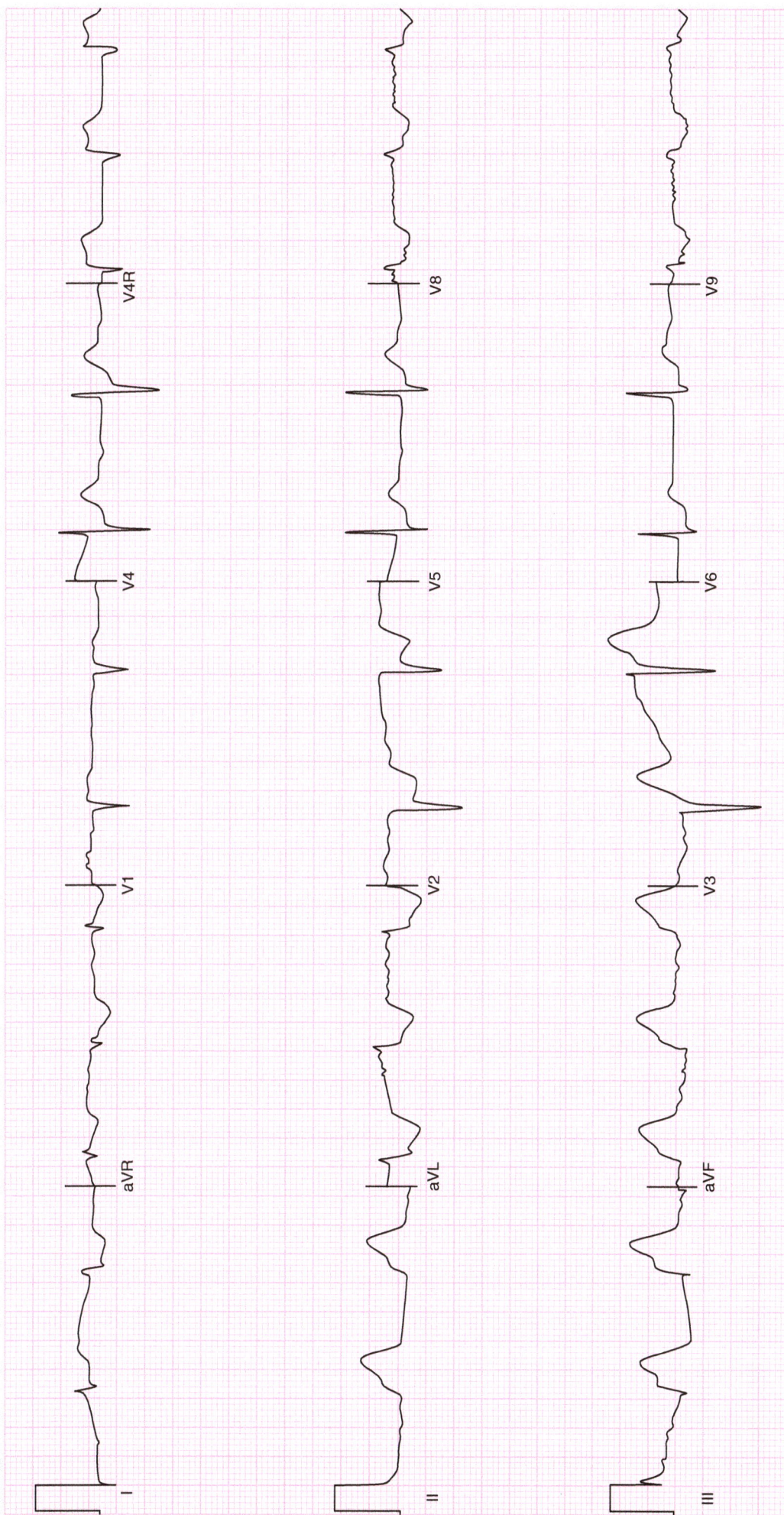

Test ECG 3.8

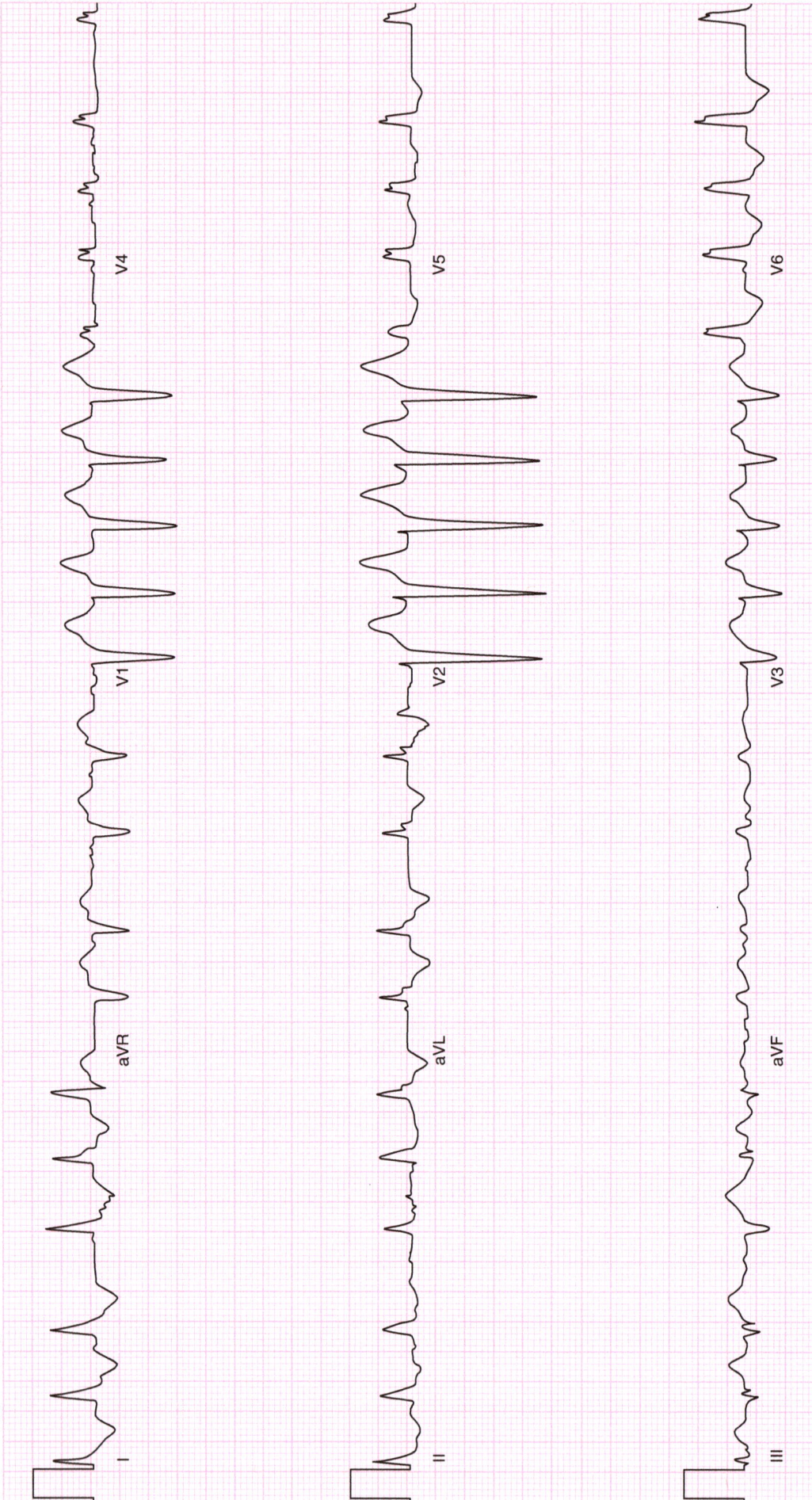

Test ECG 3.9

I

II

III

aVR

aVL

aVF

V1

V2

V3

V4

V5

V6

Test ECG 3.10

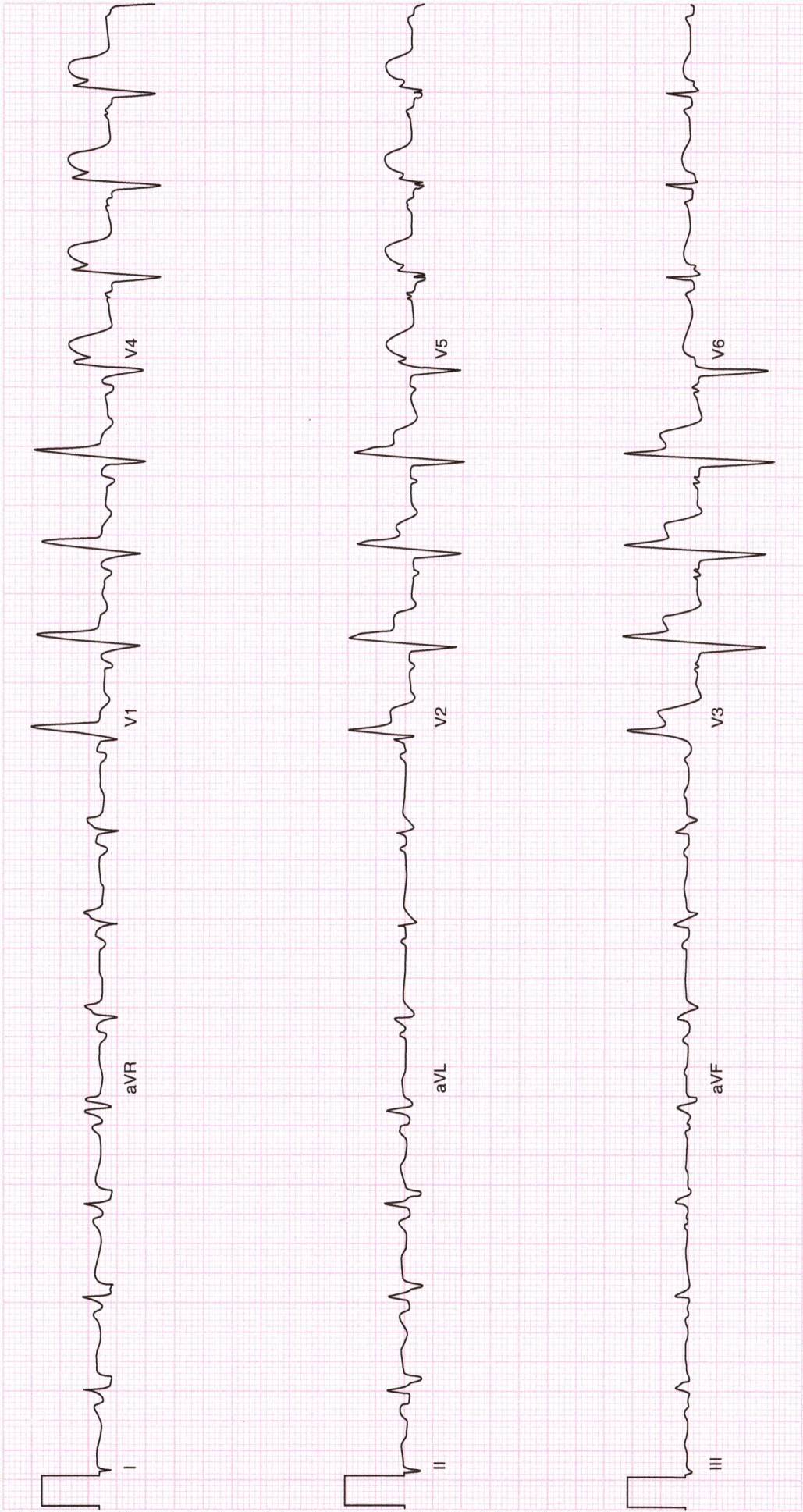

Section 3 Case Scenarios

Case Scenario 3.1	54-year-old male with chest pain

Aamir was sitting at home when he suddenly developed severe chest pain. He describes the pain as 'tight and crushing', scoring the severity as 7/10. The pain is radiating to his neck and jaw and has been getting steadily worse since it started around 30 minutes ago.

Past medical history: *High cholesterol, hypertension.*

Medication: *Ramipril, simvastatin.*

Allergies: *Penicillin.*

Social history: *Lives with partner and elderly parents. Smokes 10–15 cigarettes each day. Does not drink alcohol or use recreational drugs. Does not exercise and has a BMI of 37 (obese).*

Family history: *Older brother died of heart attack at 55 years old. Uncle died of heart attack at 60 years old.*

Review of systems: *Associated nausea.*

Examination: *Pale, cold and clammy skin. Appears short of breath. Xanthelasma around eyes. Nicotine-stained fingers. Radial pulses present.*

Clinical Observations

SpO$_2$	%	EtCO$_{2w}$	kPa	NIBP	mmHg	T°	Blood Glucose	GCS
			4.9		118			15
	95	RR	24	(91)	77	36.6°C	7.7 mmol/l	(E4 / S5 / M6)

Questions

a) **What are your differential diagnoses for Aamir?**
b) **Use the 9-step ECG interpretation tool to assess Aamir's ECG.**
c) **What rhythm is the ECG?**
d) **What is your working diagnosis?**

ECG Steps	Remember to look at every ECG lead view, not just lead II
1	What is the rate and rhythm?
2	Are there any P waves and what is their relationship with the QRS complex?
3	What is the duration and morphology of the QRS complex?
4	Is the ST segment isoelectric, depressed or elevated?
5	Are the QT intervals and T waves normal?

Clinical Steps	
6	Is the heart generating a palpable pulse of appropriate rate and providing adequate perfusion?
7	Is the rhythm unstable and at risk of deterioration?
8	Does the presenting rhythm support or change your working diagnosis?
9	Are any clinical interventions required?

Case Scenario ECG 3.1

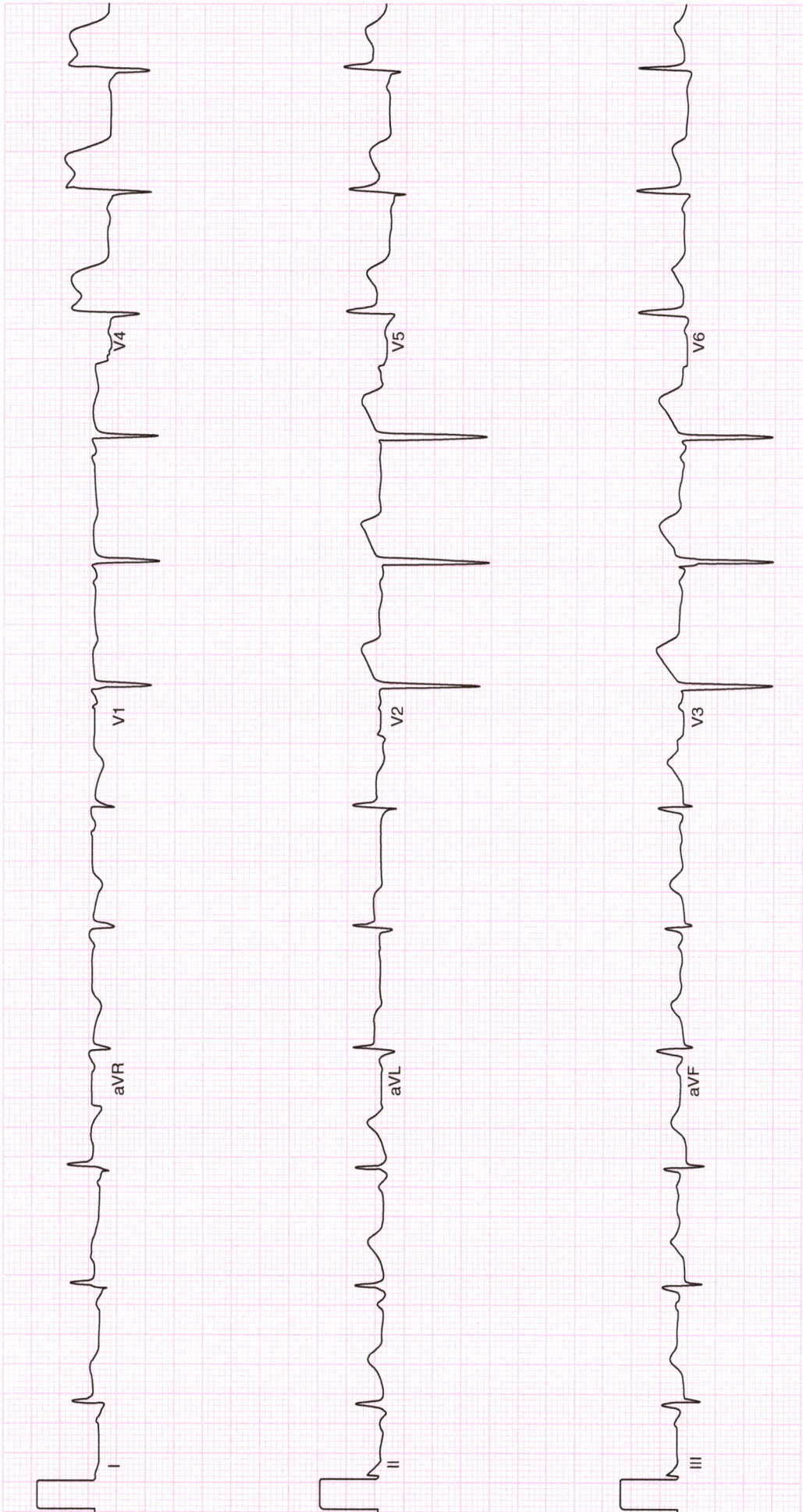

Case Scenario 3.2   71-year-old male with difficulty breathing

71-year-old Frank has been experiencing a gradual worsening of his chronic obstructive pulmonary disease over the last three months by way of increasing shortness of breath and fatigue. Today he has had a sudden exacerbation of shortness of breath, making him feel as if he cannot breathe well enough and prompting him to call for help.

Past medical history: *COPD, hypertension, high cholesterol.*

Medication: *Symbicort turbohaler 400/12, 1 puff twice a day, atorvastatin, amlodipine.*

Allergies: *None.*

Social history: *Lives alone, independent, smokes 10/day, does not drink alcohol or use illicit drugs.*

Family history: *Mother and father both died in old age, he is unsure of exact causes.*

Review of systems: *None identified.*

Examination: *Visibly short of breath. Rapid and regular radial pulse.*

Clinical Observations

SpO_2	%	$EtCO_2$	kPa	NIBP	mmHg
			4.1		118
	91	RR	28	(91)	77

T°	Blood Glucose	GCS
37.1°C	7.1 mmol/l	15 (E4 / S5 / M6)

Questions

a) What are your differential diagnoses for Frank?
b) Use the 9-step ECG interpretation tool to assess Frank's ECG.
c) What rhythm is the ECG?
d) What is your working diagnosis?

ECG Steps   Remember to look at every ECG lead view, not just lead II

1	What is the rate and rhythm?
2	Are there any P waves and what is their relationship with the QRS complex?
3	What is the duration and morphology of the QRS complex?
4	Is the ST segment isoelectric, depressed or elevated?
5	Are the QT intervals and T waves normal?

Clinical Steps

6	Is the heart generating a palpable pulse of appropriate rate and providing adequate perfusion?
7	Is the rhythm unstable and at risk of deterioration?
8	Does the presenting rhythm support or change your working diagnosis?
9	Are any clinical interventions required?

Case Scenario ECG 3.2

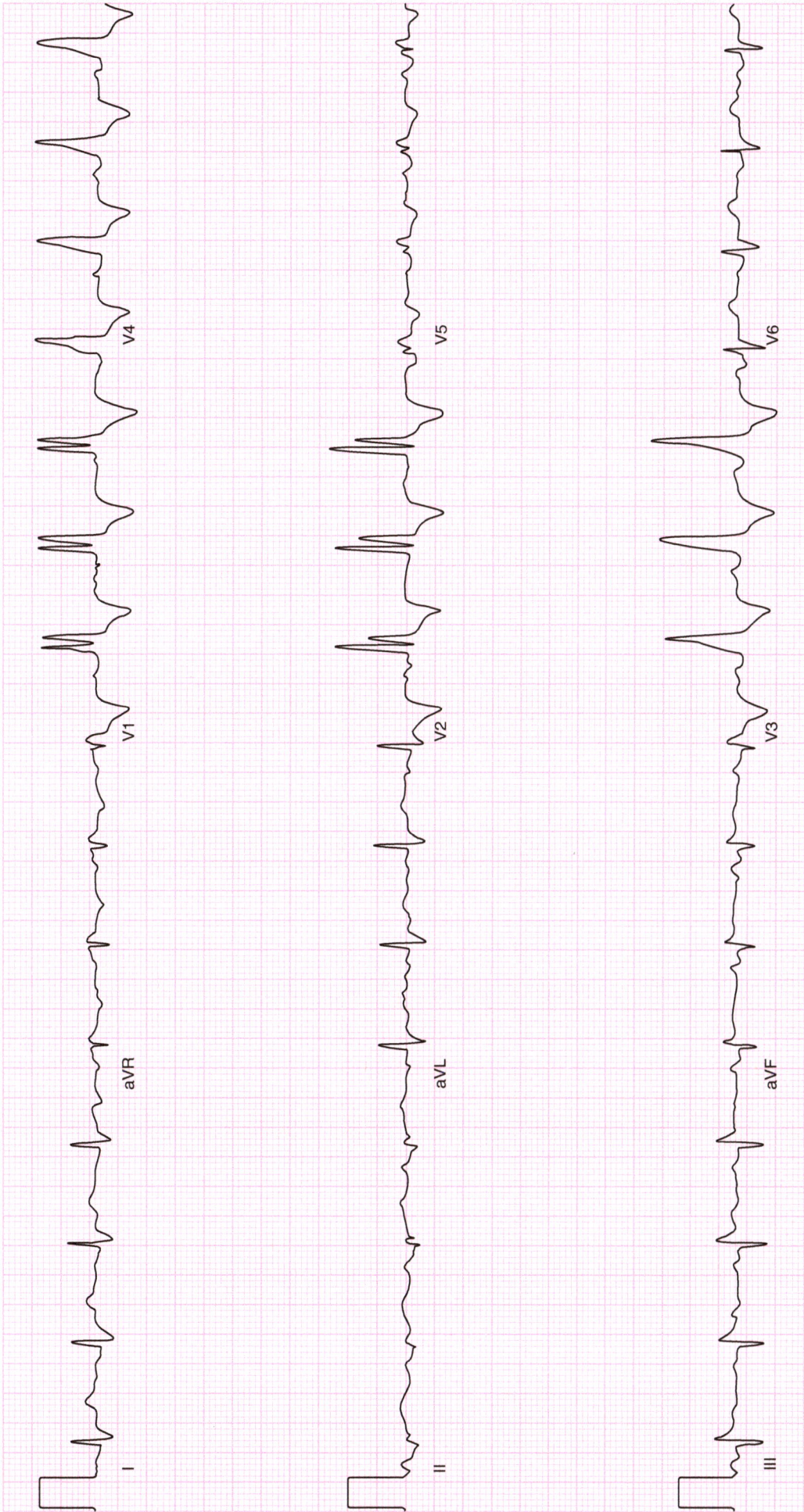

I   aVR   V1   V4

II   aVL   V2   V5

III   aVF   V3   V6

| Case Scenario 3.3 | 82-year-old female with breathing difficulty |

82-year-old Maureen was diagnosed with a lower urinary tract infection two days ago by her GP and prescribed a three-day course of trimethoprim (200 milligrams twice daily). Today she has been feeling worse, with increasing lethargy, feeling feverish and generally run down.

Past medical history: *Aortic valve replacement, left hip replacement, osteoarthritis.*

Medication: *Vitamin D, alendronate.*

Allergies: *None.*

Social history: *Lives alone, carers attend three times a day for food and personal care, does not drink alcohol, smoke or use illicit drugs.*

Family history: *Mother and father both died in old age, no siblings.*

Review of systems: *No chest pain or discomfort, no palpitations, no abdominal pain, no back pain, no difficulty breathing.*

Examination: *Rapid and regular radial pulse. Flushed and clammy.*

Clinical Observations

SpO$_2$	%	EtCO$_2$	kPa	NIBP	mmHg
			5.9		105
	95	RR	26	(73)	57

T°	Blood Glucose	GCS
37.9°C	7.6 mmol/l	15 (E4 / S5 / M6)

Questions

a) What are your differential diagnoses for Maureen?
b) Use the 9-step ECG interpretation tool to assess Maureen's ECG.
c) What rhythm is the ECG?
d) What is your working diagnosis?

ECG Steps

Remember to look at every ECG lead view, not just lead II

1	What is the rate and rhythm?
2	Are there any P waves and what is their relationship with the QRS complex?
3	What is the duration and morphology of the QRS complex?
4	Is the ST segment isoelectric, depressed or elevated?
5	Are the QT intervals and T waves normal?

Clinical Steps

6	Is the heart generating a palpable pulse of appropriate rate and providing adequate perfusion?
7	Is the rhythm unstable and at risk of deterioration?
8	Does the presenting rhythm support or change your working diagnosis?
9	Are any clinical interventions required?

Case Scenario ECG 3.3

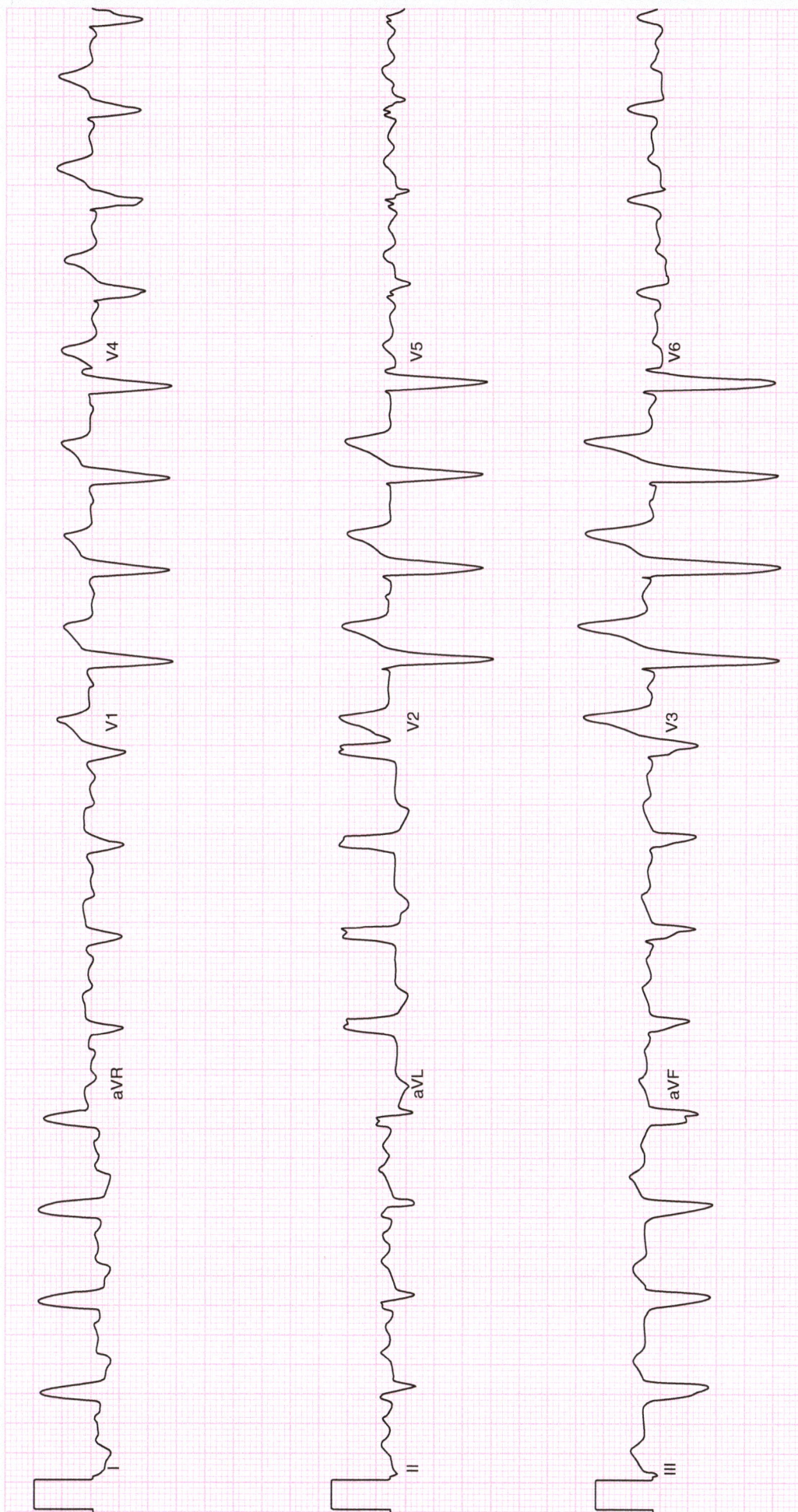

I

aVR

V1

V4

II

aVL

V2

V5

III

aVF

V3

V6

Case Scenario 3.4   63-year-old male, unwell

Alan has been unwell for three days with flu-like symptoms. He has been lethargic, feverish, nauseous and had little appetite. He has been trying to keep his fluid intake up, but he thinks it has likely been less each day than normal. He has still been taking his medications as normal; he has also been taking extra multivitamins to help his body 'fight the illness', as well as ibuprofen. Today he has felt worse, with increased fatigue, some palpitations and shortness of breath.

Past medical history: *Hypertension.*

Medication: *Losartan.*

Allergies: *None.*

Social history: *Lives with partner who is well, works as an electrician, drinks a couple of pints once or twice a week, does not smoke or use illicit drugs.*

Family history: *Mother and father both in their late 80s, two siblings, all well.*

Review of systems: *No chest pain or discomfort, no difficulty breathing, no abdominal pain, no back pain, no vomiting, no changes to bowel habits, reduced urine output and more dark than normal.*

Examination: *Strong and regular radial pulse. Flushed and clammy skin. Chest clear on auscultation.*

Clinical Observations

SpO$_2$	%	EtCO$_2$	kPa	NIBP	mmHg
			5.6		127
	95	RR	20	(104)	93

T°	Blood Glucose	GCS
38.1°C	4.4 mmol/l	15 (E4 / S5 / M6)

Questions

a) What are your differential diagnoses for Alan?
b) Use the 9-step ECG interpretation tool to assess Alan's ECG.
c) What rhythm is the ECG?
d) What is your working diagnosis?

ECG Steps	Remember to look at every ECG lead view, not just lead II
1	What is the rate and rhythm?
2	Are there any P waves and what is their relationship with the QRS complex?
3	What is the duration and morphology of the QRS complex?
4	Is the ST segment isoelectric, depressed or elevated?
5	Are the QT intervals and T waves normal?

Clinical Steps	
6	Is the heart generating a palpable pulse of appropriate rate and providing adequate perfusion?
7	Is the rhythm unstable and at risk of deterioration?
8	Does the presenting rhythm support or change your working diagnosis?
9	Are any clinical interventions required?

Case Scenario ECG 3.4

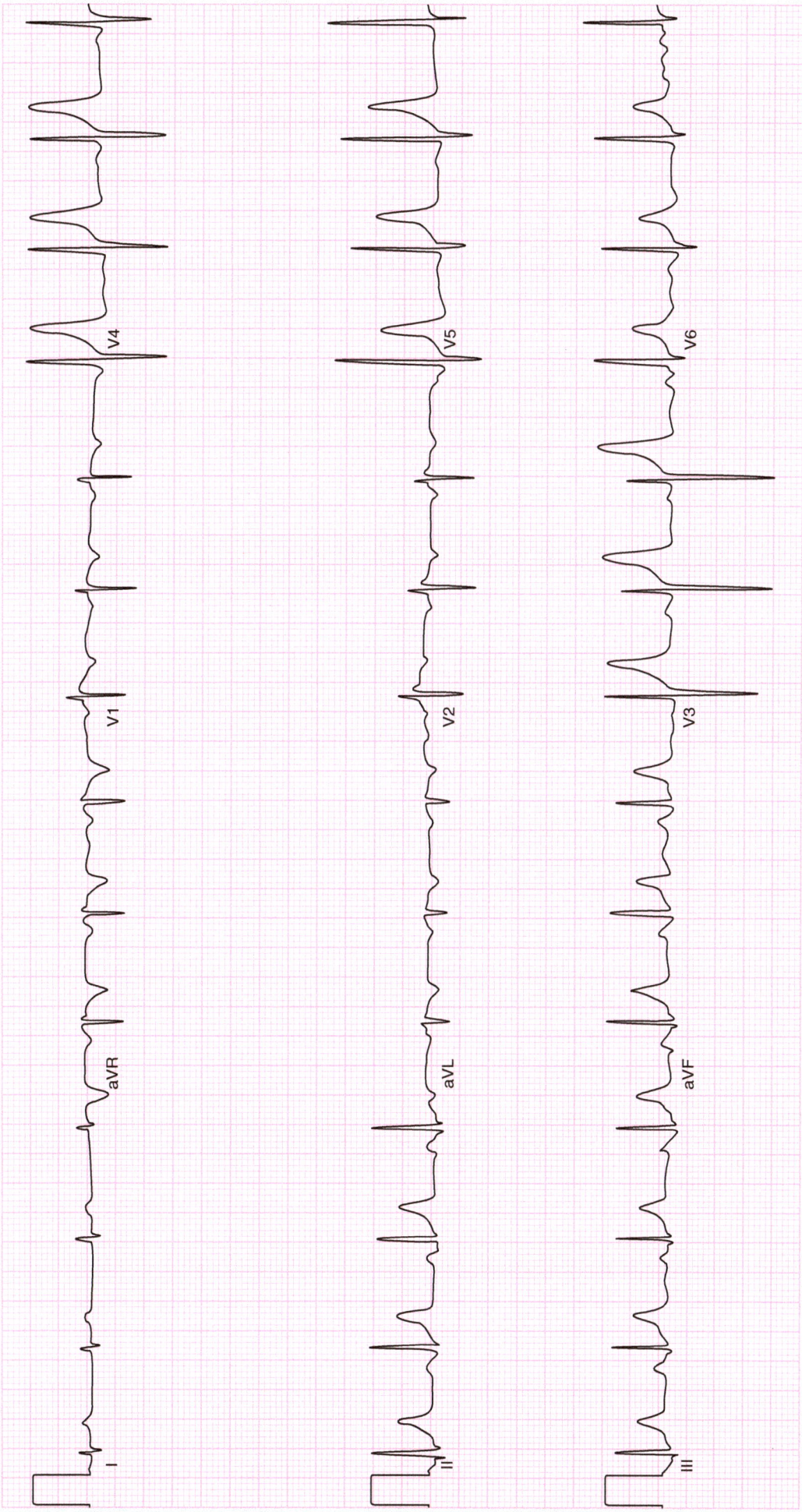

I

aVR

V1

V4

II

aVL

V2

V5

III

aVF

V3

V6

Case Scenario 3.5   78-year-old female with abdominal pain

78-year-old Judith has been suffering intermittent upper abdominal discomfort for the last two weeks. Today the discomfort has persisted and become more severe. She currently scores it as 5/10, localising it to her upper epigastric region. She struggles to describe the pain, saying it makes her feel uneasy.

Past medical history: *Type 2 diabetes, chronic kidney disease stage 3a, Raynaud's disease.*

Medication: *Metformin.*

Allergies: *None.*

Social history: *Lives with her daughter and son-in-law. Drinks a small glass of sherry before bed on most nights. Stopped smoking 10 years ago when diagnosed with diabetes. Tries to walk around the garden at least once a day for fresh air, has been struggling in recent weeks to do this, with the abdominal discomfort coming on whilst walking on some occasions.*

Family history: *Older brother died of a heart condition at 60. Younger sister alive and believed to be well.*

Review of systems: *No chest pain or discomfort, no palpitations, no back pain, no difficulty breathing. No nausea, no vomiting, no diarrhoea, no constipation, no urinary symptoms. No recent fevers.*

Examination: *Slow and weak radial pulse. Pale and clammy skin.*

Clinical Observations

SpO$_2$	%	EtCO$_2$	kPa	NIBP	mmHg
			4.9		98
	97	RR	28	(73)	64

T°	Blood Glucose	GCS
36.4°C	8.2 mmol/l	15 (E4 / S5 / M6)

Questions

- a) What are your differential diagnoses for Judith?
- b) Use the 9-step ECG interpretation tool to assess Judith's ECG.
- c) What rhythm is the ECG?
- d) What is your working diagnosis?

ECG Steps   Remember to look at every ECG lead view, not just lead II

1	What is the rate and rhythm?
2	Are there any P waves and what is their relationship with the QRS complex?
3	What is the duration and morphology of the QRS complex?
4	Is the ST segment isoelectric, depressed or elevated?
5	Are the QT intervals and T waves normal?

Clinical Steps

6	Is the heart generating a palpable pulse of appropriate rate and providing adequate perfusion?
7	Is the rhythm unstable and at risk of deterioration?
8	Does the presenting rhythm support or change your working diagnosis?
9	Are any clinical interventions required?

Case Scenario ECG 3.5

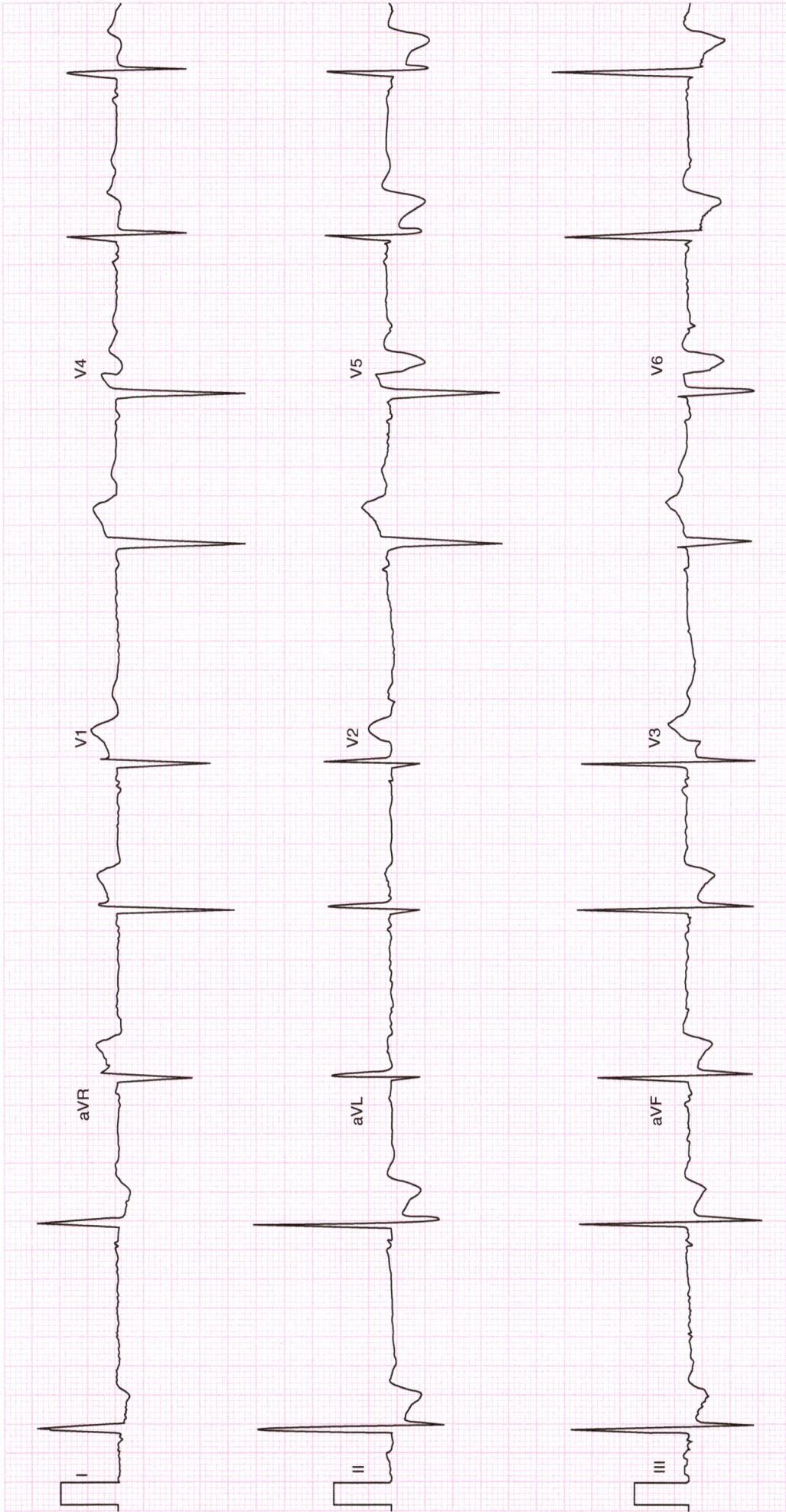

Section 3 Practice ECG Answers

Test ECG 3.1 Inferior STEMI.

Test ECG 3.2 Bradycardia and LBBB (Sgarbossa negative).

Test ECG 3.3 Anterior lateral STEMI with borderline tachycardia.

Test ECG 3.4 RBBB.

Test ECG 3.5 Hyperkalaemia.

Test ECG 3.6 Bifascicular block (RBBB + LAFB).

Test ECG 3.7 Inferior STEMI (ST depression in V1 and V2 is a sign of potential posterior infarct that would trigger obtaining a posterior ECG).

Test ECG 3.8 Right ventricular STEMI.

Test ECG 3.9 LBBB *and* AF.

Test ECG 3.10 Anterior STEMI *and* RBBB.

Section 3 Case Scenario Answers

Case Scenario 3.1 Answers	
a) What are your differential diagnoses for Aamir? *Differentials should include: Acute coronary syndrome, pulmonary embolism* **b) Use the 9-step ECG interpretation tool to assess Aamir's ECG.** **c) What rhythm is the ECG?** *Sinus rhythm with anterior and lateral STEMI.* **d) What is your working diagnosis?** *STEMI.* **Discussion**: *Aamir is presenting with classic signs and symptoms of ACS. Couple this with the ST segment elevation on his ECG which meets STEMI criteria, and the working diagnosis of STEMI is clear. Aamir has multiple risk factors which increase his risk of cardiac events. His smoking, obesity and lack of exercise in combination with a family history of cardiac events put him at high risk.*	

ECG Steps		
1	**What is the rate and rhythm?**	*The rate is around 70 beats/minute and the rhythm is regular.*
2	**Are there any P waves and what is their relationship with the QRS complex?**	*There is a P wave before every QRS complex and a QRS complex after every P wave.*
3	**What is the duration and morphology of the QRS complex?**	*The QRS complex is of normal shape and the duration is under 0.12 seconds (3 small squares).*
4	**Is the ST segment isoelectric, depressed or elevated?**	*The ST segment is displaying elevation in leads I, aVL and V2–6. There is ST segment depression in leads aVF and aVR.*
5	**Are the QT intervals and T waves normal?**	*The T wave is of normal shape and the QT interval is normal. The T waves in leads I and aVL are flattening and may become inverted.*
Clinical Steps		
6	**Is the heart generating a palpable pulse of appropriate rate and providing adequate perfusion?**	*The heart is generating a palpable pulse at an appropriate rate. The presence of radial pulses suggests adequate perfusion is currently present. This patient has hypertension, so a BP of 118/77 could be relatively hypotensive and should be monitored closely.*
7	**Is the rhythm unstable and at risk of deterioration?**	*Yes. This ECG shows active STEMI and the patient is at risk of further cardiac muscle damage or cardiac arrest.*
8	**Does the presenting rhythm support or change your working diagnosis?**	*Supports MI.*
9	**Are any clinical interventions required?**	*IV access and ACS drugs are indicated for this patient. Rapid transport with pre-alert call to activate local STEMI pathway and cath lab.*

Case Scenario 3.2   Answers

a) **What are your differential diagnoses for Frank?** *Differentials should include: Exacerbation of COPD, heart failure (congestive or right-sided), pneumonia, pulmonary embolism, acute coronary syndrome, lung cancer.*

b) **Use the 9-step ECG interpretation tool to assess Frank's ECG.**

c) **What rhythm is the ECG?** *RBBB.*

d) **What is your working diagnosis?** *Worsening shortness of breath likely due to exacerbation of COPD, though cannot exclude heart failure, pneumonia or other potential causes.*

Discussion: *Frank's ECG shows right bundle branch block. We can see slurring S waves in the lateral leads I and V6. The 'typical' RSR complex in V1 is also present. This ECG finding fits with Frank's presentation; we know that RBBB can be caused by COPD due to the associated right ventricular strain. We must also consider that the cause of this RBBB may be due to another underlying co-morbidity that has not yet been identified. In addition, we do not know if Frank has had RBBB previously diagnosed or if this is a new presentation.*

ECG Steps

1	**What is the rate and rhythm?**	*The rate is around 90 beats/minute and the rhythm is regular.*
2	**Are there any P waves and what is their relationship with the QRS complex?**	*There is a P wave before every QRS complex and a QRS complex after every P wave.*
3	**What is the duration and morphology of the QRS complex?**	*The QRS complex is of RBBB morphology and the duration is (just) over 0.12 seconds (3 small squares).*
4	**Is the ST segment isoelectric, depressed or elevated?**	*The ST segment is displaying some depression in leads V1–V4.*
5	**Are the QT intervals and T waves normal?**	*The T wave is inverted in the precordial leads. The QT interval is normal.*

Clinical Steps

6	**Is the heart generating a palpable pulse of appropriate rate and providing adequate perfusion?**	*The heart is generating a palpable pulse at an appropriate rate. The presence of radial pulses suggests adequate perfusion is currently present. This patient has diagnosed hypertension, so a BP of 118/77 could be relatively hypotensive and should be monitored closely.*
7	**Is the rhythm unstable and at risk of deterioration?**	*No.*
8	**Does the presenting rhythm support or change your working diagnosis?**	*Does not impact diagnosis though could support respiratory cause.*
9	**Are any clinical interventions required?**	*The ECG does not specifically require any interventions. Frank does, however, need treatment and transport for his respiratory presentation.*

Case Scenario 3.3   Answers

a) **What are your differential diagnoses for Maureen?** *Differentials should include: Urinary sepsis, pyelonephritis.*

b) **Use the 9-step ECG interpretation tool to assess Maureen's ECG.**

c) **What rhythm is the ECG?** *LBBB (Sgarbossa negative).*

d) **What is your working diagnosis?** *Urinary sepsis.*

Discussion: *Maureen is presenting with symptoms of sepsis; this fits with her recent history of urinary tract infection. Her ECG shows LBBB which has not been previously diagnosed. She does not have any cardiac symptoms and her history of cardiac surgery and age could explain the presence of the LBBB. But we must also consider that, being female and of advanced age, Maureen is at increased risk of experiencing an atypical or silent MI. In this situation the balance of probability would point to the LBBB being an incidental finding. The LBBB is Sgarbossa negative which further reassures us that the chances of Maureen having an acute cardiac event at this time are low. In this case, Maureen will be transported to hospital for further care due to sepsis, so the finding of LBBB can be passed on to the hospital.*

ECG Steps		
1	What is the rate and rhythm?	*The rate is around 95 beats/minute and the rhythm is regular.*
2	Are there any P waves and what is their relationship with the QRS complex?	*There is a P wave before every QRS complex and a QRS complex after every P wave.*
3	What is the duration and morphology of the QRS complex?	*The QRS complex is of LBBB morphology and the duration is greater than 0.12 seconds (3 small squares).*
4	Is the ST segment isoelectric, depressed or elevated?	*The ST segment is displaying elevation associated with LBBB. It does not meet Sgarbossa criteria.*
5	Are the QT intervals and T waves normal?	*The T wave is of normal shape for LBBB and the QT interval is normal.*
Clinical Steps		
6	Is the heart generating a palpable pulse of appropriate rate and providing adequate perfusion?	*The heart is generating a palpable pulse at an appropriate rate. The presence of radial pulses suggests adequate perfusion is currently present.*
7	Is the rhythm unstable and at risk of deterioration?	*No. The rhythm is stable.*
8	Does the presenting rhythm support or change your working diagnosis?	*Does not impact the working diagnosis for this patient.*
9	Are any clinical interventions required?	*No interventions are required based on this ECG. The patient requires treatment and transport for sepsis.*

Case Scenario 3.4   Answers

a) What are your differential diagnoses for Alan? *Differentials should include: flu, chest infection, urinary tract infection, urinary sepsis, pyelonephritis, hyperkalaemia.*

b) Use the 9-step ECG interpretation tool to assess Alan's ECG.

c) What rhythm is the ECG? *Sinus rhythm with hyperkalaemia.*

d) What is your working diagnosis? *Hyperkalaemia and flu/infection.*

Discussion: *Alan has given us several clues in his history that suggest he is at risk of hyperkalaemia. He is medicated with Losartan, an angiotensin receptor blocker, which belongs to a group of medications that can cause hyperkalaemia. The same applies to NSAIDs; he has been taking ibuprofen since becoming unwell. He has also been taking additional vitamin supplements which could potentially contain potassium. Finally, his illness has caused a potential reduced fluid intake, reflected in reduced urine output. All of these findings should raise concerns that there is a risk of hyperkalaemia. His ECG supports this concern and assists us in making a working diagnosis. The tall, peaked T waves are a sign of hyperkalaemia.*

ECG Steps		
1	**What is the rate and rhythm?**	*The rate is around 75 beats/minute and the rhythm is regular.*
2	**Are there any P waves and what is their relationship with the QRS complex?**	*There is a P wave before every QRS complex and a QRS complex after every P wave.*
3	**What is the duration and morphology of the QRS complex?**	*The QRS complex is of normal morphology and the duration is less than 0.12 seconds (3 small squares).*
4	**Is the ST segment isoelectric, depressed or elevated?**	*The ST segment is mostly isoelectric, with some J point elevation in V3–V5.*
5	**Are the QT intervals and T waves normal?**	*The T waves are peaked and showing signs of hyperkalaemia. The QT interval is normal.*
Clinical Steps		
6	**Is the heart generating a palpable pulse of appropriate rate and providing adequate perfusion?**	*The heart is generating a palpable pulse at an appropriate rate. The presence of radial pulses suggests adequate perfusion is currently present.*
7	**Is the rhythm unstable and at risk of deterioration?**	*No. The rhythm is stable.*
8	**Does the presenting rhythm support or change your working diagnosis?**	*Suggests hyperkalaemia.*
9	**Are any clinical interventions required?**	*No interventions are required based on this ECG alone. However, the patient requires transport to further care due to signs of hyperkalaemia.*

Case Scenario 3.5	Answers

a) **What are your differential diagnoses for Judith?** *Differentials should include: acute coronary syndrome, abdominal pathology, pneumonia.*
b) **Use the 9-step ECG interpretation tool to assess Judith's ECG.**
c) **What rhythm is the ECG?** *Sinus bradycardia with STEMI equivalent.*
d) **What is your working diagnosis?** *ACS – STEMI equivalent.*
Discussion: *Judith is presenting with diffuse symptoms of intermittent upper abdominal discomfort. The worsening of symptoms today raises our concern, along with Judith's history. She has risk factors for ACS and for silent or atypical ACS presentation (page 94). Initially, her ECG may give us the impression of ACS due to the clear ST depression in the inferior and lateral leads, but this ST depression, in combination with the ST segment elevation in leads aVR and V1, is a worrying indication that she may have obstruction of the left main coronary artery or the left anterior descending artery. Her intermittent symptoms over recent weeks could suggest worsening stenosis of the culprit coronary artery, with the worsening symptoms today suggesting that occlusion has occurred.*

ECG Steps		
1	What is the rate and rhythm?	*The rate is around 50 beats/minute and the rhythm is irregular.*
2	Are there any P waves and what is their relationship with the QRS complex?	*There is a P wave before every QRS complex and a QRS complex after every P wave.*
3	What is the duration and morphology of the QRS complex?	*The QRS complex is of high amplitude in all leads and the duration is less than 0.12 seconds (3 small squares).*
4	Is the ST segment isoelectric, depressed or elevated?	*The ST segment is displaying elevation in leads aVR, V1 and V2. There is widespread downward-sloping ST segment depression in lateral and inferior leads.*
5	Are the QT intervals and T waves normal?	*The T wave is inverted alongside leads with ST depression. Multiple leads have biphasic T waves.*
Clinical Steps		
6	Is the heart generating a palpable pulse of appropriate rate and providing adequate perfusion?	*The heart is generating a palpable pulse, though the pulse is weak and the rate is bradycardic.*
7	Is the rhythm unstable and at risk of deterioration?	*Yes, signs of STEMI equivalent suggest there is active coronary artery occlusion.*
8	Does the presenting rhythm support or change your working diagnosis?	*Supports, ACS – STEMI equivalent.*
9	Are any clinical interventions required?	*IV access, ACS drugs and rapid transport with pre-alert to activate cath lab are indicated for this patient.*

References

1. A. West, 'Pain in chest', in *French's Index of Differential Diagnosis*. Boca Raton: CRC Press, 2016.

2. M. L. Ashwath and S. Gandhi, 'ST-elevation myocardial infarction', in *BMJ Best Practice* [Online]. London: BMJ Publishing Group, 2018.

3. N. I. Nikolaou et al., 'European Resuscitation Council guidelines for resuscitation 2015 section 8. Initial management of acute coronary syndromes', *Resuscitation*, vol. 95, 2015, pp. 264–277.

4. British Heart Foundation, *Cardiovascular Disease Statistics*, 2014. Available: https://www.bhf.org.uk/informationsupport/publications/statistics/cardiovascular-disease-statistics-2014.

5. J. Kendall, 'Acute coronary syndromes', in *Royal College of Emergency Medicine Learning* [Online]. London: RCEM, 2018.

6. S. Goodacre et al., 'The healthcare burden of acute chest pain', *Heart*, vol. 91, 2005, pp. 229–230.

7. Joint Royal College Ambulance Liaison Committee and Association of Ambulance Chief Executives, *JRCALC Clinical Guidelines 2019*. Bridgwater: Class Professional Publishing, 2019.

8. T. Quinn et al., 'Effects of prehospital 12-lead ECG on processes of care and mortality in acute coronary syndrome: a linked cohort study from the Myocardial Ischaemia National Audit Project', *Heart*, vol. 100, no. 12, 2014, pp. 944–950.

9. J. Kendall and I. Hancock, 'Chest pain syndromes', in *Royal College of Emergency Medicine Learning* [Online]. London: RCEM, 2019.

10. G. R. Nimmo and T. Walsh, 'Critical illness', in *Davidson's Principles and Practices of Medicine*. Edinburgh: Churchill Livingstone, 2014.

11. T. Standl, 'The nomenclature, definition and distinction of types of shock', *Continuing Medical Education*, vol. 115, no. 45, 2014, pp. 757–768.

12. F. G. Bonanno, 'Clinical pathology of the shock syndromes', *Journal of Emergency Trauma and Shock*, vol. 4, no. 2, 2011, pp. 233–243.

13. C. Vahdatpour, D. Collins and S. Goldberg, 'Cardiogenic shock', *Journal of the American Heart Association*, vol. 8, no. 8, 2019.

14. National Institute for Health and Care Excellence, 'Chest pain of recent onset', *NICE Clinical Guideline 95*. London: NICE, 2016.

15. A. G. Japp and C. Robertson, eds., *Macleod's Clinical Diagnosis*. Edinburgh: Churchill Livingstone, 2013.

16. C. S. Deen, 'Non-ST-elevation myocardial infarction', in *BMJ Best Practice* [Online]. London: BMJ Publishing Group, 2018.

17. D. E. Mohrman and L. J. Heller, *Cardiovascular Physiology*, 9th edn. New York: McGraw-Hill, 2018.

18. A. R. Houghton and D. Gray, 'Electrocardiography', in J. Firth, C. Conlon and T. Cox, eds., *Oxford Textbook of Medicine*, 6th edn. Oxford: Oxford University Press, 2020.

19. M. Roffi et al., '2015 ESC guidelines for the management of acute coronary syndromes in patients presenting without persistent ST-segment elevation', *European Heart Journal*, vol. 37, no. 3, 2015, pp. 267–315.

20. S. W. Yusuf, 'Unstable angina', in *BMJ Best Practice* [Online]. London: BMJ Publishing Group, 2019.

21. K. Thygesen et al., 'Universal definition of myocardial infarction: Kristian Thygesen, Joseph S. Alpert and Harvey D. White on behalf of the Joint ESC/ACCF/AHA/WHF Task Force for the Redefinition of Myocardial Infarction', *European Heart Journal*, vol. 28, no. 20, 2007, pp. 2525–2538.

22. M. Ahmed, 'Acute coronary syndrome – explained by a cardiologist' [Online], 2018. Available: https://myheart.net/articles/acute-coronary-syndrome-explained-by-a-cardiologist/.

23. K. Thygesen et al., 'Fourth universal definition of myocardial infarction (2018)', *European Heart Journal*, vol. 40, no. 3, 2018, pp. 237–269.

24. R. J. de Winter et al., 'A new ECG sign of proximal LAD occlusion', *New England Journal of Medicine*, vol. 359, no. 19, 2008, pp. 2071–2073.

25. T. Garcia, *12-Lead ECG: The Art of Interpretation*, 2nd edn. Burlington: Jones and Bartlett Learning, 2013.

26. C. de Zwaan, F. W. Bar and H. J. Wellens, 'Characteristic electrocardiographic pattern indicating a critical stenosis high in left anterior descending coronary artery in patients admitted because of impending myocardial infarction', *American Heart Journal*, vol. 103, 1982, pp. 730–736.

27. T. Pollehn et al., 'The electrocardiographic differential diagnosis of ST-segment depression', *Emergency Medical Journal*, vol. 19, 2002, pp. 129–135.

28. T. Phalen and B. Aehlert, *The 12-Lead ECG in Acute Coronary Syndromes*, 4th edn. Maryland Heights: Elsevier Mosby JEMS, 2018.

29. D. E. Newby, N. R. Grubb and A. Bradbury, 'Cardiovascular disease', in *Davidson's Principles and Practices of Medicine*, 22nd edn. Edinburgh: Churchill Livingstone, 2014.

30. A. L. Goldberger, 'Electrocardiography', in *Harrison's Principles of Internal Medicine*, 20th edn. New York: McGraw-Hill, 2018.

31. B. Ibanez et al., '2017 ESC guidelines for the management of acute myocardial infarction in patients presenting with ST-segment elevation', *European Heart Journal*, vol. 39, no. 2, 2017, pp. 119–177.

32. J. Kendall, 'Management of STEMI and its complications', in *Royal College of Emergency Medicine Learning* [Online]. London: RCEM, 2019.

33. A. J. Camm and N. Bunce, 'Cardiovascular disease', in P. Kumar and M. Clark, eds., *Clinical Medicine*, 7th edn. Edinburgh: Saunders Elsevier, 2009, pp. 717–720.

34. A. Mentias et al., 'Outcomes of ischaemic mitral regurgitation in anterior versus inferior ST-elevation myocardial infarction', *Open Heart*, vol. 3, 2016, pp. 1–8.

35. K. Wu, 'Pericarditis', in *BMJ Best Practice* [Online]. London: BMJ Publishing Group, 2019.

36. L. Dare, 'Pericarditis', in *Royal College of Emergency Medicine Learning* [Online]. London: RCEM, 2018.

37. J. Edhouse, W. J. Brady and F. Morris, 'ABC of clinical electrocardiography acute myocardial infarction – part II', *BMJ*, vol. 524, 2002, pp. 963–966.

38. D. Kireyev et al., 'Clinical utility of aVR – the neglected electrocardiographic lead', *Annals of Noninvasive Electrocardiology*, vol. 15, no. 2, 2010, pp. 175–180.

39. J. T. Tikkanen et al., 'Long-term outcome associated with early repolarization on electrocardiography', *New England Journal of Medicine*, vol. 361, no. 26, 2009, pp. 2529–2537.

40. R. G. Hiss, L. E. Lamb and M. F. Allen, 'Electrocardiographical findings in 67,375 asymptomatic subjects', *American Journal of Cardiology*, vol. 6, 1960, pp. 200–231.

41. L. Dare, 'ST-elevation without infarction', in *Royal College of Emergency Medicine Learning* [Online]. London: RCEM, 2019.

42. Y. Mizusawa and A. A. M. Wilde, 'Brugada syndrome', *Circulation: Arrhythmia and Electrophysiology*, vol. 5, no. 3, 2012, pp. 606–616.

43. C. Antzelevitch et al., 'Brugada syndrome: 1992–2002', *Journal of the American College of Cardiology*, vol. 41, no. 10, 2003, pp. 1665–1671.

44. F. Morris and W. Brady, 'ABC of clinical electrocardiography: acute myocardial infarction – part I', *BMJ*, vol. 324, 2002, pp. 831–834.

45. M. R. Ginks et al., 'Cardiac arrhythmias', in J. Firth, C. Conlon and T. Cox, eds., *Oxford Textbook of Medicine*, 6th edn. Oxford: Oxford University Press, 2020.

46. S. W. Yusuf, 'Acute exacerbation of congestive heart failure', in *BMJ Best Practice* [Online]. London: BMJ Publishing Group, 2018.

47. V. Henson, 'Cardiogenic pulmonary oedema', in *Royal College of Emergency Medicine Learning* [Online]. London: RCEM, 2017.

48. P. Ponikowski et al., '2016 ESC guidelines for the diagnosis and treatment of acute and chronic heart failure', *European Heart Journal*, vol. 37, 2016, pp. 2129–2200.

49. P. M. Seferovic et al., 'Heart failure in cardiomyopathies: a position paper from the Heart Failure Association of the European Society of Cardiology', *European Journal of Heart Failure*, vol. 21, 2019, pp. 553–576.

50. S. M. Stevens, S. C. Woller and G. V. Fontaine, 'Pulmonary embolism', in *BMJ Best Practice* [Online]. London: BMJ Publishing Group, 2018.

51. A. Wakai, 'Pulmonary hypertension and right heart failure', in *Royal College of Emergency Medicine Learning* [Online]. London: RCEM, 2018.

52. S. W. Smith et al., 'Diagnosis of ST-elevation myocardial infarction in the presence of left bundle branch block with the ST-elevation to S-wave ratio in a modified Sgarbossa rule', *Annals of Emergency Medicine*, vol. 60, no. 6, 2012, pp. 766–776.

53. E. B. Sgarbossa et al., 'Electrocardiographic diagnosis of evolving acute myocardial infarction in the presence of left bundle-branch block', *The New England Journal of Medicine*, vol. 334, no. 8, 1996, pp. 481–487.

54. D. H. Do et al., 'Electrocardiographic right ventricular strain precedes hypoxic pulseless electrical activity cardiac arrests: looking beyond pulmonary embolism', *Resuscitation*, vol. 151, 2020, pp. 127–134.

55. S. Konstantinides et al., '2019 ESC guidelines for the diagnosis and management of acute pulmonary embolism developed in collaboration with the European Respiratory Society (ERS)', *European Heart Journal*, vol. 41, no. 4, 2019, pp. 543–603.

56. P. T. Reid and J. A. Innes, 'Respiratory disease', in *Davidson's Principles and Practice of Medicine*, 22nd edn. Edinburgh: Churchill Livingstone, 2014.

57. E. Boey, S. Teo and K. Poh, 'Electrocardiographic findings in pulmonary embolism', *Singapore Medical Journal*, vol. 56, no. 10, 2015, pp. 533–537.

58. A. French, 'Cardiac implantable devices', in *Royal College of Emergency Medicine Learning* [Online]. London: RCEM, 2013.

59. M. Brignole et al., '2013 ESC guidelines on cardiac pacing and cardiac resynchronization therapy', *European Heart Journal*, vol. 34, 2013, pp. 2281–2329.

60. A. Parfitt and E. Townsend, 'Disorders of potassium balance', in *Royal College of Emergency Medicine Learning* [Online]. London: RCEM, 2019.

61. B. T. Montague, J. R. Ouellette and G. K. Buller, 'Retrospective review of the frequency of ECG changes in hyperkalemia', *Clinical Journal of the American Society of Nephrology*, vol. 3, no. 2, 2008, pp. 324–330.

62. T. J. McDonald, R. A. Oram and B. Vaidya, 'Investigating hyperkalaemia in adults', *BMJ*, vol. 351, 2015, h4762.

63. P. O. Ettinger, T. J. Regan and H. A. Oldewurtel, 'Hyperkalemia, cardiac conduction, and the electrocardiogram: a review', *American Heart Journal*, vol. 88, no. 3, 1974, pp. 360–371.

64. M. J. Field et al., 'Clinical biochemistry and metabolism', in *Davidson's Principles and Practices of Medicine*, 22nd edn. Edinburgh: Churchill Livingstone, 2014.

65. M. M. Yaqoob, 'Water, electrolytes and acid-base balance', in P. Kumar and M. Clark, eds., *Clinical Medicine*, 7th edn. Edinburgh: Saunders Elsevier, 2009.

66. T. Gregory and M. Smith, 'Cardiovascular complications of brain injury', *Continuing Education in Anaesthesia Critical Care & Pain*, vol. 12, no. 2, 2012, pp. 67–71.

67. S. Purushothaman et al., 'Study of ECG changes and its relation to mortality in cases of cerebrovascular accidents', *Journal of Natural Science, Biology and Medicine*, vol. 5, no. 2, 2014, pp. 434–436.

68. S. Chatterjee, 'ECG changes in subarachnoid haemorrhage: a synopsis', *Netherlands Heart Journal*, vol. 19, no. 1, 2011, pp. 31–34.

Consolidation Practice ECGs and Case Scenarios

Practice ECGs Set 1

Practice ECG 1.1

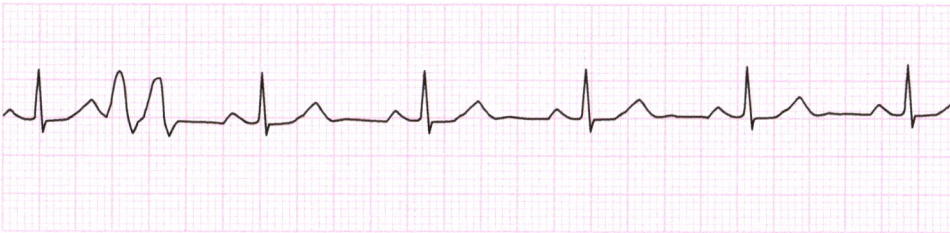

Practice ECG 1.2

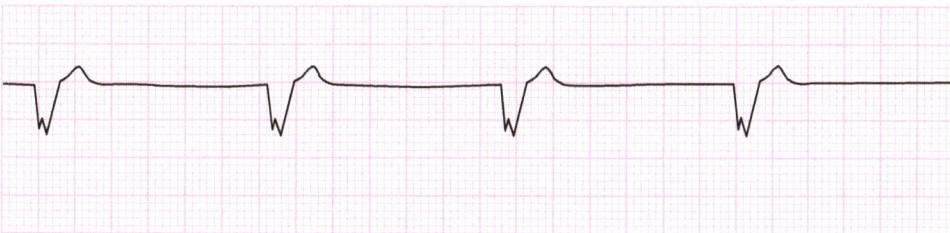

Practice ECG 1.3

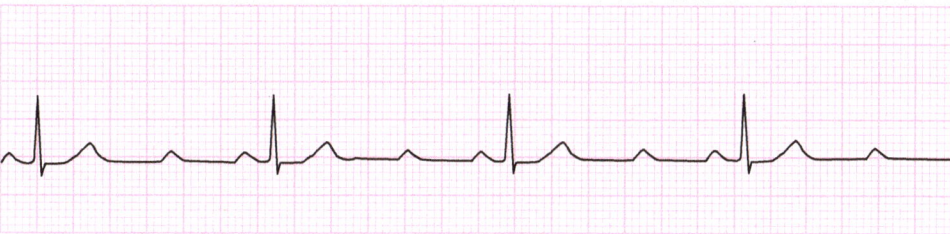

Practice ECG 1.4

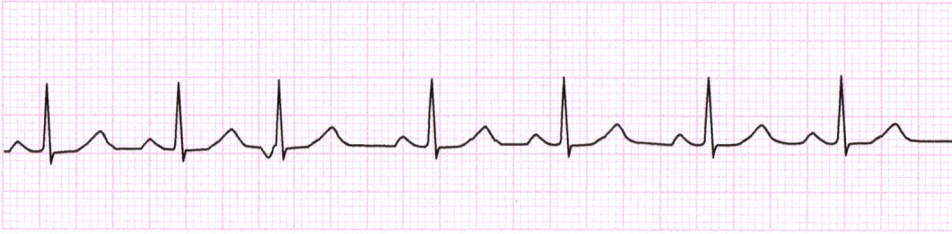

Practice ECG 1.5

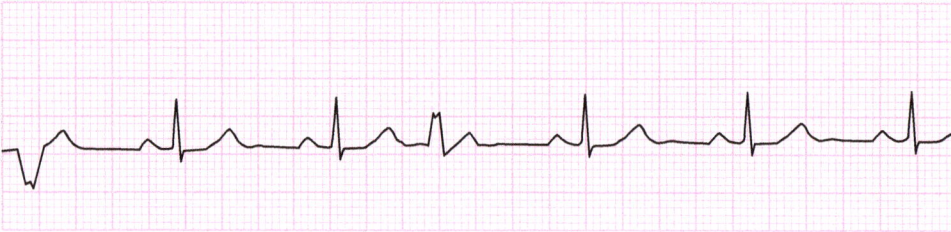

Practice ECG 1.6

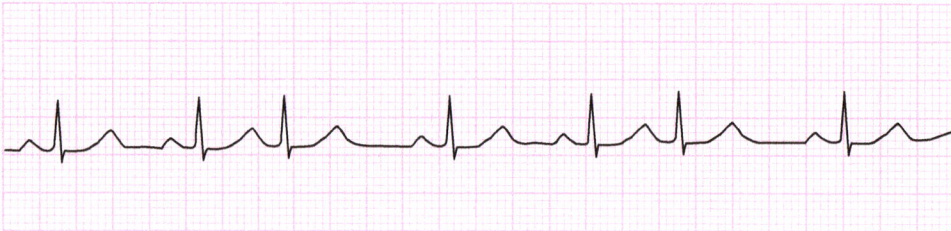

Practice ECG 1.7

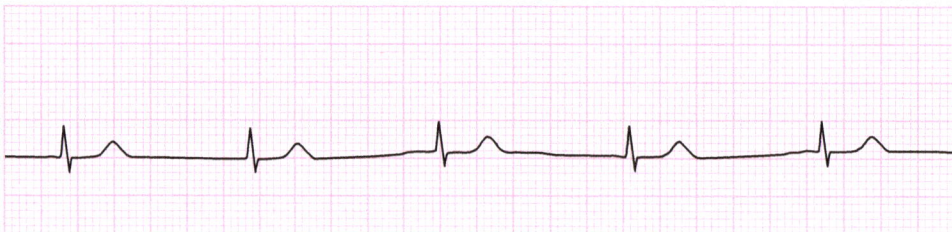

Practice ECG 1.8

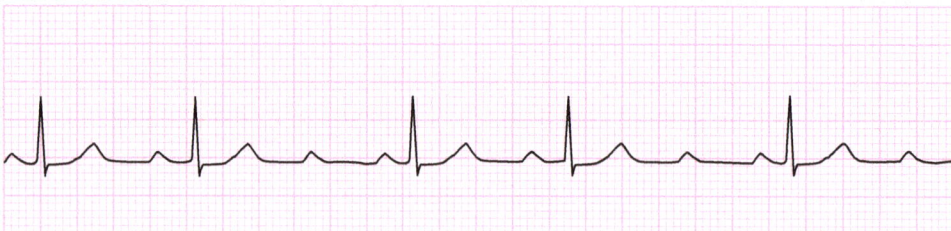

Practice ECG 1.9

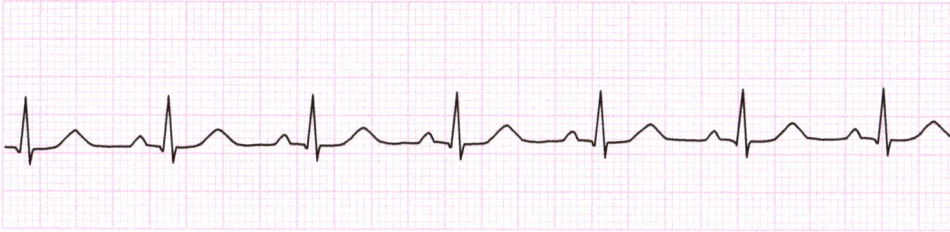

Practice ECG 1.10

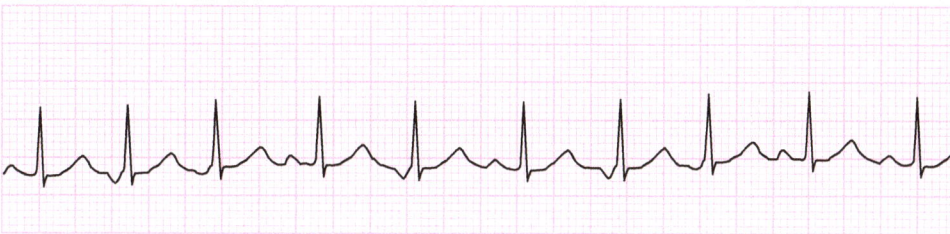

Practice ECGs Set 2

Practice ECG 2.1

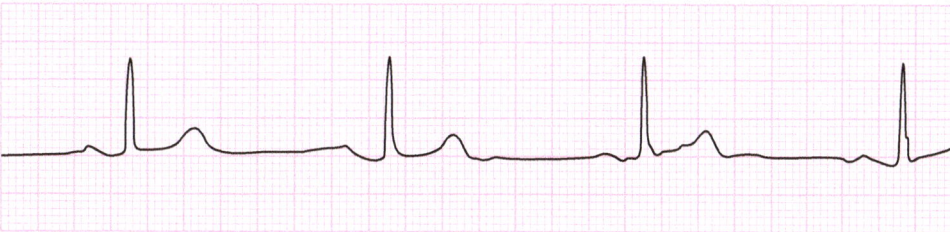

Practice ECG 2.2

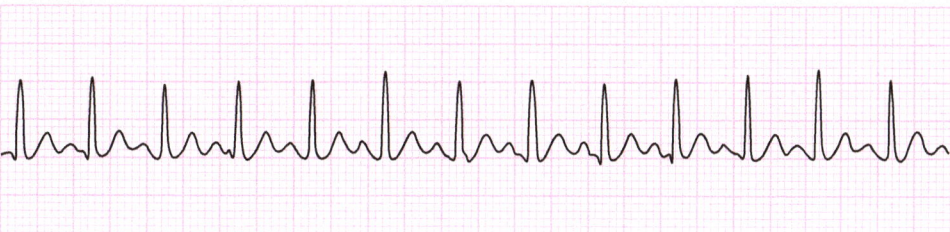

Practice ECG 2.3

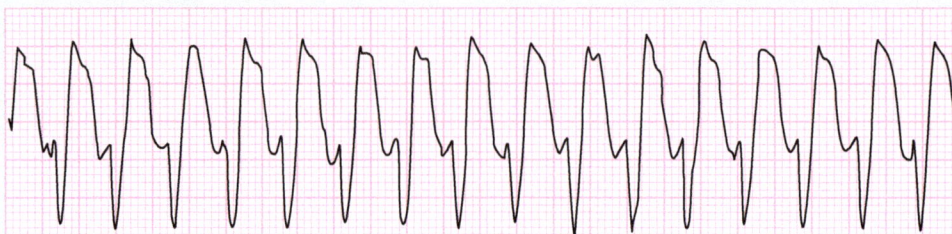

Practice ECG 2.4

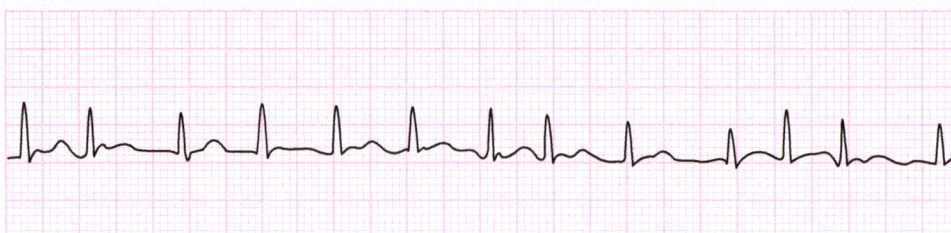

Practice ECG 2.5

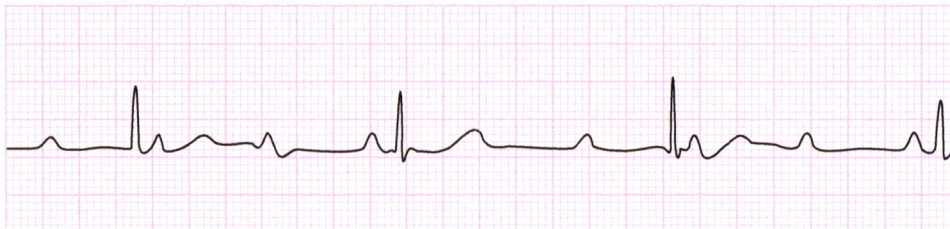

Practice ECG 2.6

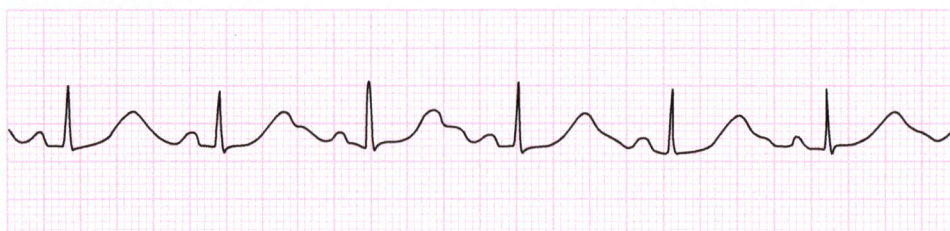

Practice ECG 2.7

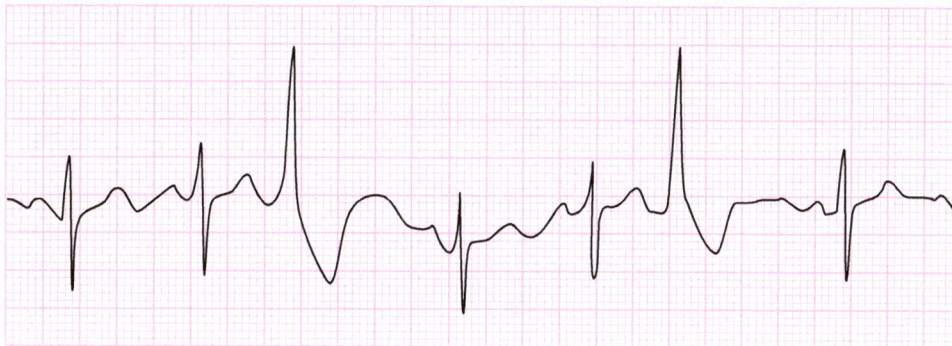

Practice ECG 2.8

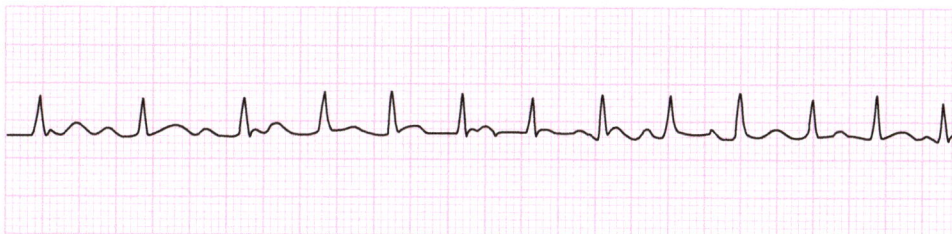

Practice ECG 2.9

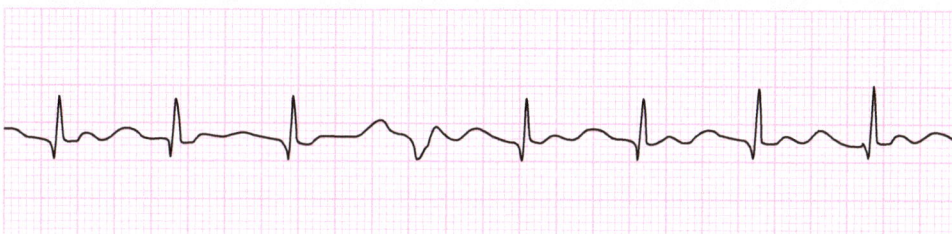

Practice ECG 2.10

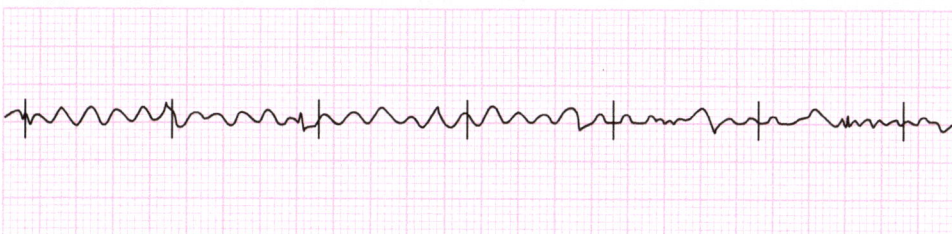

Practice ECG 3.1

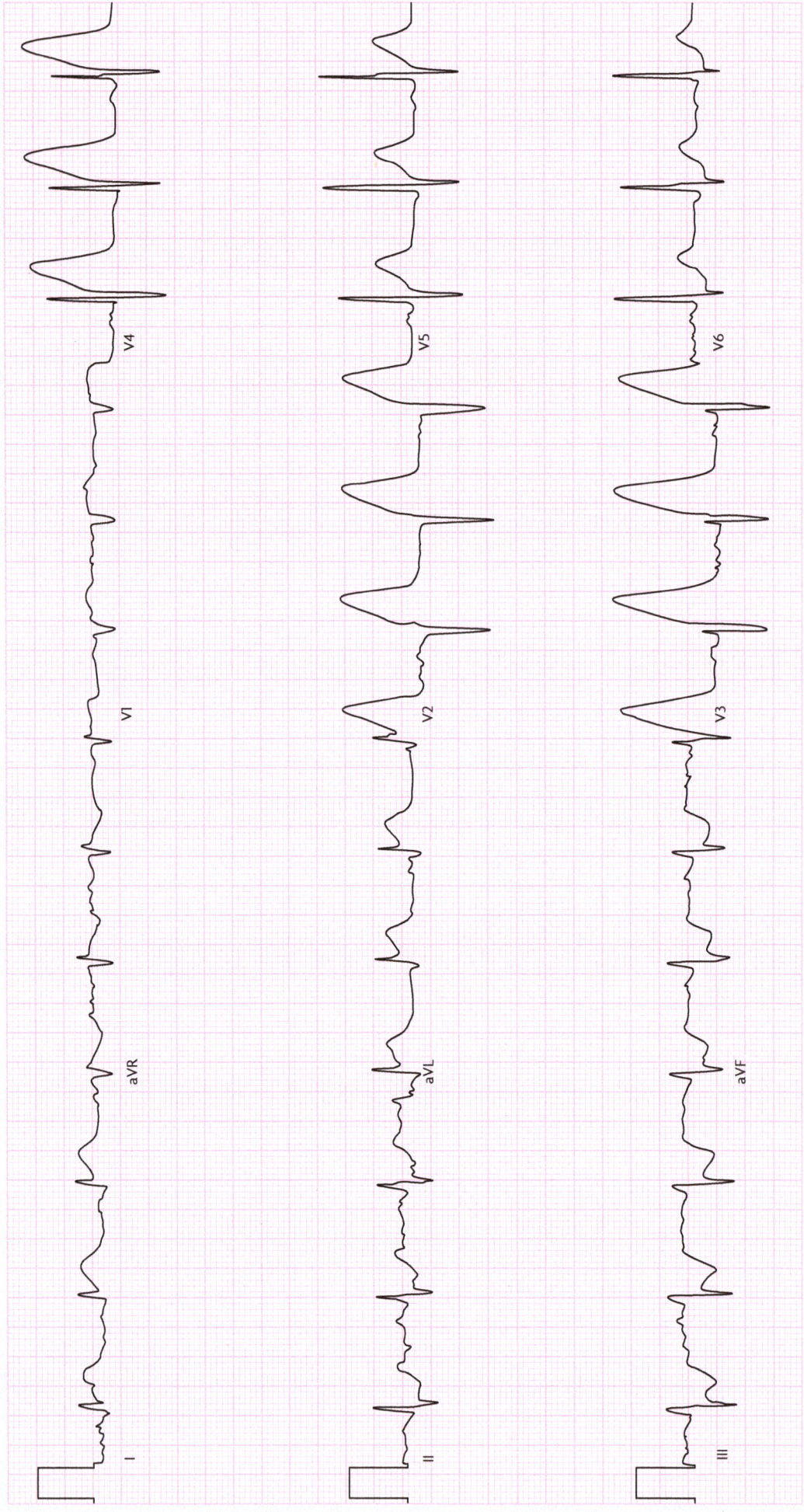

Practice ECG 3.2

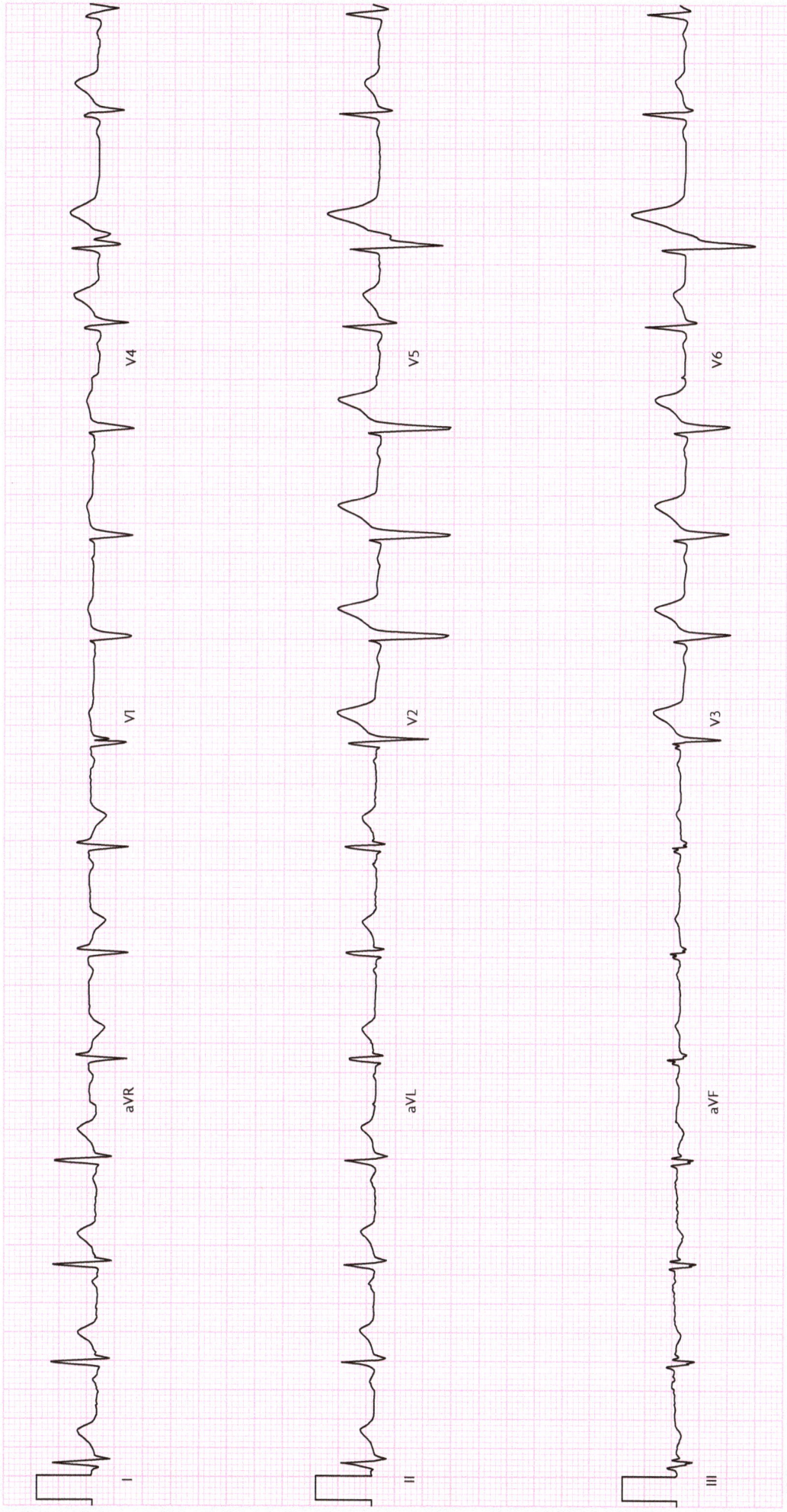

Practice ECG 3.3

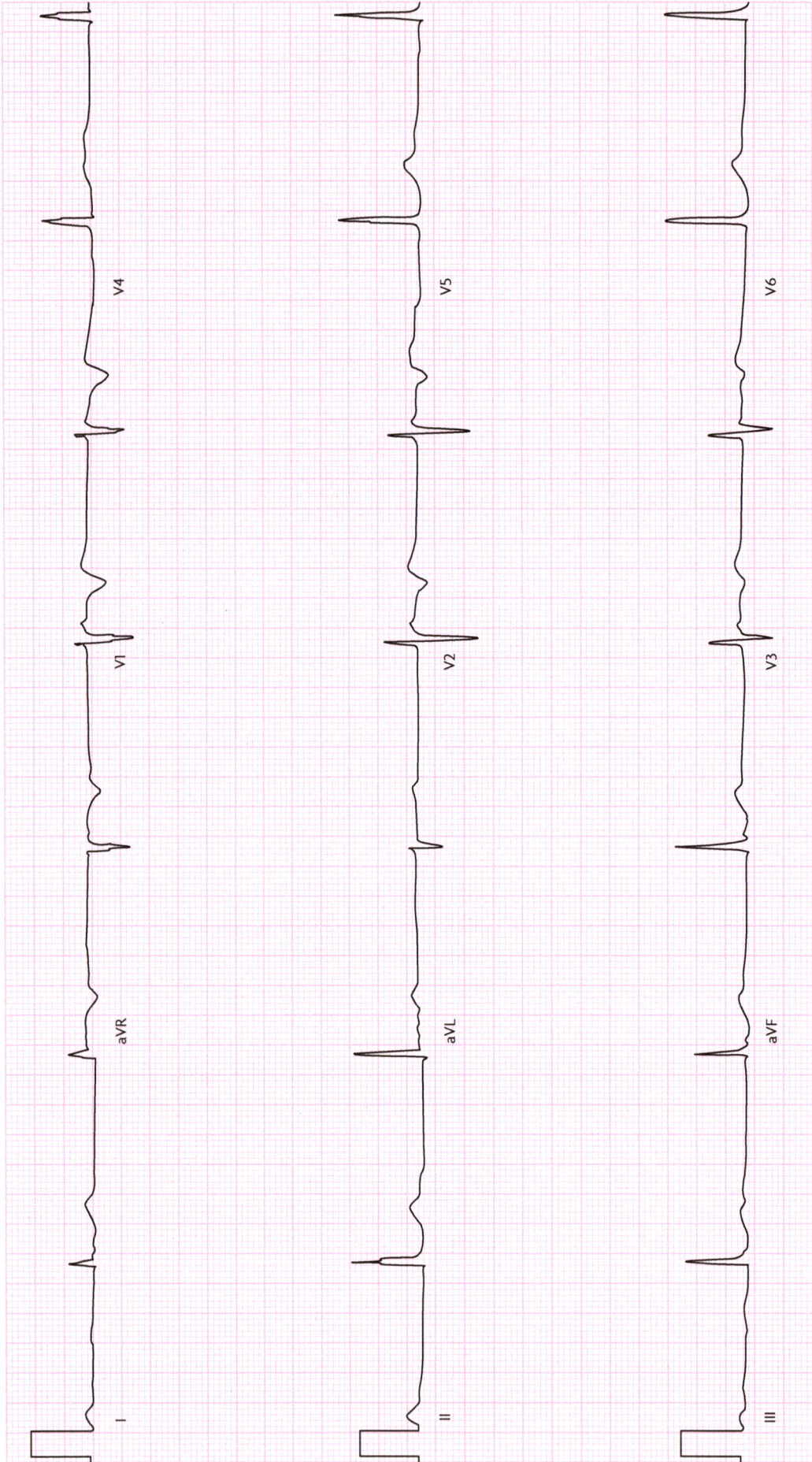

Practice ECG 3.4

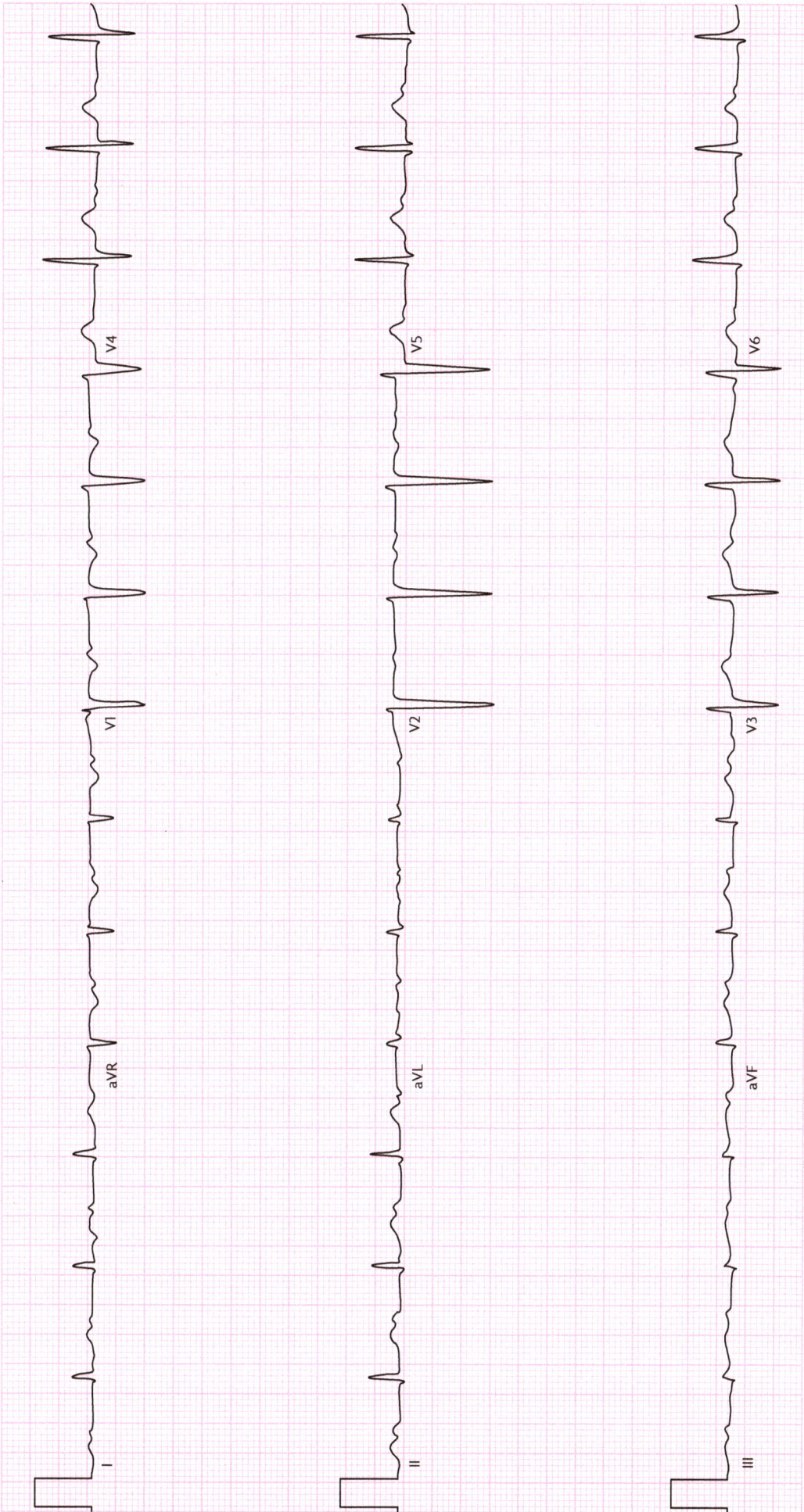

I

II

III

aVR

aVL

aVF

V1

V2

V3

V4

V5

V6

Practice ECG 3.5

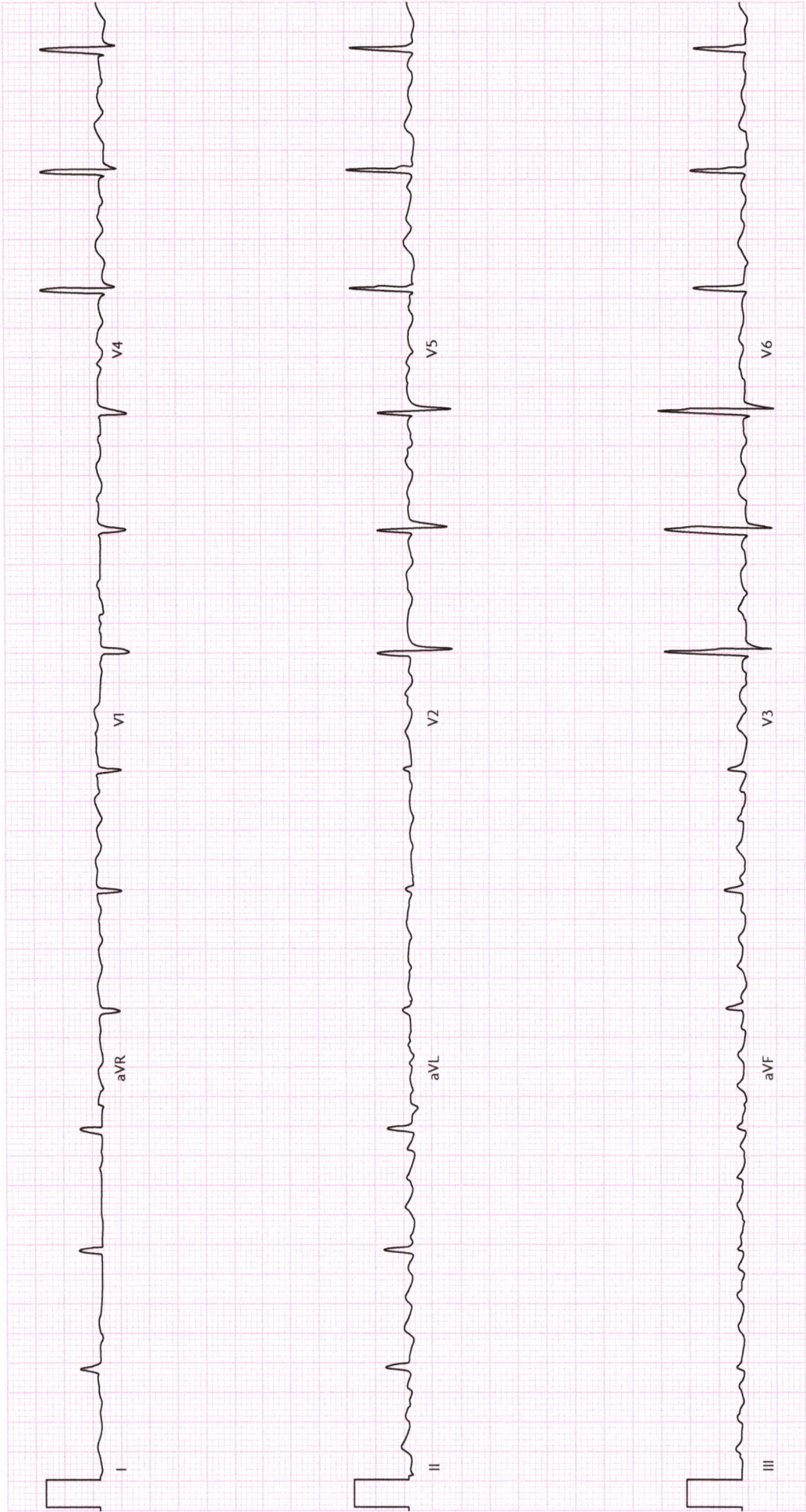

I

II

III

aVR

aVL

aVF

V1

V2

V3

V4

V5

V6

Practice ECG 3.6

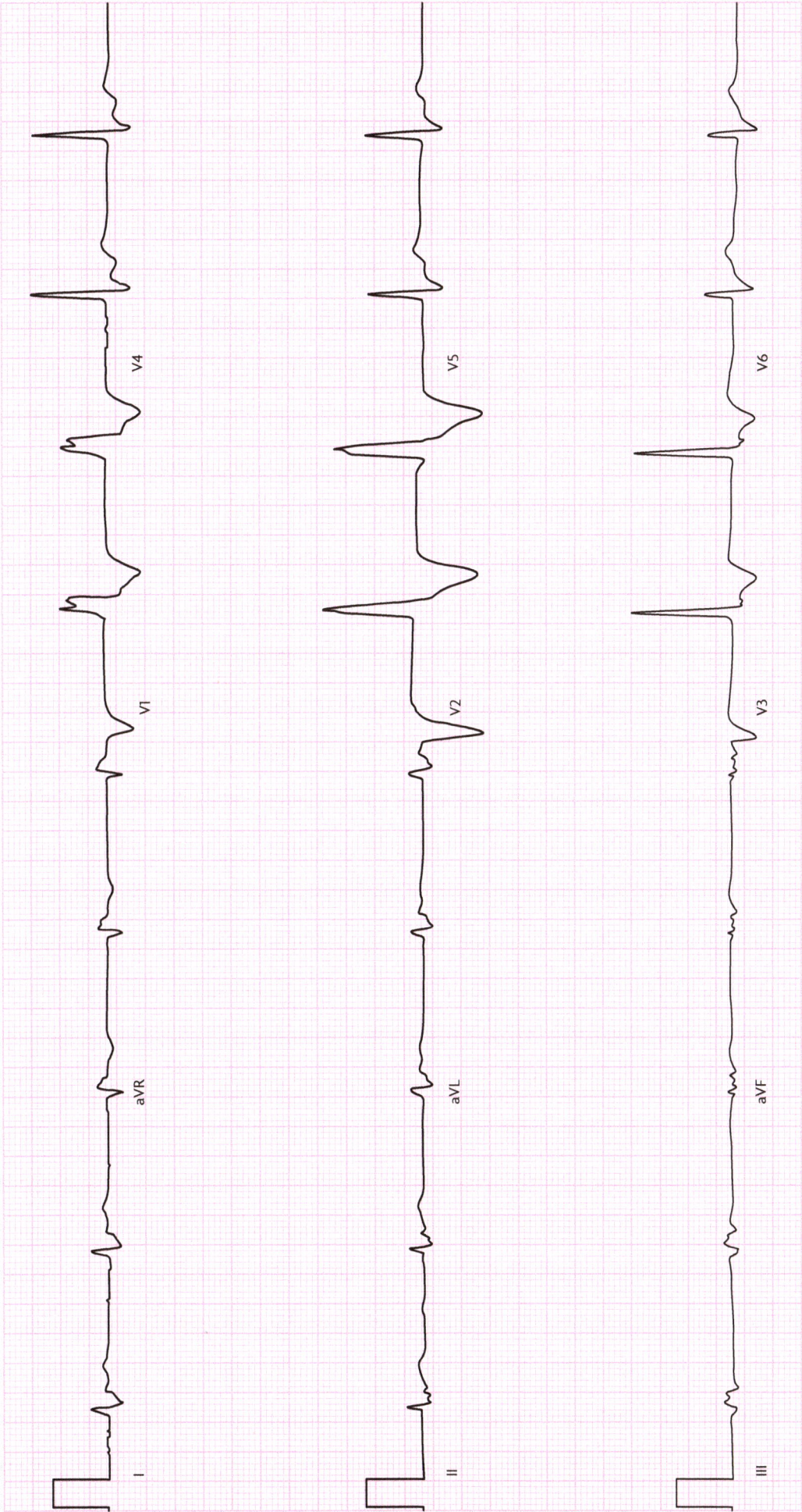

I

II

III

aVR

aVL

aVF

V1

V2

V3

V4

V5

V6

Practice ECG 3.7

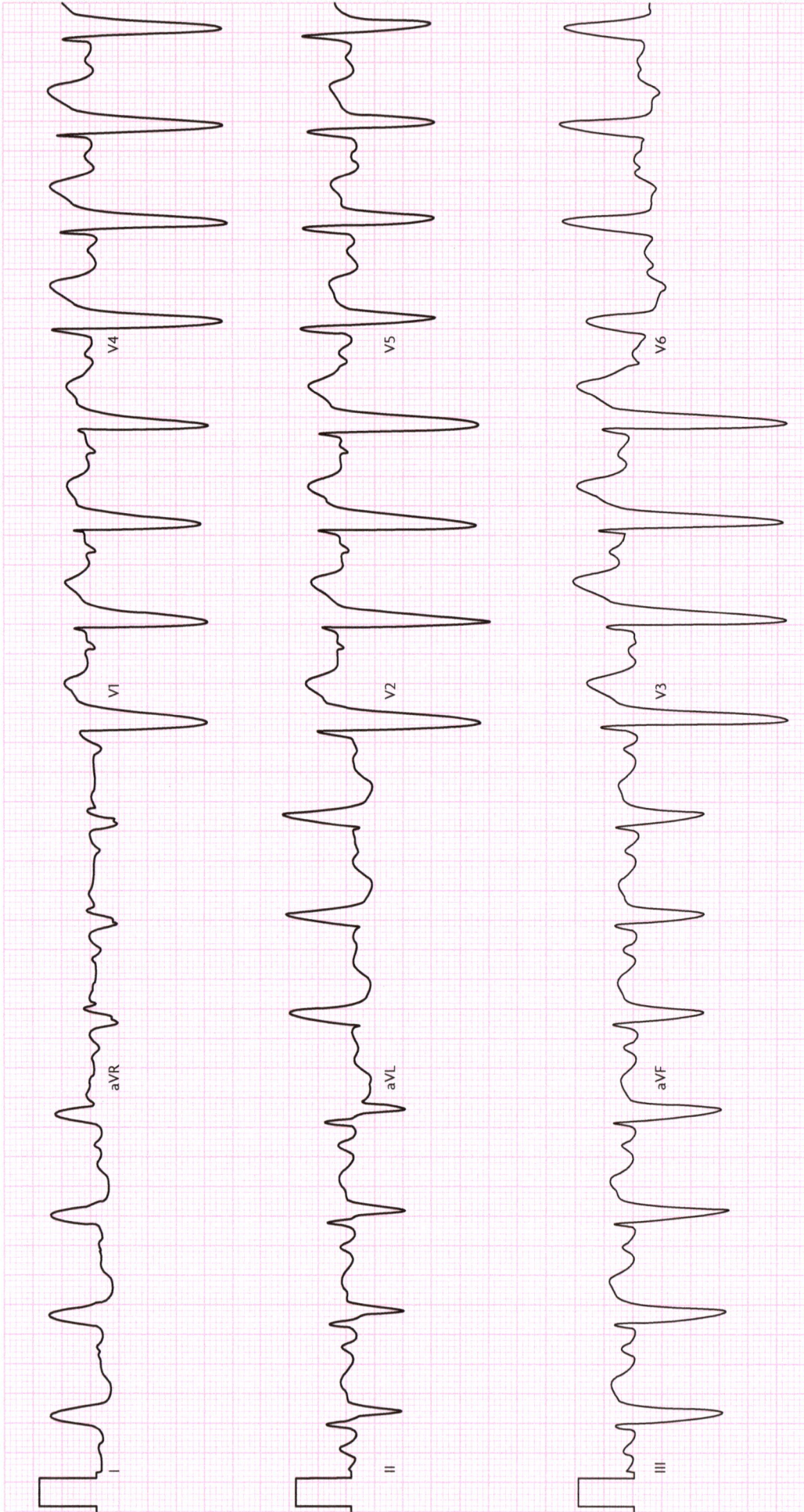

Practice ECG 3.8

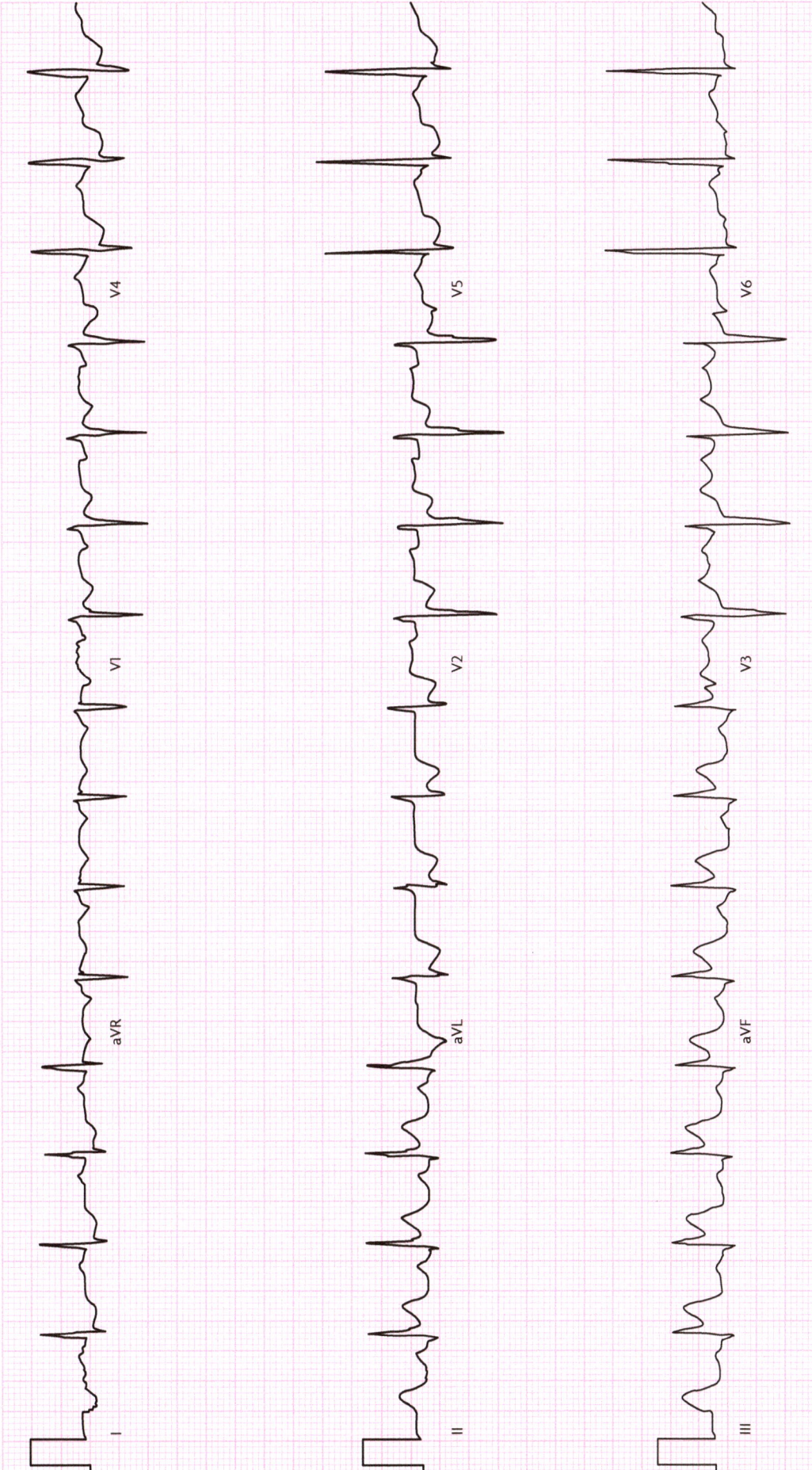

I

II

III

aVR

aVL

aVF

V1

V2

V3

V4

V5

V6

Practice ECG 3.9

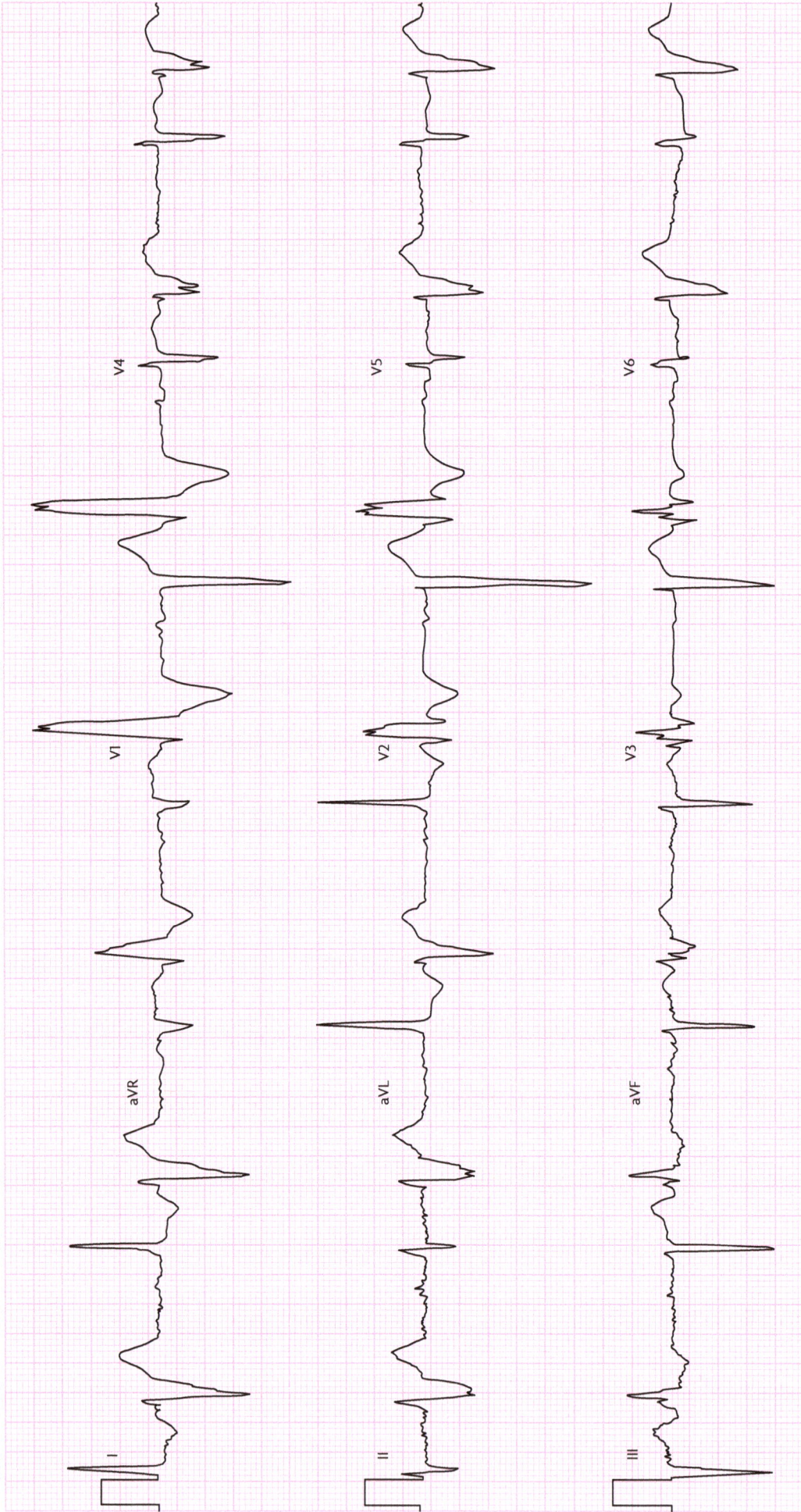

Practice ECG 3.10

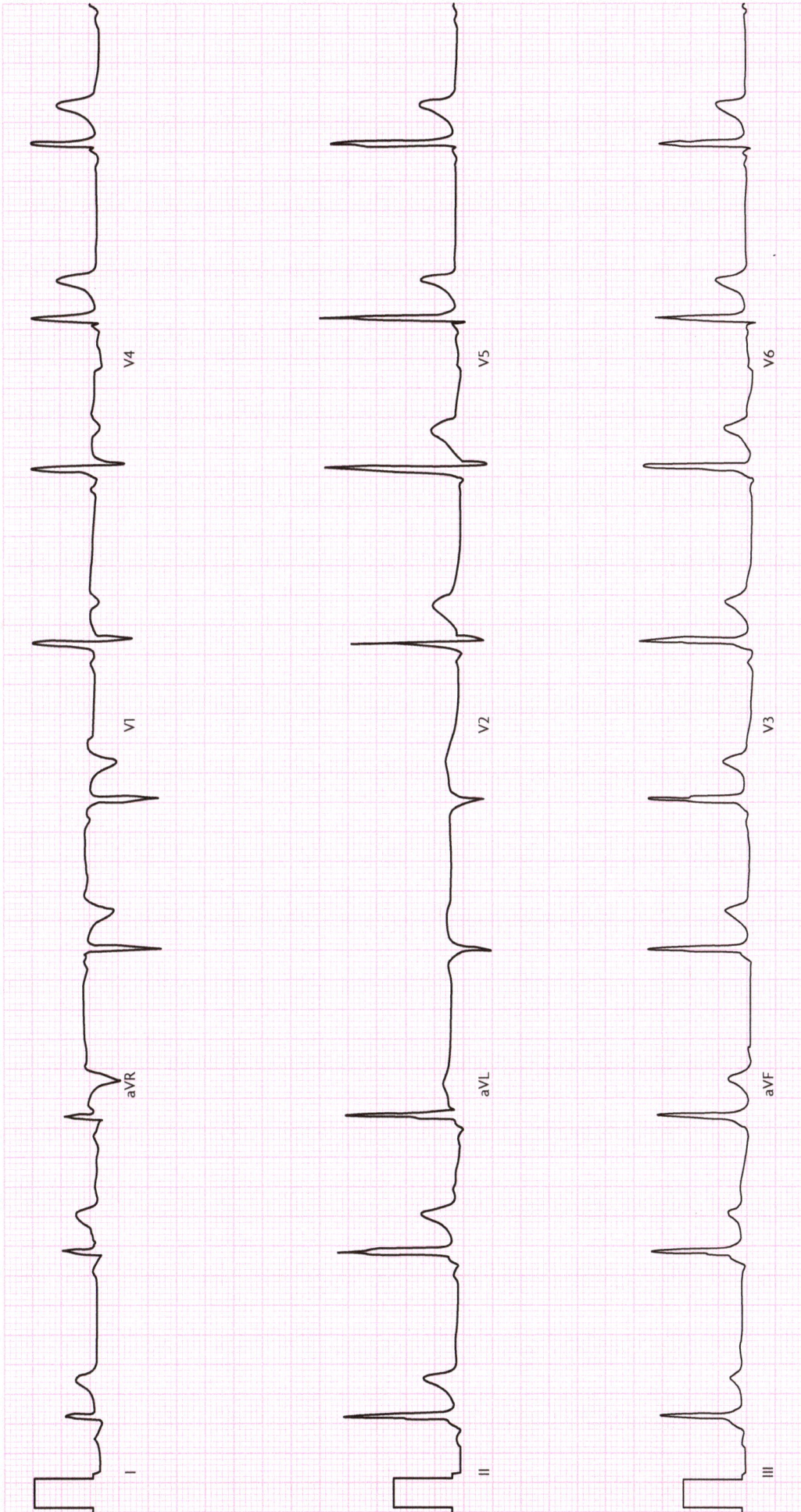

Practice ECGs Set 4

Practice ECG 4.1

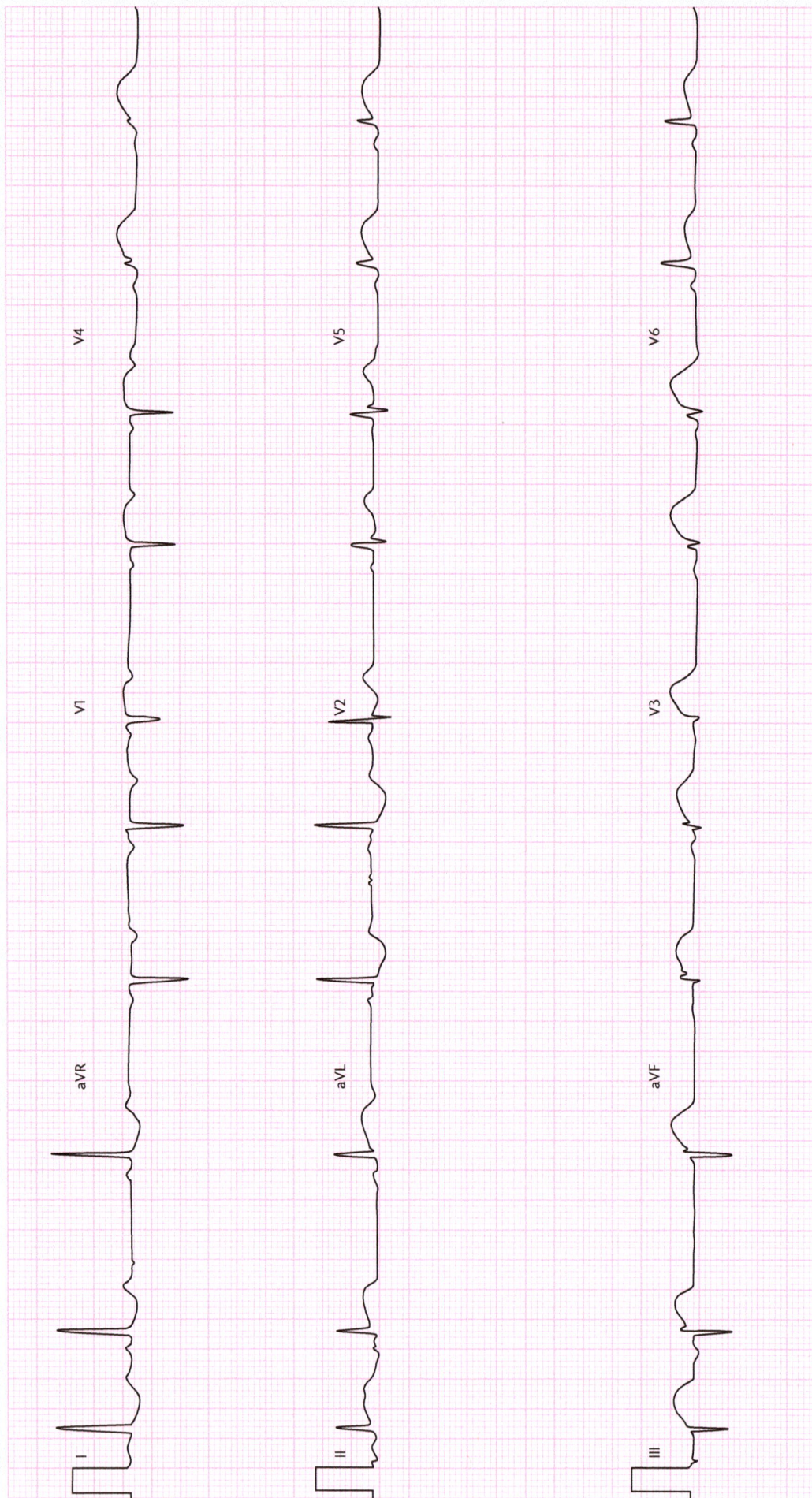

Practice ECG 4.2

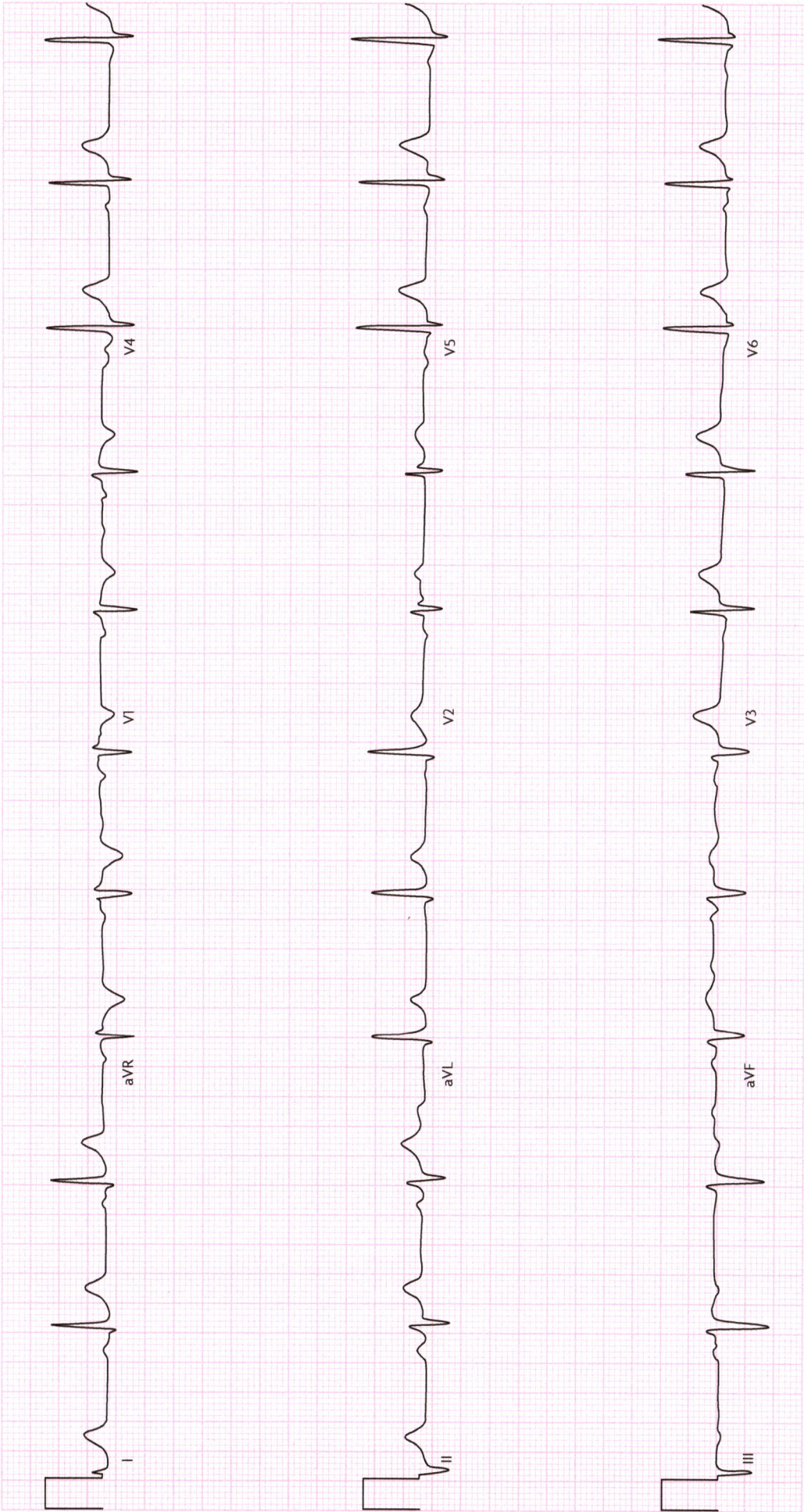

Practice ECG 4.3

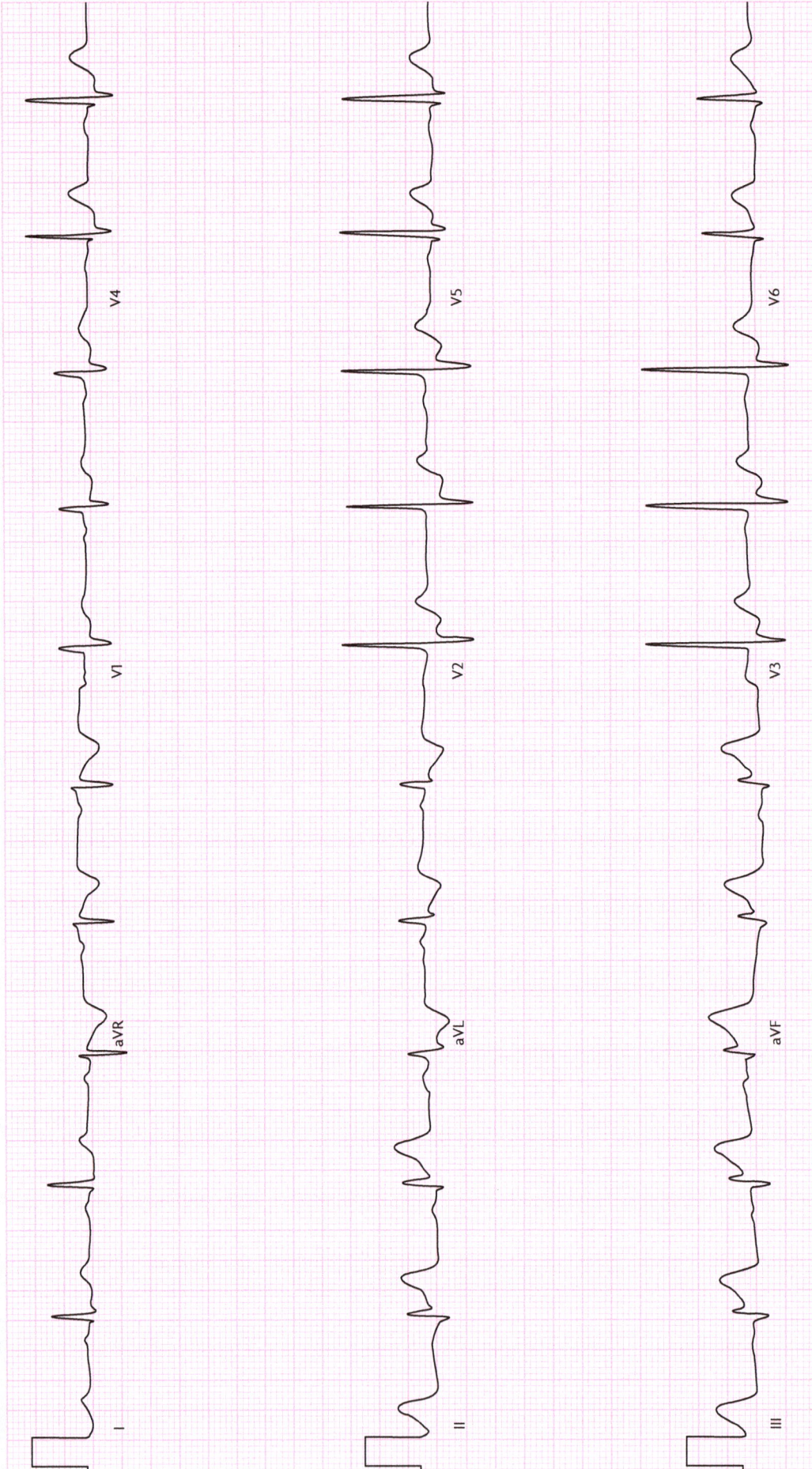

Practice ECG 4.4

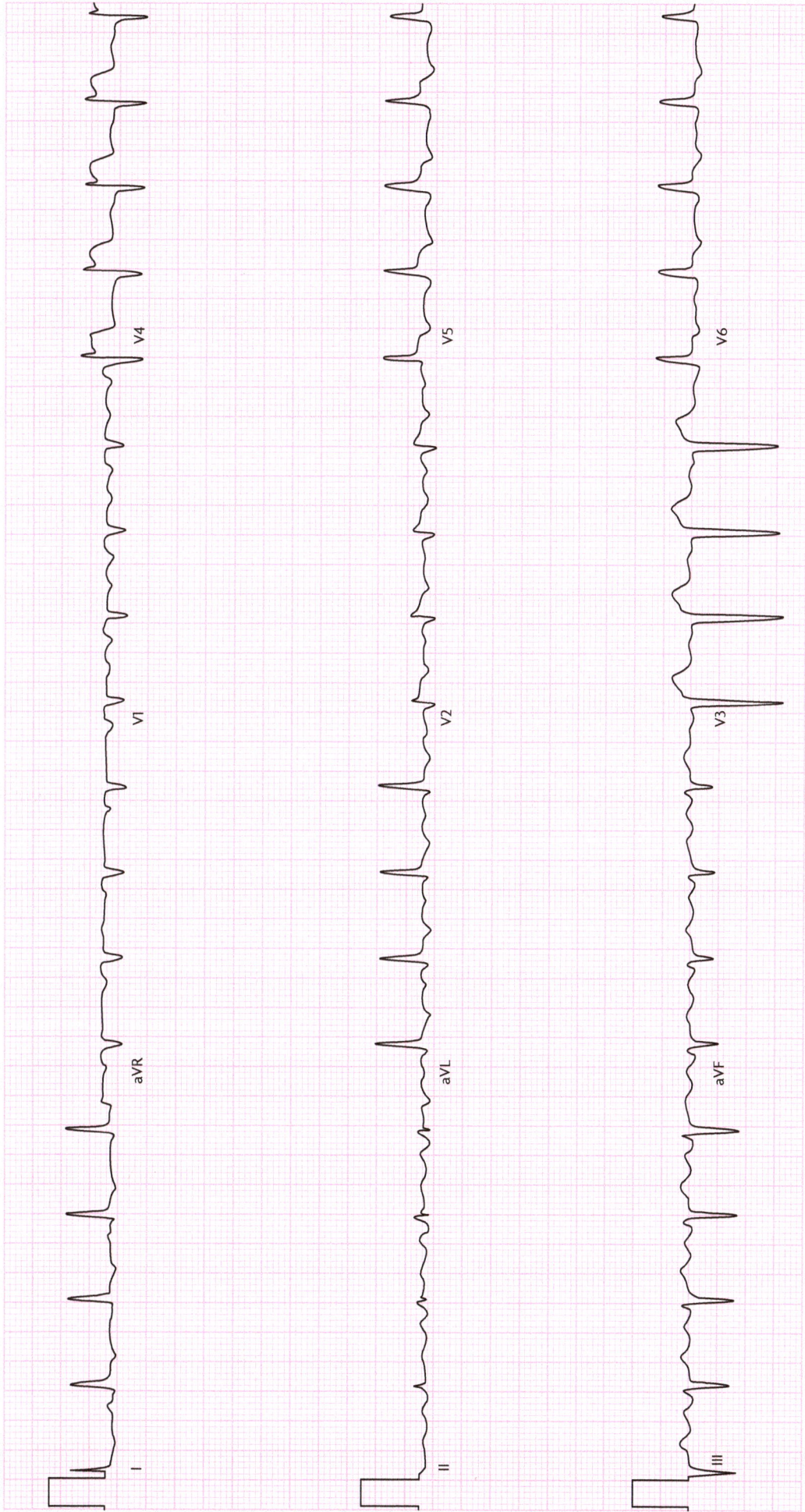

Practice ECG 4.5

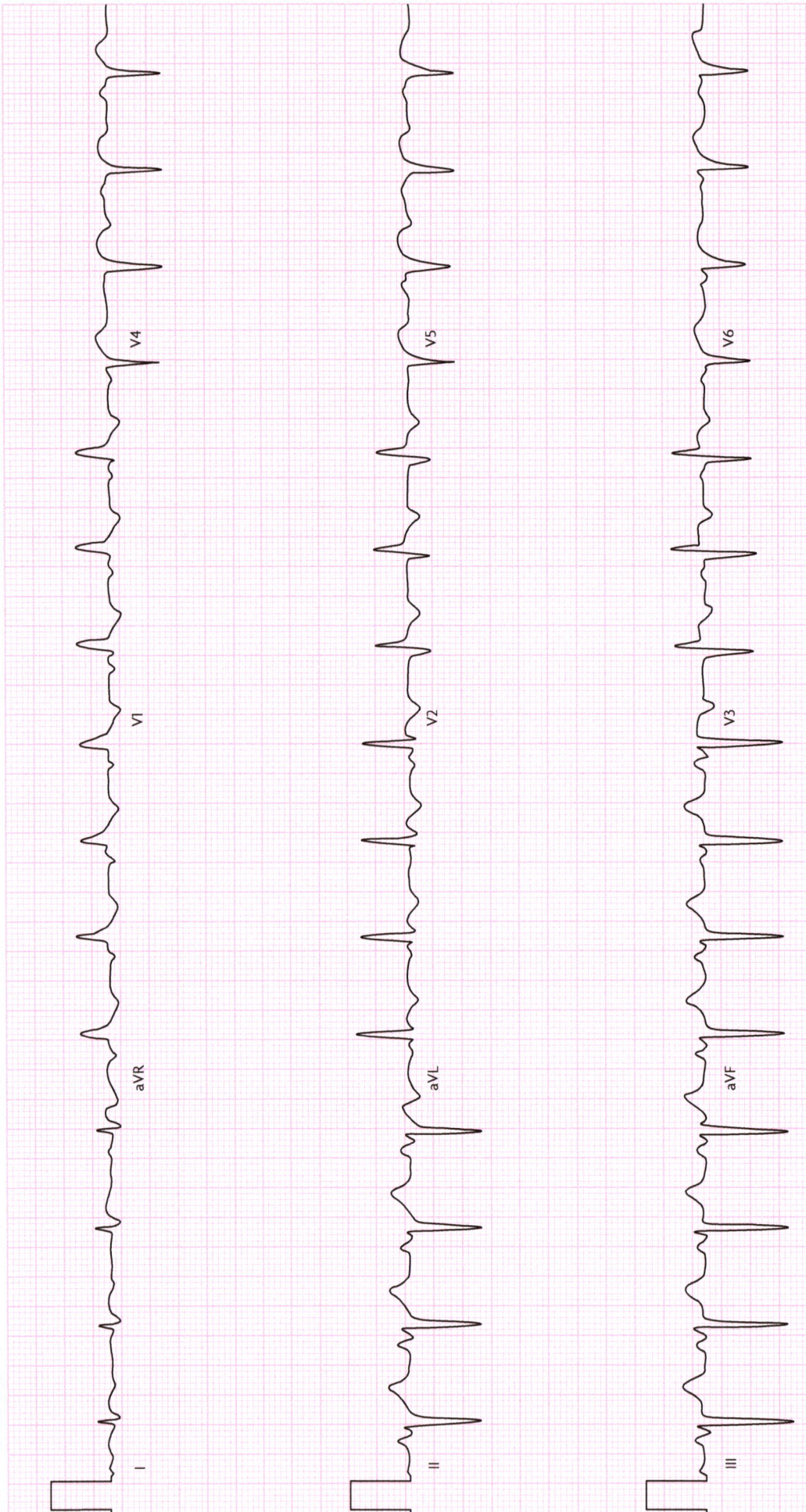

I

aVR

V1

V4

II

aVL

V2

V5

III

aVF

V3

V6

Practice ECG 4.6

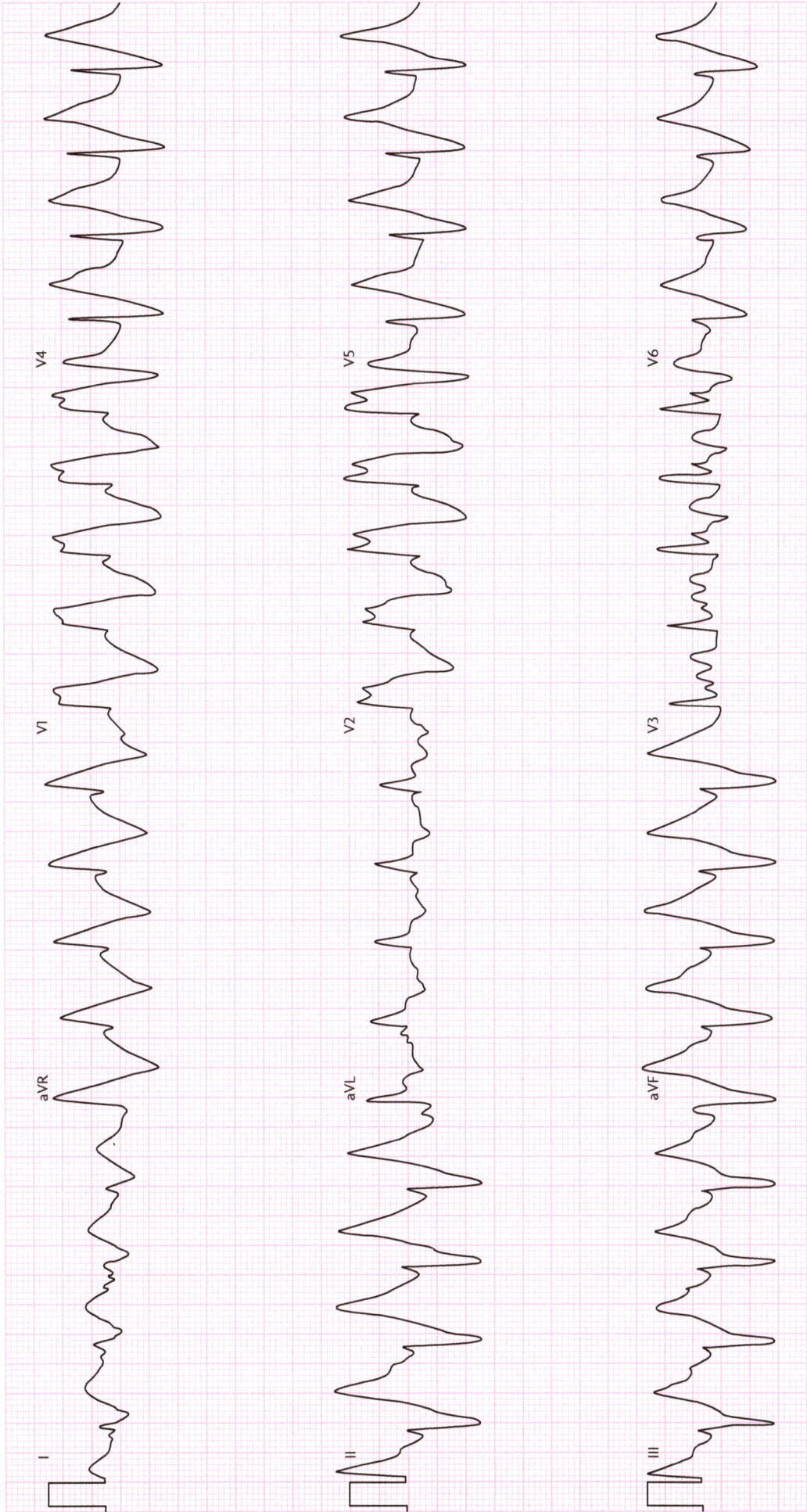

Practice ECG 4.7

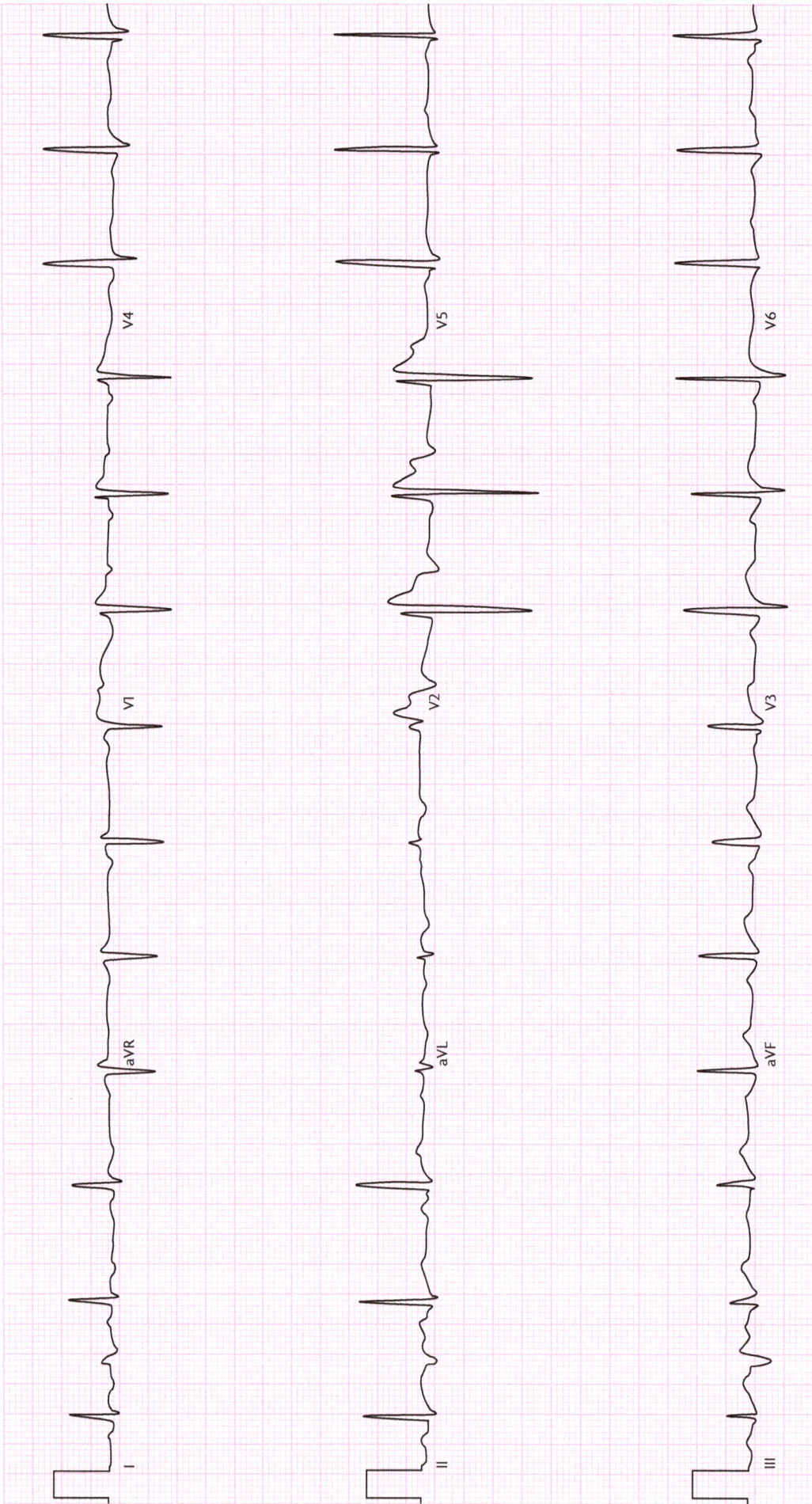

Practice ECG 4.8

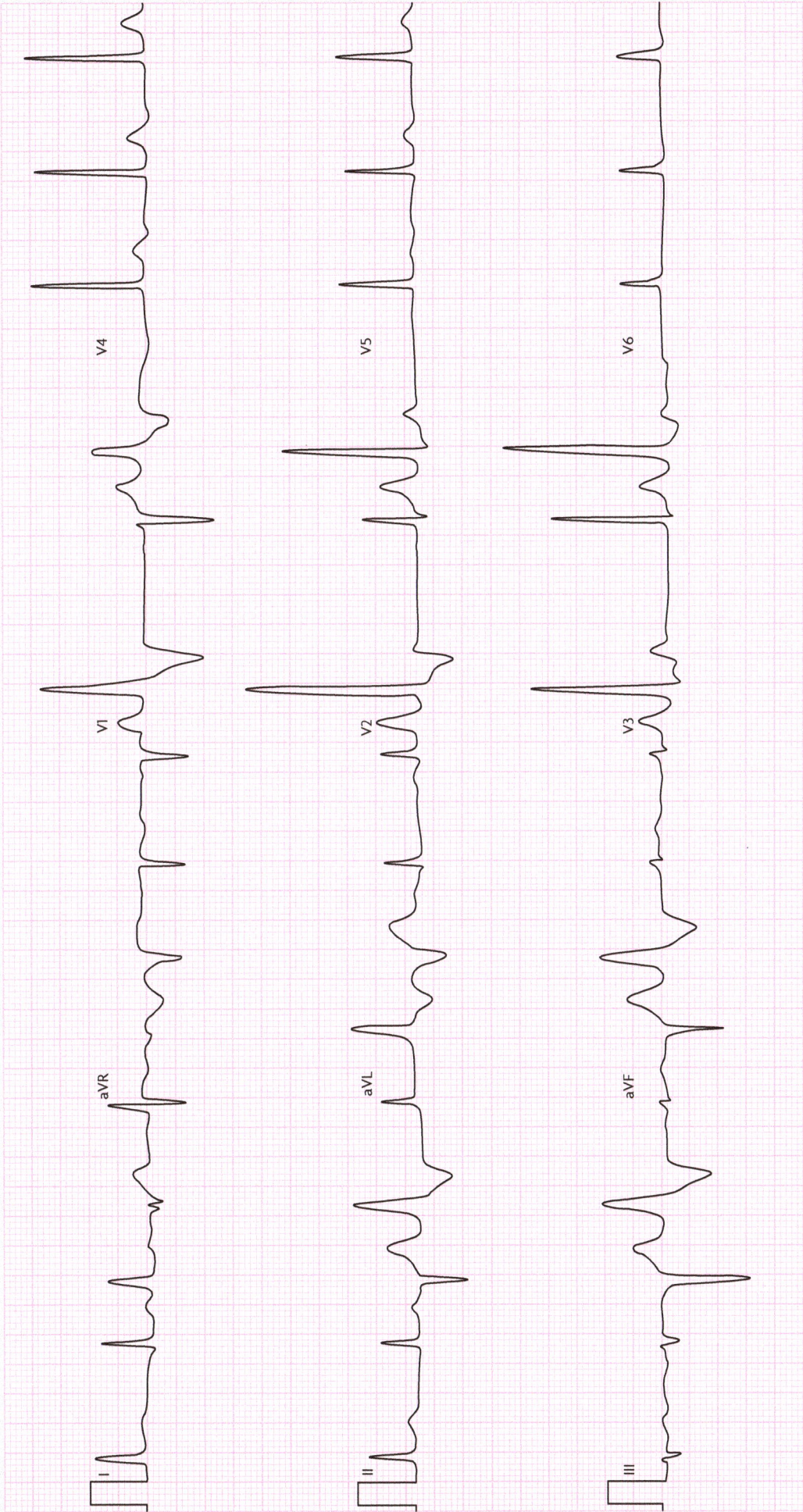

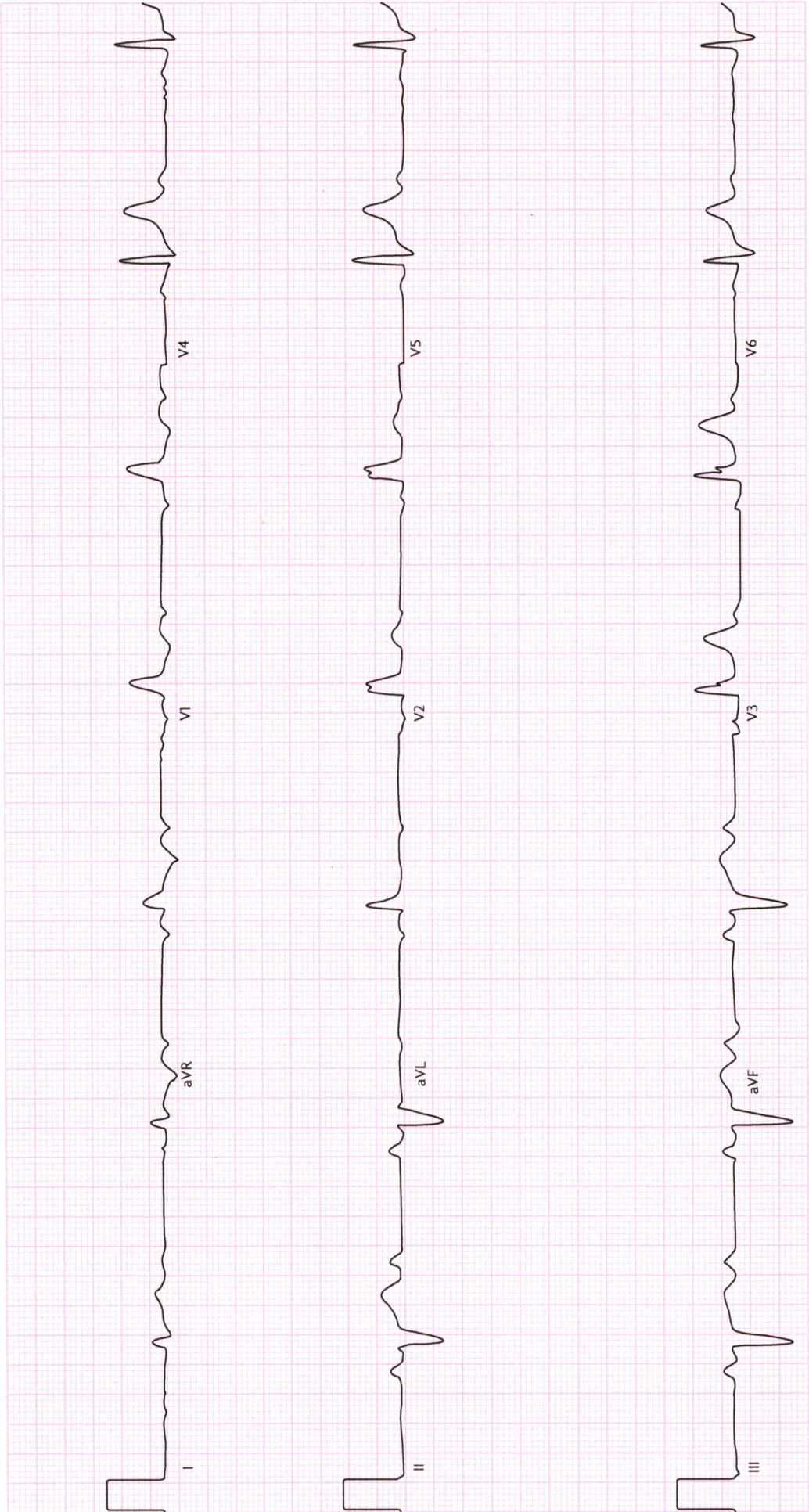

Practice ECG 4.10

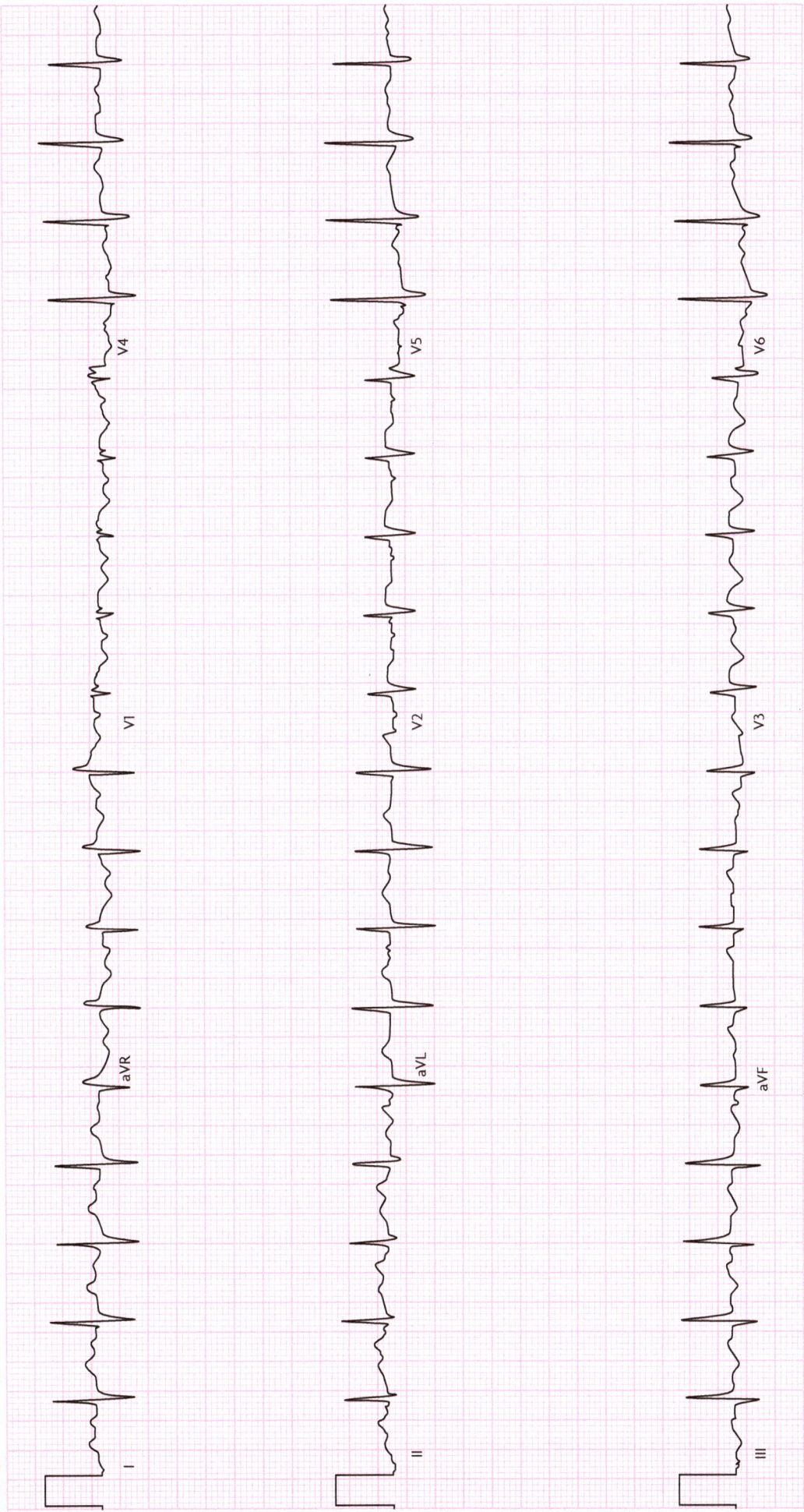

I

II

III

aVR

aVL

aVF

V1

V2

V3

V4

V5

V6

Practice ECG 5.1

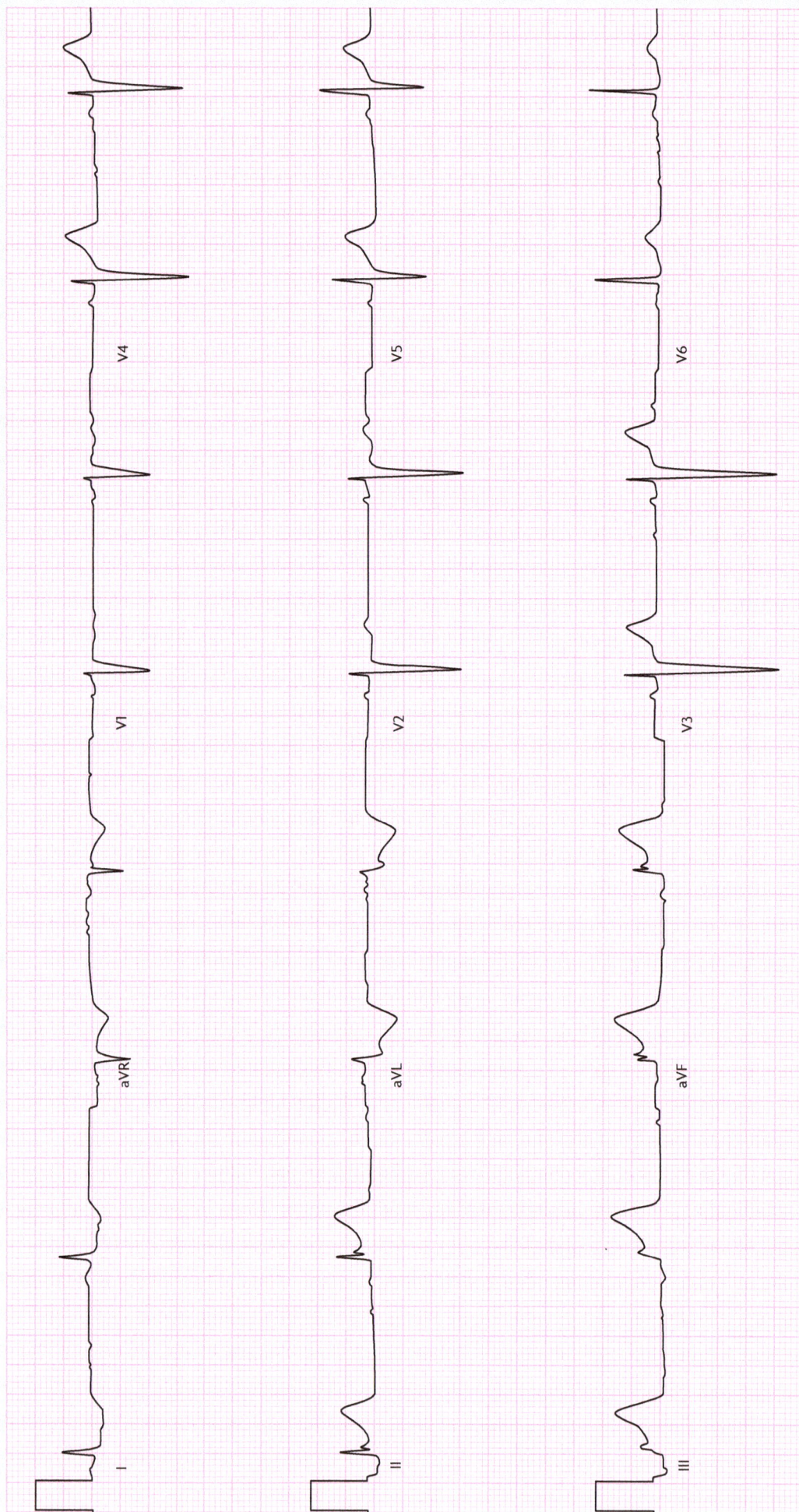

Practice ECG 5.2

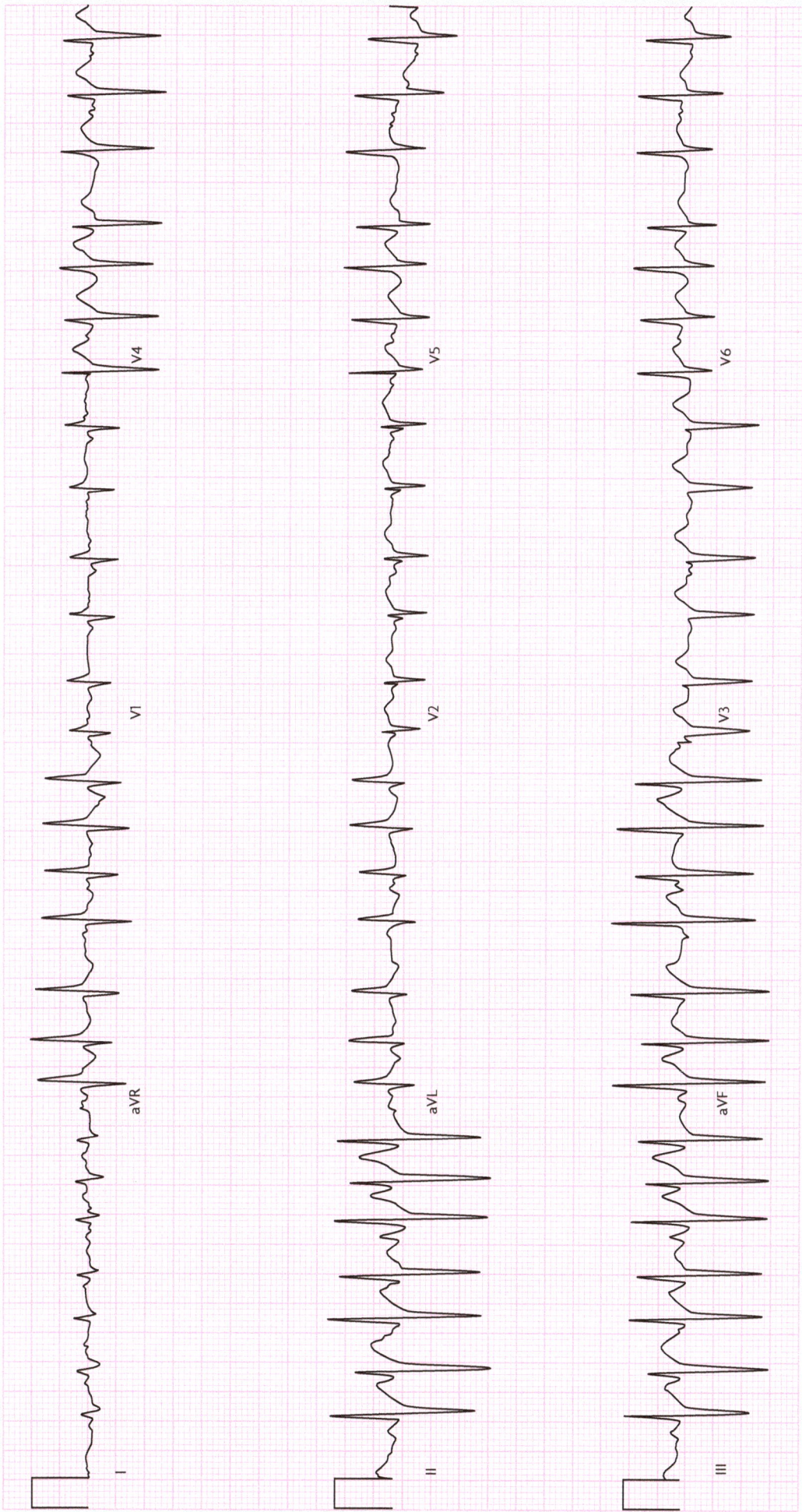

Practice ECG 5.3

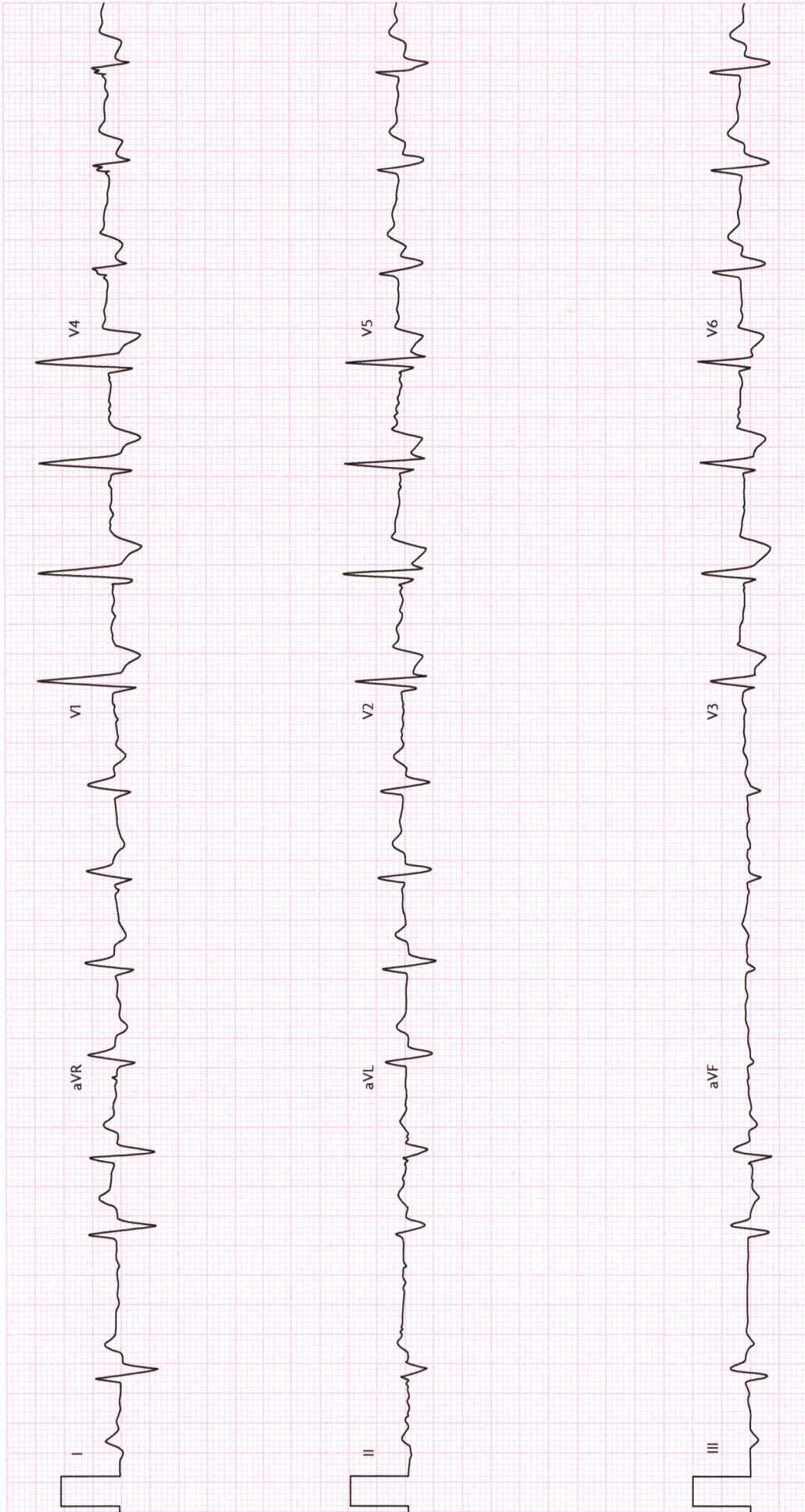

I

II

III

aVR

aVL

aVF

V1

V2

V3

V4

V5

V6

Practice ECG 5.4

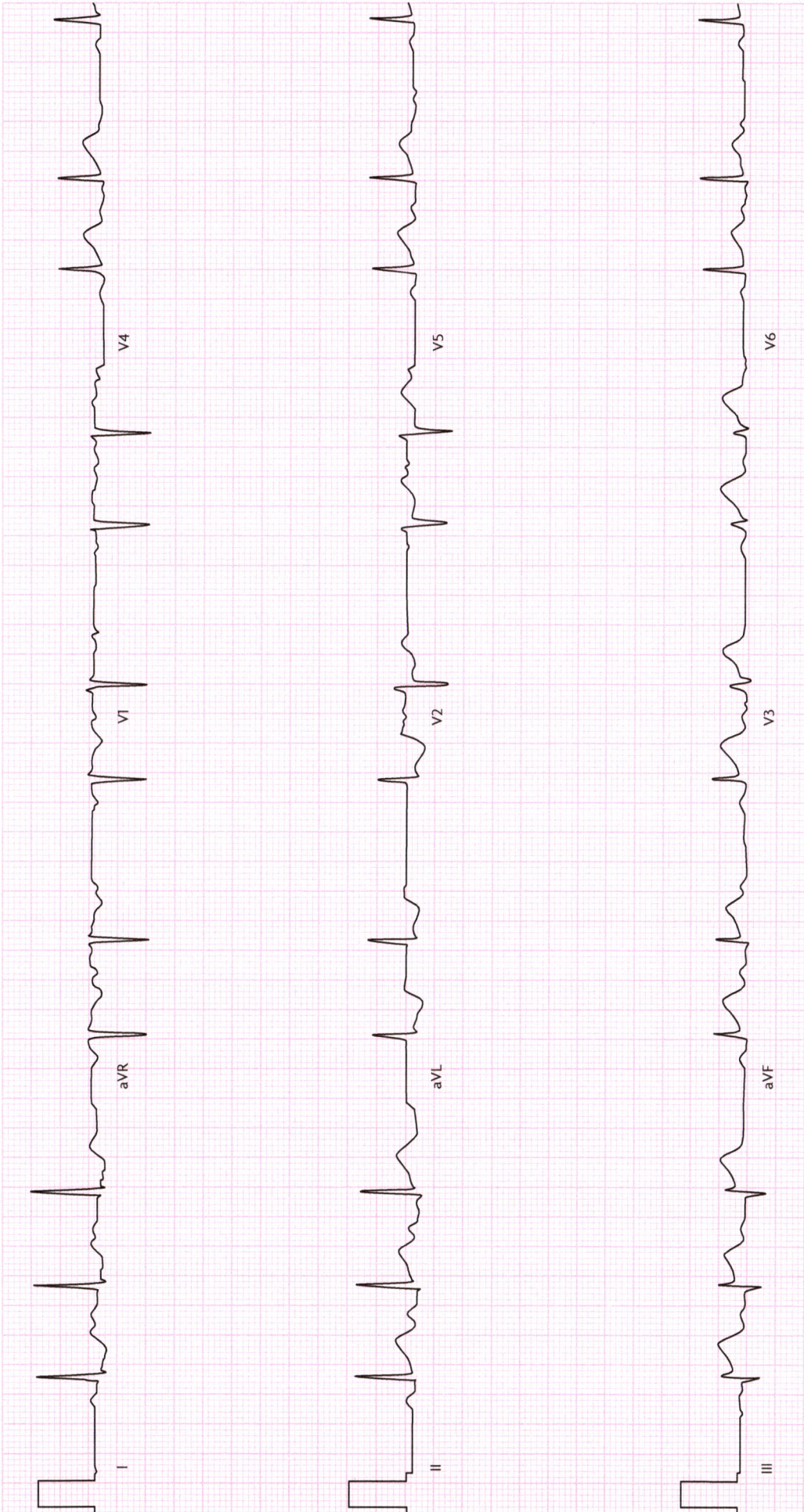

Practice ECG 5.5

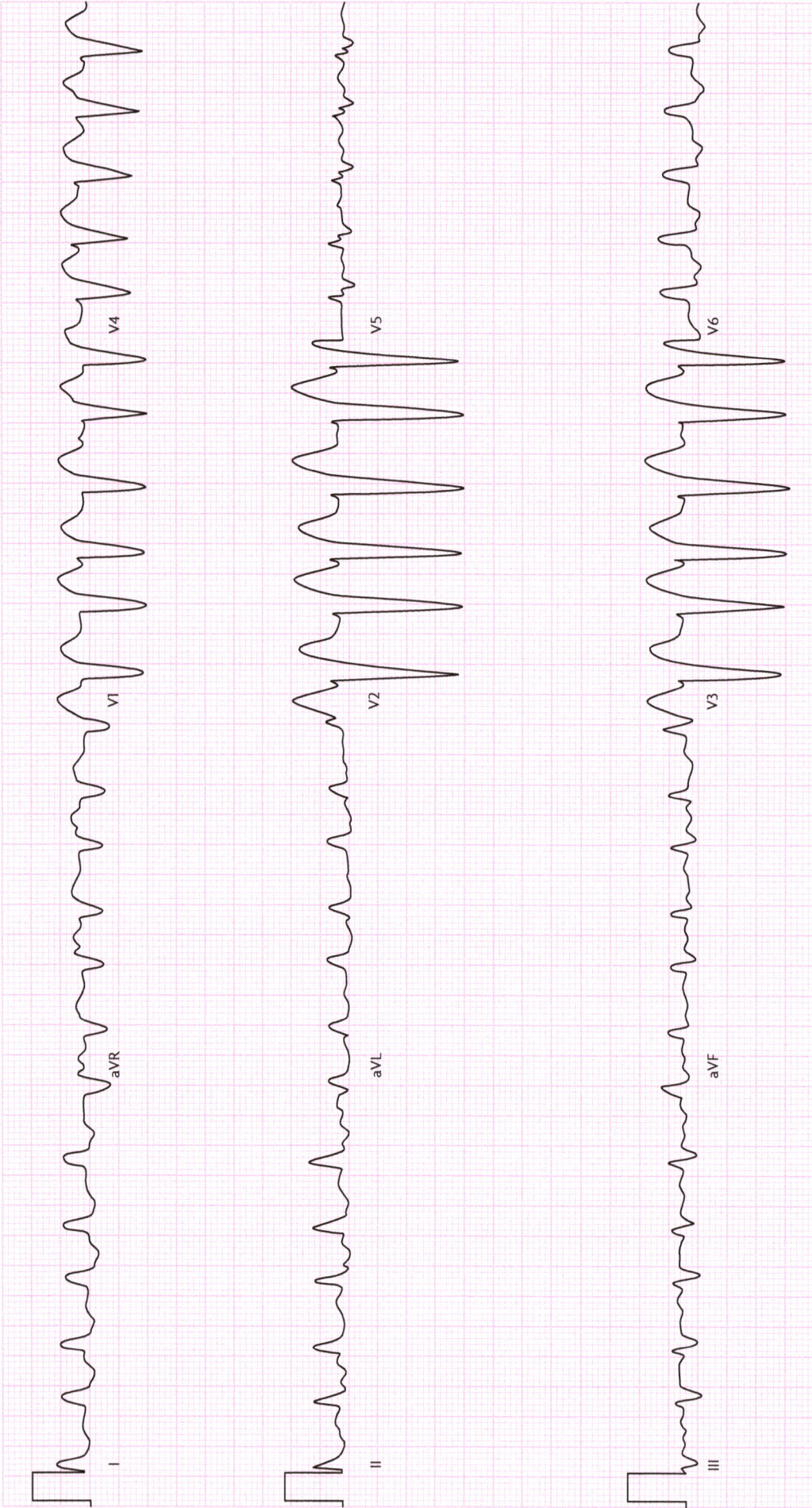

I

aVR

v1

v4

II

aVL

v2

v5

III

aVF

v3

v6

Practice ECG 5.6

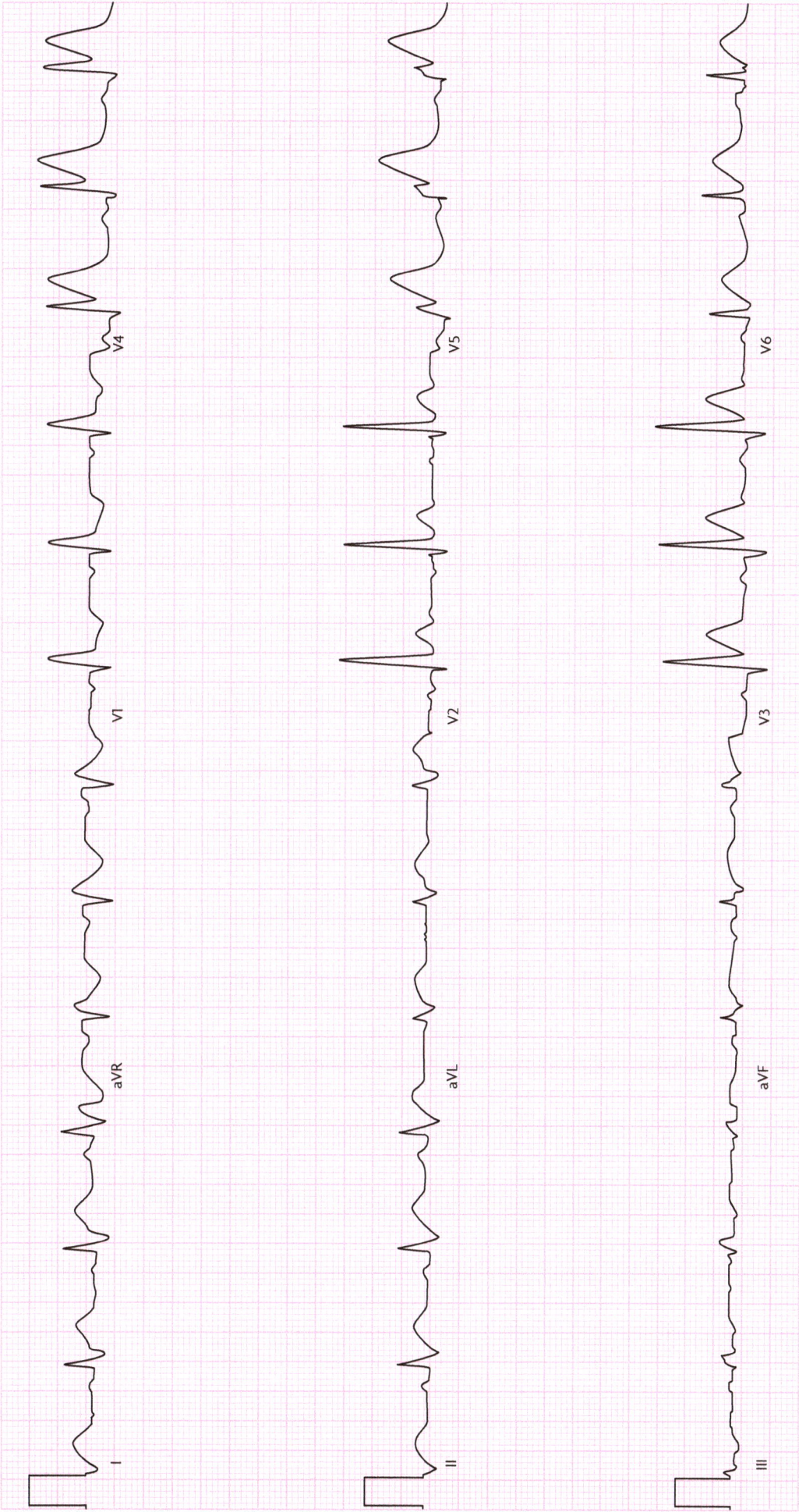

I

aVR

V1

V4

II

aVL

V2

V5

III

aVF

V3

V6

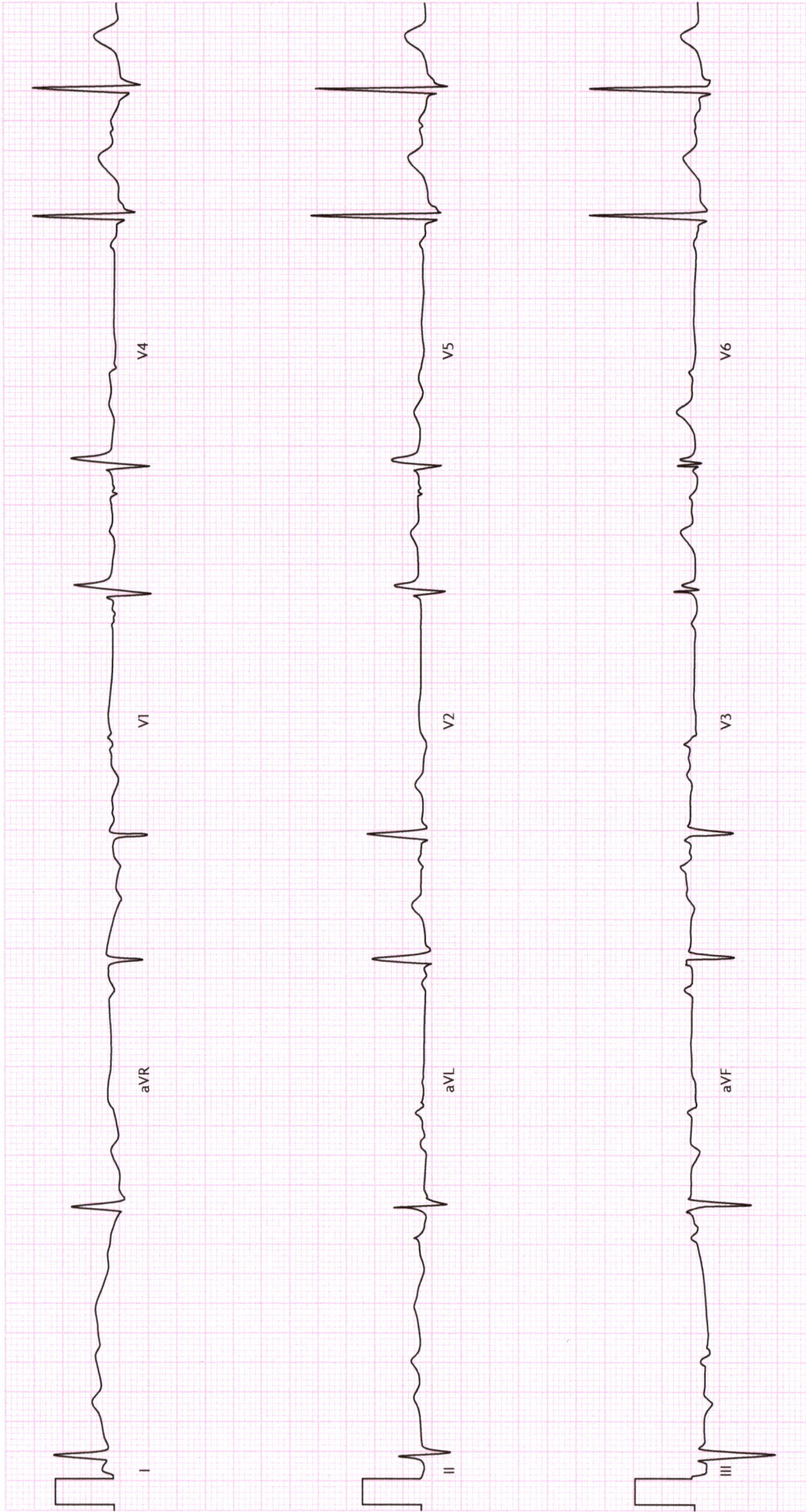

Practice ECG 5.8

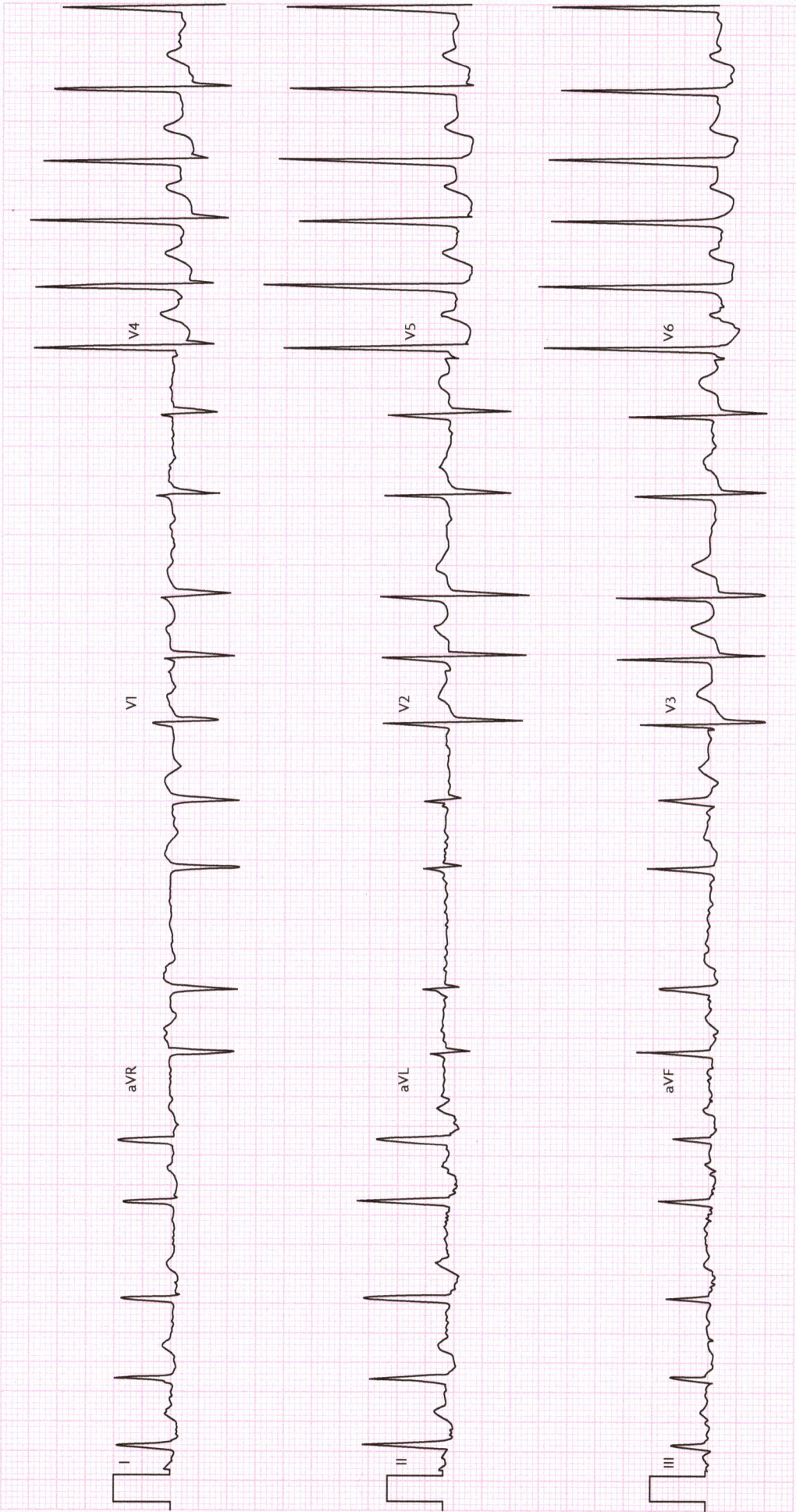

I

II

III

aVR

aVL

aVF

V1

V2

V3

V4

V5

V6

Practice ECG 5.9

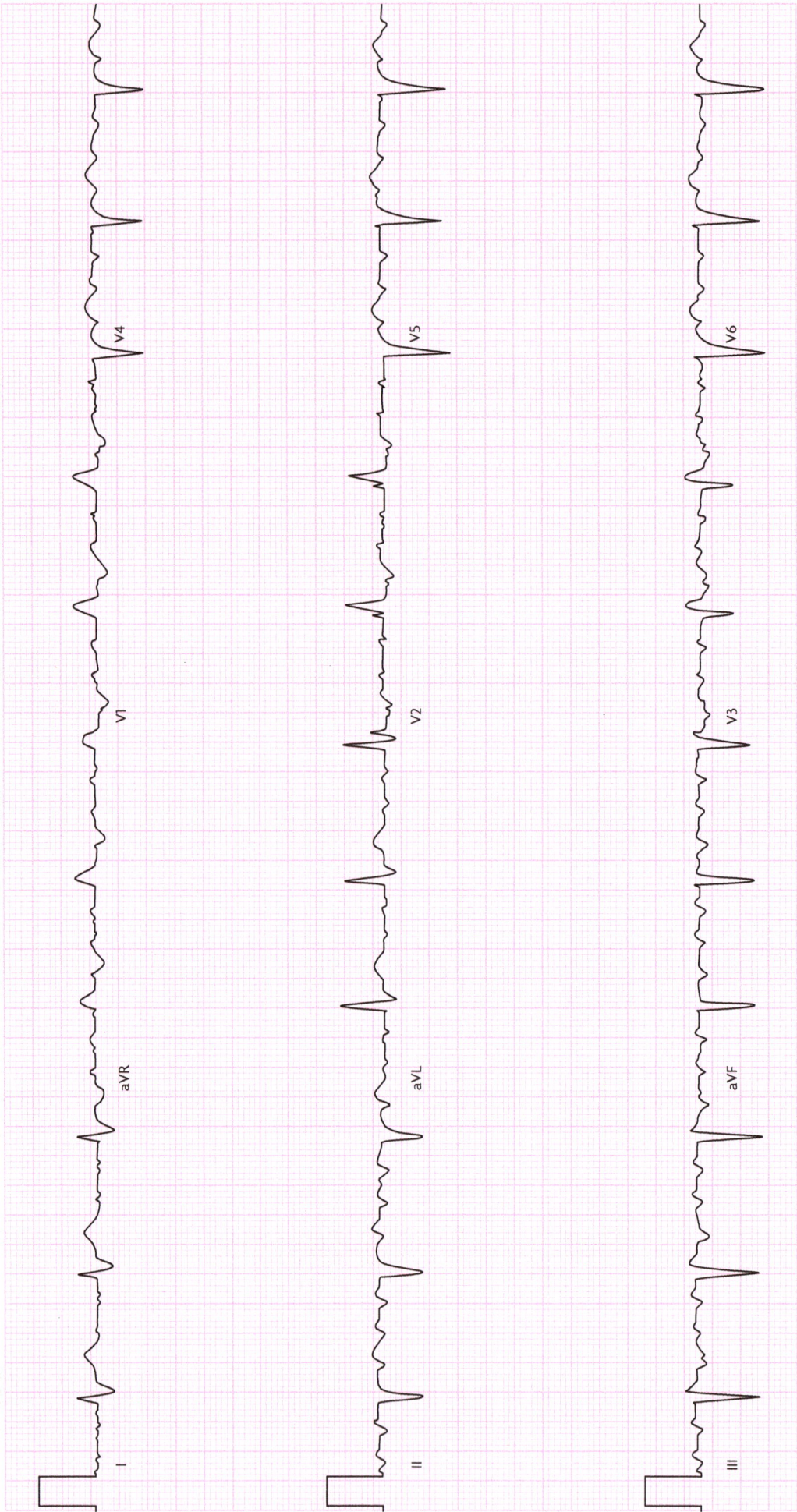

Practice ECG 5.10

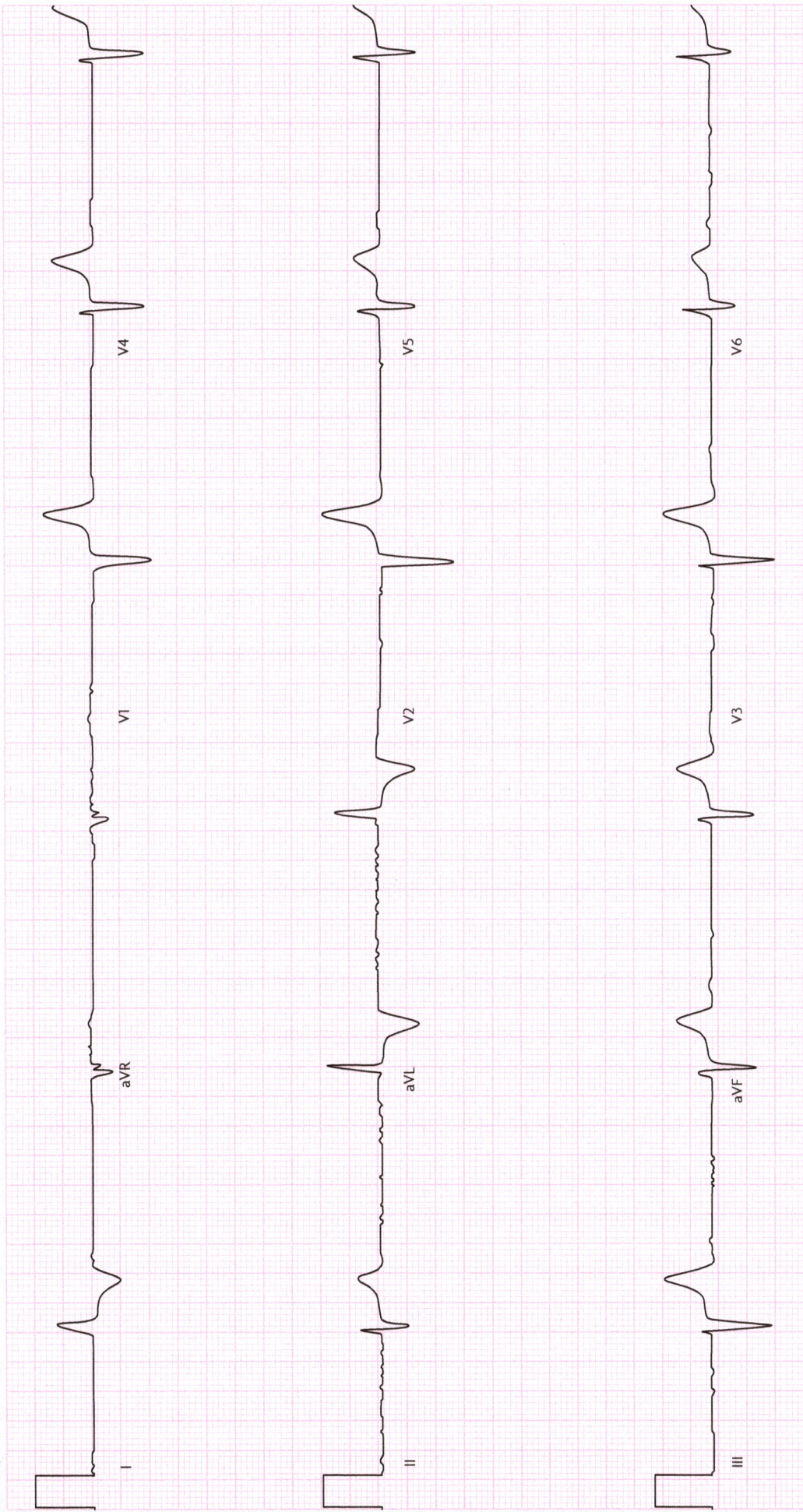

I

II

III

aVR

aVL

aVF

V1

V2

V3

V4

V5

V6

Practice ECG Answers

Set 1

Practice ECG 1.1 Couplets.

Practice ECG 1.2 Idioventricular rhythm.

Practice ECG 1.3 2nd degree type 2 AV block.

Practice ECG 1.4 Premature atrial contraction.

Practice ECG 1.5 Multifocal PVCs.

Practice ECG 1.6 Premature junctional contraction.

Practice ECG 1.7 Junctional rhythm.

Practice ECG 1.8 2nd degree type 1 AV block.

Practice ECG 1.9 Sinus rhythm.

Practice ECG 1.10 Multifocal atrial tachycardia.

Set 2

Practice ECG 2.1 Sinus bradycardia.

Practice ECG 2.2 Sinus tachycardia.

Practice ECG 2.3 Ventricular tachycardia.

Practice ECG 2.4 Atrial fibrillation.

Practice ECG 2.5 3rd degree AV block.

Practice ECG 2.6 Long QT syndrome.

Practice ECG 2.7 Trigeminy.

Practice ECG 2.8 Atrial fibrillation.

Practice ECG 2.9 Unifocal premature ventricular contraction.

Practice ECG 2.10 Ventricular fibrillation with pacing spikes visible.

Set 3

Practice ECG 3.1 STEMI anterior lateral.

Practice ECG 3.2 Sinus rhythm with PVC.

Practice ECG 3.3 Junctional rhythm.

Practice ECG 3.4 1st degree AV block.

Practice ECG 3.5 Atrial flutter.

Practice ECG 3.6 Accelerated idioventricular rhythm.

Practice ECG 3.7 Left bundle branch block.

Practice ECG 3.8 STEMI inferior with signs of posterior.

Practice ECG 3.9 Bigeminy.

Practice ECG 3.10 Wolff-Parkinson-White syndrome.

Set 4

Practice ECG 4.1 STEMI inferior lateral (with PAC).

Practice ECG 4.2 Left anterior fascicular block.

Practice ECG 4.3 STEMI inferior with signs of posterior.

Practice ECG 4.4 STEMI anterior.

Practice ECG 4.5 Bifascicular block.

Practice ECG 4.6 Hyperkalaemia and tachycardia.

Practice ECG 4.7 Brugada.

Practice ECG 4.8 Bigeminy.

Practice ECG 4.9 Trifascicular block.

Practice ECG 4.10 Right ventricular strain pattern S1 Q3 T3.

Set 5

Practice ECG 5.1 STEMI inferior and bradycardia.

Practice ECG 5.2 Multifocal atrial tachycardia.

Practice ECG 5.3 Right bundle branch block and ST segment depression.

Practice ECG 5.4 STEMI inferior and 2nd degree type 1 AV block.

Practice ECG 5.5 Left bundle branch block and atrial fibrillation.

Practice ECG 5.6 STEMI anterior and right bundle branch block.

Practice ECG 5.7 Incomplete right bundle branch block and 2nd degree type 2 AV block.

Practice ECG 5.8 Atrial fibrillation with rapid ventricular response and ST segment depression.

Practice ECG 5.9 Right bundle branch block and atrial flutter.

Practice ECG 5.10 Junctional rhythm in absolute bradycardia with hyperkalaemia.

Case Scenarios Set 1

Case Scenario 4.1.1	64-year-old male, collapsed

You are called to an office building for Vincent, who has reportedly collapsed at work. When you arrive on site a member of staff meets you and takes you to where Vincent collapsed, on the 12th floor. In the lift the member of staff tells you that Vincent was in a meeting when he became 'white as a sheet' and started to sweat profusely. He slumped in his chair and 'sort of half fell asleep'. They could not get any sense out of him; he quietly mumbled if they asked him anything.

You arrive in the conference room to find it empty but for Vincent, a first aider and one of Vincent's colleagues. Vincent is lying in the recovery position; he is indeed semi-conscious and unable to answer any questions. There is little more history to be obtained; what little you have has been given by his colleague.

Past medical history: *Unknown, although they believe he does have some medical history as he takes medication at work and has missed some days of work in recent years for hospital and doctors' appointments.*

Medication: *Simvastatin, aspirin, GTN (glyceryl trinitrate) spray, nicotine patches and gum are all found in his work bag, along with half a packet of cigarettes.*

Allergies: *Unknown*

Social history: *Lives alone, leaves the office several times a day to smoke although trying to give up. Appears overweight.*

Family history: *Unknown.*

Review of systems: *Unable.*

Examination: *Slow and weak radial pulse. Cold, clammy skin.*

Clinical Observations

SpO$_2$	%	EtCO$_2$	kPa	NIBP	mmHg	T°	Blood Glucose	GCS
			6.1		87			12
	94	RR	14	(58)	43	35.9°C	7.9 mmol/l	(E3 / S3 / M6)

Questions

a) What are your differential diagnoses for Vincent?
b) Use the 9-step ECG interpretation tool to assess Vincent's ECG.
c) What rhythm is the ECG?
d) What is your working diagnosis?

ECG Steps	Remember to look at every ECG lead view, not just lead II
1	What is the rate and rhythm?
2	Are there any P waves and what is their relationship with the QRS complex?
3	What is the duration and morphology of the QRS complex?
4	Is the ST segment isoelectric, depressed or elevated?
5	Are the QT intervals and T waves normal?

Clinical Steps	
6	Is the heart generating a palpable pulse of appropriate rate and providing adequate perfusion?
7	Is the rhythm unstable and at risk of deterioration?
8	Does the presenting rhythm support or change your working diagnosis?
9	Are any clinical interventions required?

Case Scenario ECG 4.1.1

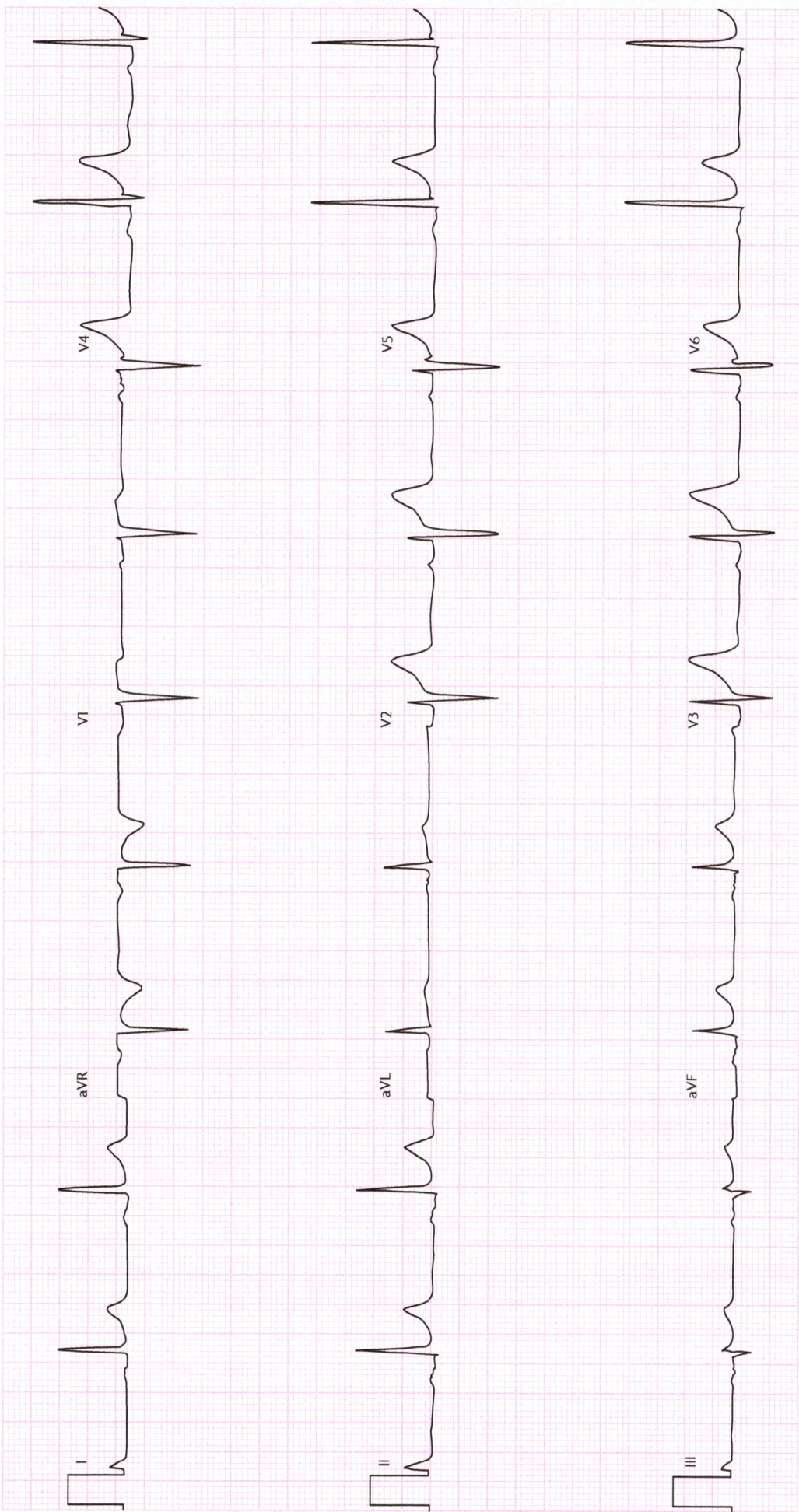

Case Scenario 4.1.2	62-year-old female with palpitations

Prisha has been experiencing intermittent palpitations for several days. Today they have lasted longer than before and she has started to feel anxious, short of breath and as if she is going to pass out. She describes the feeling as being 'as though her heart is racing, even though she is sitting still'. You note that Prisha appears to be very anxious and distressed, and is breathing rapidly.

Past medical history: *Anxiety, high cholesterol.*

Medication: *Aspirin, simvastatin.*

Allergies: *None*

Social history: *Lives with husband and three adult children, does not drink alcohol, smoke or use illicit drugs. Is a stay-at-home parent.*

Family history: *Father died of heart attack at 53, older brother survived heart attack at 47.*

Review of systems: *No chest pain or discomfort, no abdominal pain, no back pain, no difficulty breathing.*

Examination: *Rapid and regular radial pulse. Good, clear air entry on auscultation of lungs.*

Clinical Observations

SpO$_2$	%	EtCO$_2$	kPa	NIBP	mmHg	T°	Blood Glucose	GCS
	99	RR	5.1 / 28	(85)	118 / 69	36.7°C	7.6 mmol/l	15 (E4 / S5 / M6)

Questions

a) What are your differential diagnoses for Prisha?
b) Use the 9-step ECG interpretation tool to assess Prisha's ECG.
c) What rhythm is the ECG?
d) What is your working diagnosis?

ECG Steps
Remember to look at every ECG lead view, not just lead II

1	What is the rate and rhythm?
2	Are there any P waves and what is their relationship with the QRS complex?
3	What is the duration and morphology of the QRS complex?
4	Is the ST segment isoelectric, depressed or elevated?
5	Are the QT intervals and T waves normal?

Clinical Steps

6	Is the heart generating a palpable pulse of appropriate rate and providing adequate perfusion?
7	Is the rhythm unstable and at risk of deterioration?
8	Does the presenting rhythm support or change your working diagnosis?
9	Are any clinical interventions required?

Case Scenario ECG 4.1.2

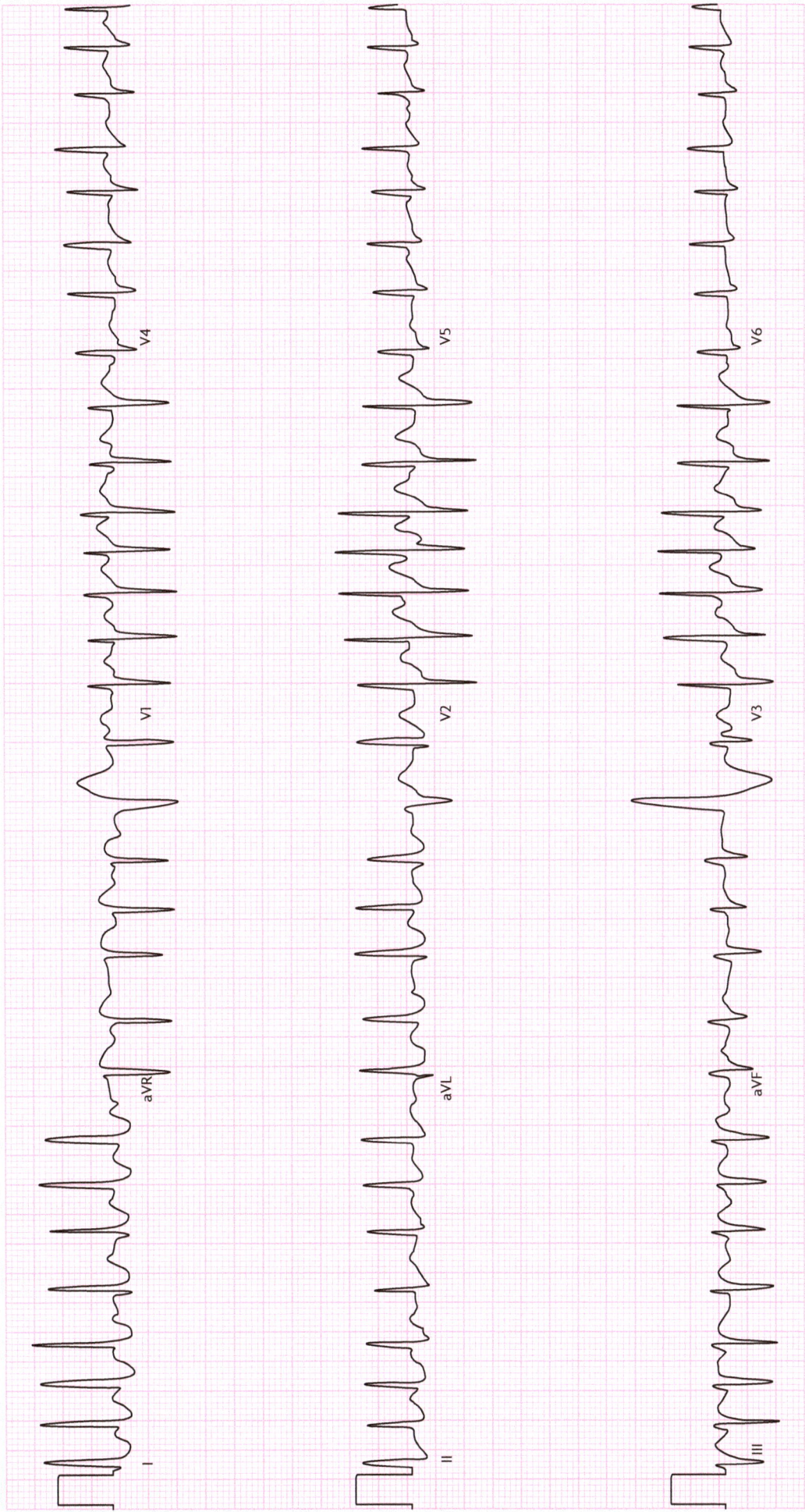

I aVR V1 V4

II aVL V2 V5

III aVF V3 V6

Case Scenario 4.1.3	21-year-old male, fall while cycling

21-year-old Pedro was riding his bicycle home from work and rushing to try and beat his personal best. Pedro swerved to avoid a pedestrian who had stepped into the road, causing Pedro to lose control and fall from his bike.

A non-paramedic crew arrived at the scene and found Pedro still lying in the road where he had fallen. His left lower leg is clearly fractured. He is in a lot of pain; he scores it as 9/10 and is very distressed. No other injuries are found except for some minor abrasions to his hands. The crew have called for paramedic support for pain relief. While waiting for your arrival they have obtained an ECG.

Past medical history: *Usually well.*

Medication: *None.*

Allergies: *None.*

Social history: *Lives with flatmates from university. Currently in his final year. Drinks regularly and smokes occasionally at weekends. No illicit drug use. Pedro is trying to lose weight and get fitter by cycling. He is moderately overweight.*

Family history: *Mother survived breast cancer five years ago. Father in poor health due to obesity.*

Review of systems: *Nothing identified.*

Examination: *Radial pulse present, regular and strong. Obvious fracture to left lower leg. No other injuries or concerns identified on primary and secondary survey.*

Clinical Observations

SpO$_2$	%	EtCO$_2$	kPa	NIBP	mmHg	T°	Blood Glucose	GCS
			5.2		141			15
	99	RR	24	(109)	93	35.9°C	5.2 mmol/l	(E4 / S5 / M6)

Questions

a) **Use the 9-step ECG interpretation tool to assess Pedro's ECG.**
b) **What rhythm is the ECG?**

ECG Steps	Remember to look at every ECG lead view, not just lead II
1	What is the rate and rhythm?
2	Are there any P waves and what is their relationship with the QRS complex?
3	What is the duration and morphology of the QRS complex?
4	Is the ST segment isoelectric, depressed or elevated?
5	Are the QT intervals and T waves normal?

Clinical Steps	
6	Is the heart generating a palpable pulse of appropriate rate and providing adequate perfusion?
7	Is the rhythm unstable and at risk of deterioration?
8	Does the presenting rhythm support or change your working diagnosis?
9	Are any clinical interventions required?

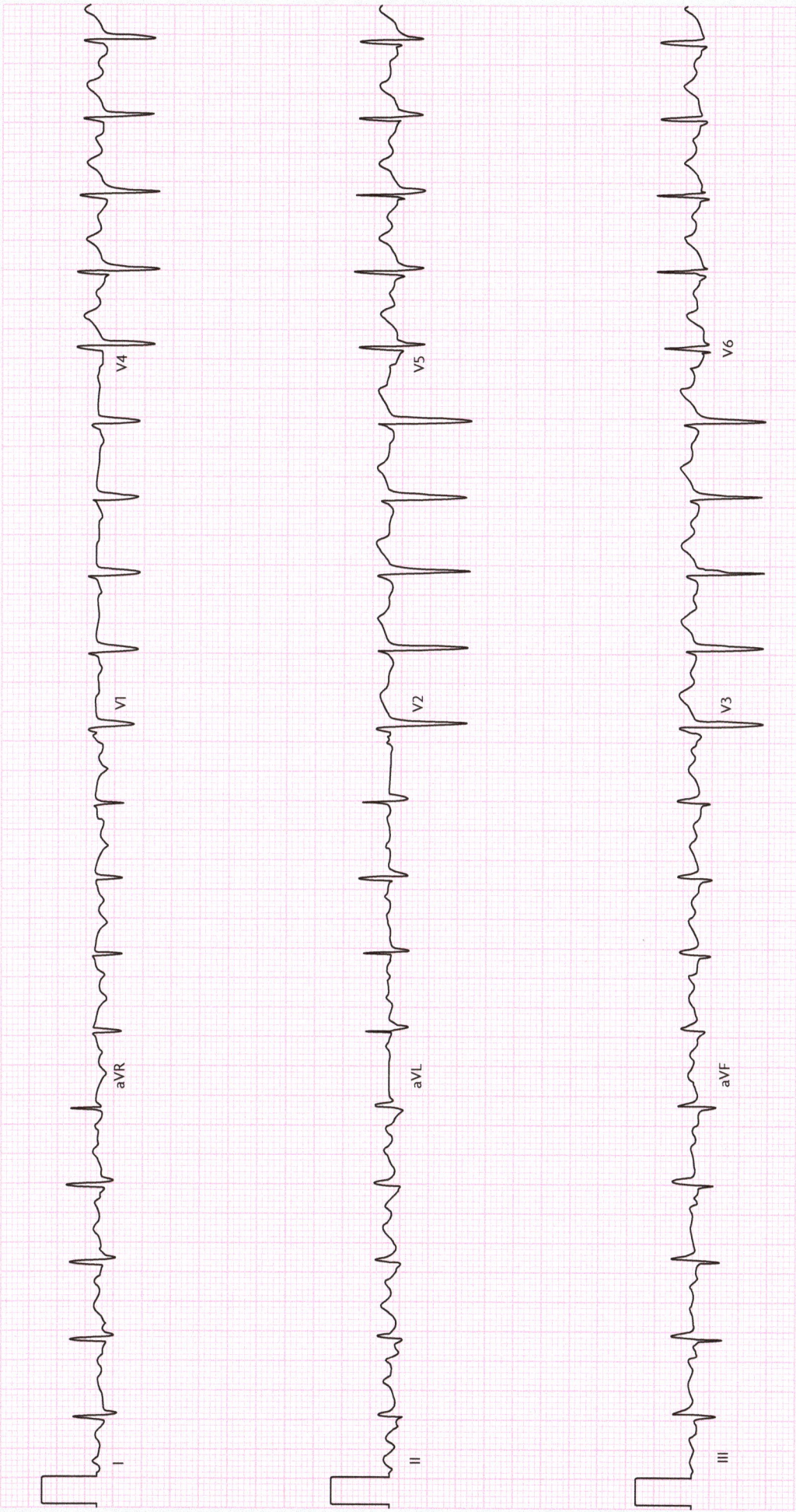

Case Scenario ECG 4.1.3

Case Scenario 4.1.4   52-year-old female, collapsed

Karen has been found by her colleagues in a collapsed state at work. She is in the bathroom and was last seen about 30 minutes ago. Colleagues say she appeared to be well and didn't complain of anything when they last saw her. She appears to have been incontinent of urine and has irregular respirations.

Past medical history: *Unknown.*

Medication: *Unknown.*

Allergies: *Unknown.*

Social history: *Unknown.*

Family history: *Unknown.*

Review of systems: *Unable.*

Examination: *Irregular radial pulse. Irregular respirations.*

Clinical Observations

SpO$_2$	%	EtCO$_2$	kPa	NIBP	mmHg
			6.2		209
	96	RR	14	(148)	117

T°	Blood Glucose	GCS
35.9°C	6.6 mmol/l	5 (E1 / S1 / M3)

Questions

a) **What are your differential diagnoses for Karen?**
b) **Use the 9-step ECG interpretation tool to assess Karen's ECG.**
c) **What rhythm is the ECG?**
d) **What is your working diagnosis?**

ECG Steps   Remember to look at every ECG lead view, not just lead II

1	What is the rate and rhythm?
2	Are there any P waves and what is their relationship with the QRS complex?
3	What is the duration and morphology of the QRS complex?
4	Is the ST segment isoelectric, depressed or elevated?
5	Are the QT intervals and T waves normal?

Clinical Steps

6	Is the heart generating a palpable pulse of appropriate rate and providing adequate perfusion?
7	Is the rhythm unstable and at risk of deterioration?
8	Does the presenting rhythm support or change your working diagnosis?
9	Are any clinical interventions required?

Case Scenario ECG 4.1.4

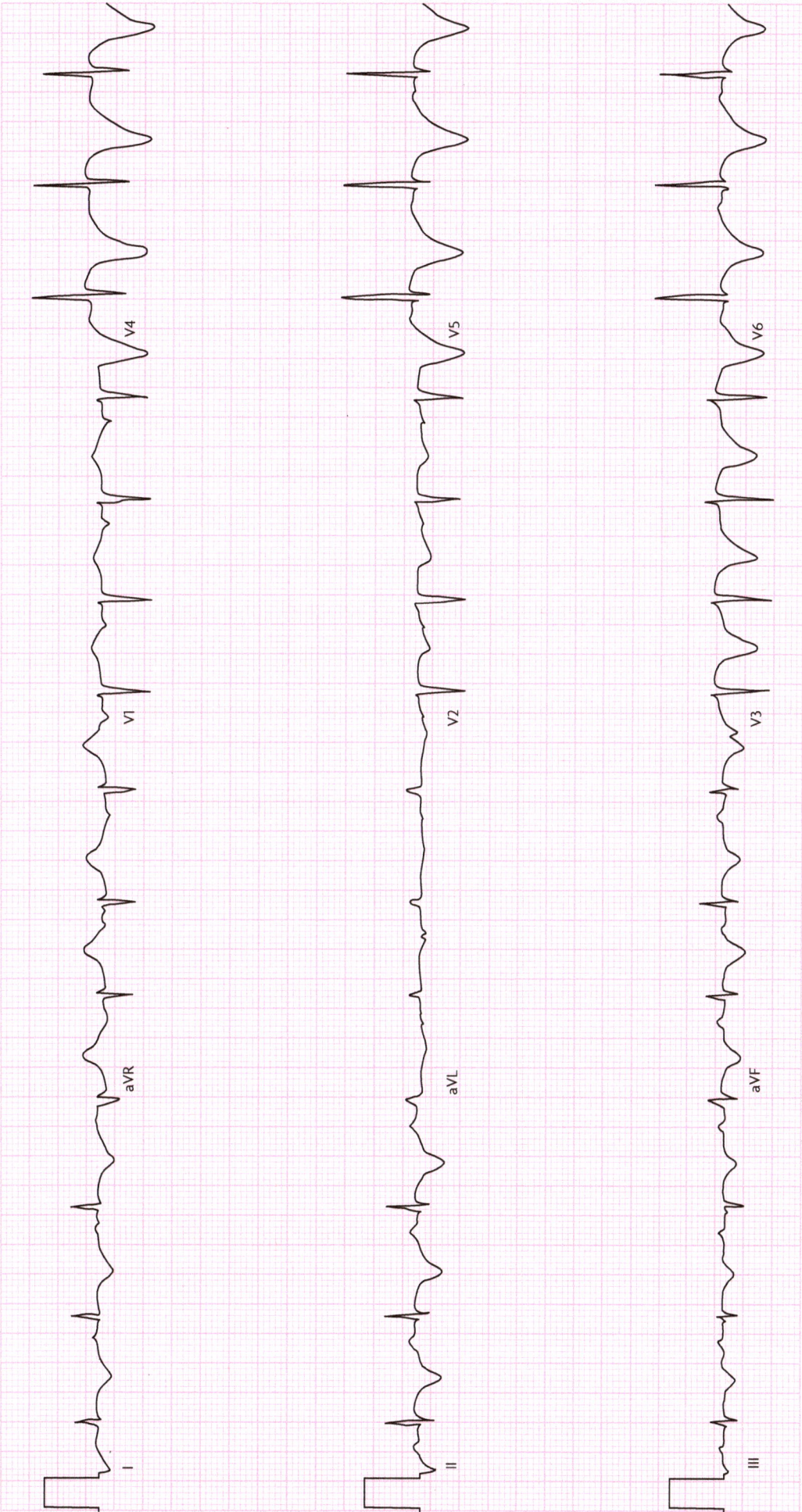

Case Scenario 4.1.5	23-year-old female having seizure

Marta was attending an appointment at her GP practice for a 12-lead ECG as she has been experiencing short episodes of palpitations over recent weeks. During the appointment she experienced palpitations and became unresponsive, with several seconds of what the nurse reported as 'seizure-like activity'. She has now recovered and is feeling fine. She states that she cannot remember quite what happened today.

The nurse managed to capture an ECG whilst Marta was unresponsive.

Past medical history: *None.*

Medication: *None.*

Allergies: *None.*

Social history: *Lives with flatmates. Works as a barista whilst studying for her master's degree. She does not drink alcohol, smoke or use illicit drugs.*

Family history: *Mother, father and older brother are all well, unsure what caused her grandparents' deaths.*

Review of systems: *No chest pain or discomfort, no abdominal pain, no back pain, no difficulty breathing.*

Examination: *Regular radial pulse.*

Clinical Observations

SpO₂	%	EtCO₂	kPa	NIBP	mmHg
			5.0		115
	100	RR	20	(80)	63

T°	Blood Glucose	GCS
36.4°C	6.9 mmol/l	15 (E4 / S5 / M6)

Questions

a) What are your differential diagnoses for Marta?
b) Use the 9-step ECG interpretation tool to assess Marta's ECG.
c) What rhythm is the ECG?
d) What is your working diagnosis?

ECG Steps

Remember to look at every ECG lead view, not just lead II

1	What is the rate and rhythm?
2	Are there any P waves and what is their relationship with the QRS complex?
3	What is the duration and morphology of the QRS complex?
4	Is the ST segment isoelectric, depressed or elevated?
5	Are the QT intervals and T waves normal?

Clinical Steps

6	Is the heart generating a palpable pulse of appropriate rate and providing adequate perfusion?
7	Is the rhythm unstable and at risk of deterioration?
8	Does the presenting rhythm support or change your working diagnosis?
9	Are any clinical interventions required?

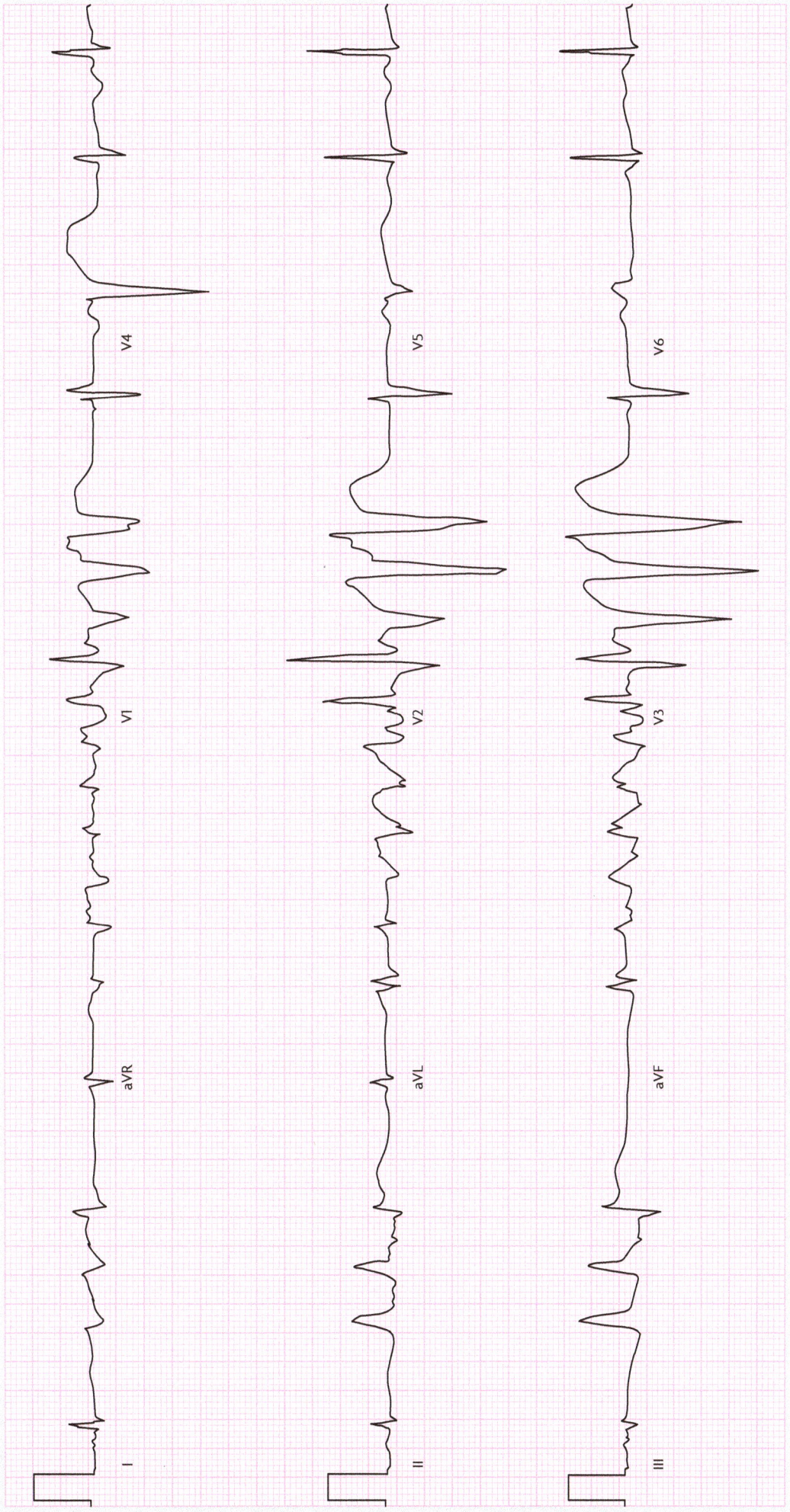

Case Scenarios Set 2

Case Scenario 4.2.1	17-year-old female with breathing difficulties

Alisha was on her way to college when she started to feel anxious, have palpitations and feel as if she couldn't breathe. Initially, she went to the bathroom to sit down but then started to feel faint. A teacher found her and took her to the first aid room, where she is now semi-recumbent on the couch. Alisha describes her palpitations as though her heart is racing and going to 'jump out of her chest'. Her breathing feels a little better now that she is sitting but she still feels short of breath and anxious.

Past medical history: *None.*

Medication: *None.*

Allergies: *None.*

Social history: *Lives with parents and younger brother, does not drink alcohol, smoke or use illicit drugs. Studying for her final year of college, with exams approaching.*

Family history: *Mother and father both well.*

Review of systems: *No chest pain or discomfort, no abdominal pain, no back pain, no difficulty breathing.*

Examination: *Rapid and regular radial pulse.*

Clinical Observations

SpO$_2$	%	EtCO$_2$	kPa	NIBP	mmHg		T$^\circ$	Blood Glucose	GCS
	100	RR	4.9 25	(75)	101 62		36.5°C	6.6 mmol/l	15 (E4 / S5 / M6)

Questions

a) What are your differential diagnoses for Alisha?
b) Use the 9-step ECG interpretation tool to assess Alisha's ECG.
c) What rhythm is the ECG?
d) What is your working diagnosis?

ECG Steps	Remember to look at every ECG lead view, not just lead II
1	What is the rate and rhythm?
2	Are there any P waves and what is their relationship with the QRS complex?
3	What is the duration and morphology of the QRS complex?
4	Is the ST segment isoelectric, depressed or elevated?
5	Are the QT intervals and T waves normal?

Clinical Steps	
6	Is the heart generating a palpable pulse of appropriate rate and providing adequate perfusion?
7	Is the rhythm unstable and at risk of deterioration?
8	Does the presenting rhythm support or change your working diagnosis?
9	Are any clinical interventions required?

Case Scenario ECG 4.2.1

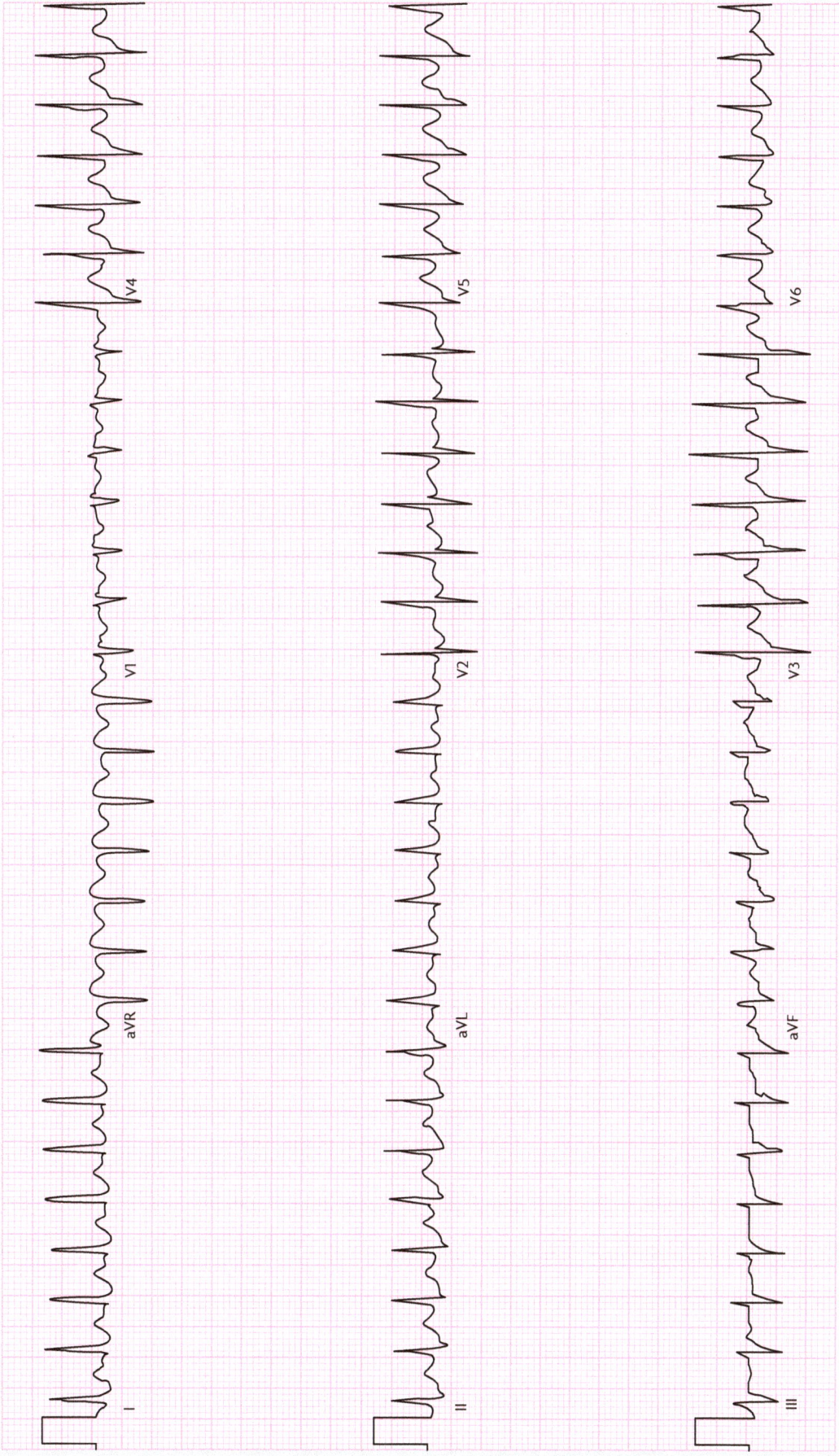

aVR   V1   V4

aVL   V2   V5

aVF   V3   V6

I

II

III

Case Scenario 4.2.2 — 31-year-old male with chest pain

Harry has recovered from a viral respiratory infection in the last few days. He has, however, been feeling worse again since yesterday. For the last four hours he has developed worsening, sharp chest pain in the centre of his chest. He scores the pain as 6/10. It also radiates to his back. He was feeling feverish during the night.

Past medical history: *None.*

Medication: *None.*

Allergies: *None.*

Social history: *Lives alone, does not drink alcohol, smoke or use illicit drugs. Works as a personal trainer. Exercises regularly and eats a healthy diet.*

Family history: *Mother, father and older sister all well.*

Review of systems: *No palpitations, no abdominal pain, no difficulty breathing, no nausea or vomiting, no diarrhoea or constipation, no urinary symptoms.*

Examination: *Rapid and regular radial pulse. Flushed and clammy. Pain worse when lying flat on his back. Lungs clear on auscultation.*

Clinical Observations

SpO$_2$	%	EtCO$_2$	kPa	NIBP	mmHg
			5.2		115
	96	RR	20	(84)	68

T$^°$	Blood Glucose	GCS
38.2°C	8.2 mmol/l	15 (E4 / S5 / M6)

Questions

a) **What are your differential diagnoses for Harry?**
b) **Use the 9-step ECG interpretation tool to assess Harry's ECG.**
c) **What rhythm is the ECG?**
d) **What is your working diagnosis?**

ECG Steps

Remember to look at every ECG lead view, not just lead II

1	**What is the rate and rhythm?**
2	**Are there any P waves and what is their relationship with the QRS complex?**
3	**What is the duration and morphology of the QRS complex?**
4	**Is the ST segment isoelectric, depressed or elevated?**
5	**Are the QT intervals and T waves normal?**

Clinical Steps

6	**Is the heart generating a palpable pulse of appropriate rate and providing adequate perfusion?**
7	**Is the rhythm unstable and at risk of deterioration?**
8	**Does the presenting rhythm support or change your working diagnosis?**
9	**Are any clinical interventions required?**

Case Scenario ECG 4.2.2

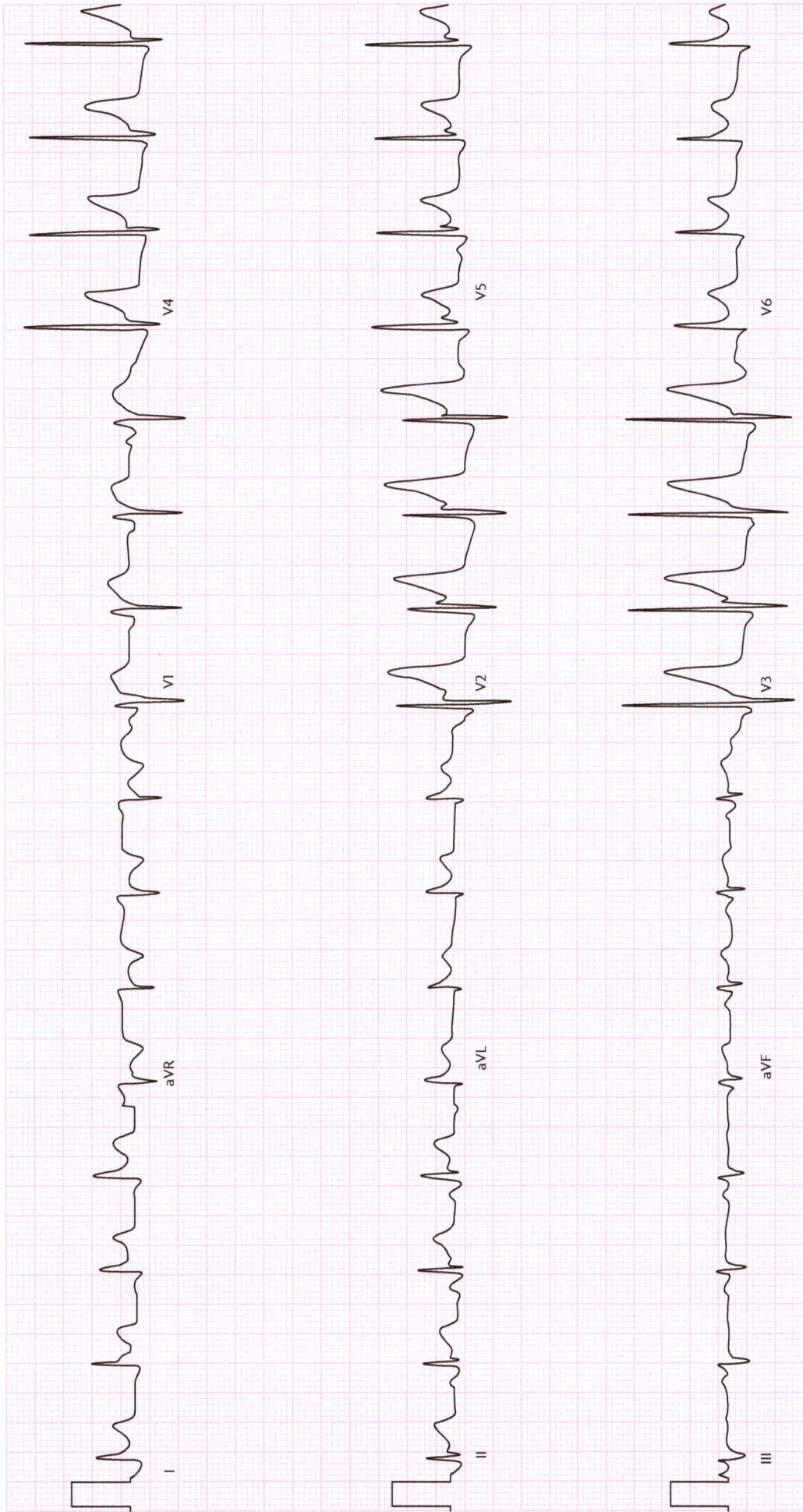

Case Scenario 4.2.3   19-year-old female with breathing difficulties

Melissa was at university when she started to feel anxious and short of breath. She started to experience pins and needles in her hands and feel dizzy. She feared she would pass out so she sat down in the corridor. A member of staff came to help her and called an ambulance.

When you arrive, Melissa is sitting in a private tutorial room with a first aider. She says she is already starting to feel better. She is no longer dizzy and the pins and needles have resolved as well. She still feels a little short of breath and anxious. She has been well recently with no illnesses. She is in her first year at university and exams are coming up.

Past medical history: *None.*

Medication: *None.*

Allergies: *None.*

Social history: *Lives in student accommodation. Drinks several alcoholic drinks several times a week, does not smoke or use illicit drugs.*

Family history: *Mother and father both well, no siblings.*

Review of systems: *No chest pain or discomfort, no palpitations, no abdominal pain, no back pain, no difficulty breathing. No recent illness.*

Examination: *Regular radial pulse. Flushed. Lungs clear on auscultation. Heart sounds S1+S2+0.*

Clinical Observations

SpO_2	%	$EtCO_2$	kPa	NIBP	mmHg	T°	Blood Glucose	GCS
			4.7		118	36.5°C	7.5 mmol/l	15
	100	RR	24	(85)	77			(E4 / S5 / M6)

Questions

a) **What are your differential diagnoses for Melissa?**
b) **Use the 9-step ECG interpretation tool to assess Melissa's ECG.**
c) **What rhythm is the ECG?**
d) **What is your working diagnosis?**

ECG Steps   Remember to look at every ECG lead view, not just lead II

1	What is the rate and rhythm?
2	Are there any P waves and what is their relationship with the QRS complex?
3	What is the duration and morphology of the QRS complex?
4	Is the ST segment isoelectric, depressed or elevated?
5	Are the QT intervals and T waves normal?

Clinical Steps

6	Is the heart generating a palpable pulse of appropriate rate and providing adequate perfusion?
7	Is the rhythm unstable and at risk of deterioration?
8	Does the presenting rhythm support or change your working diagnosis?
9	Are any clinical interventions required?

Case Scenario ECG 4.2.3

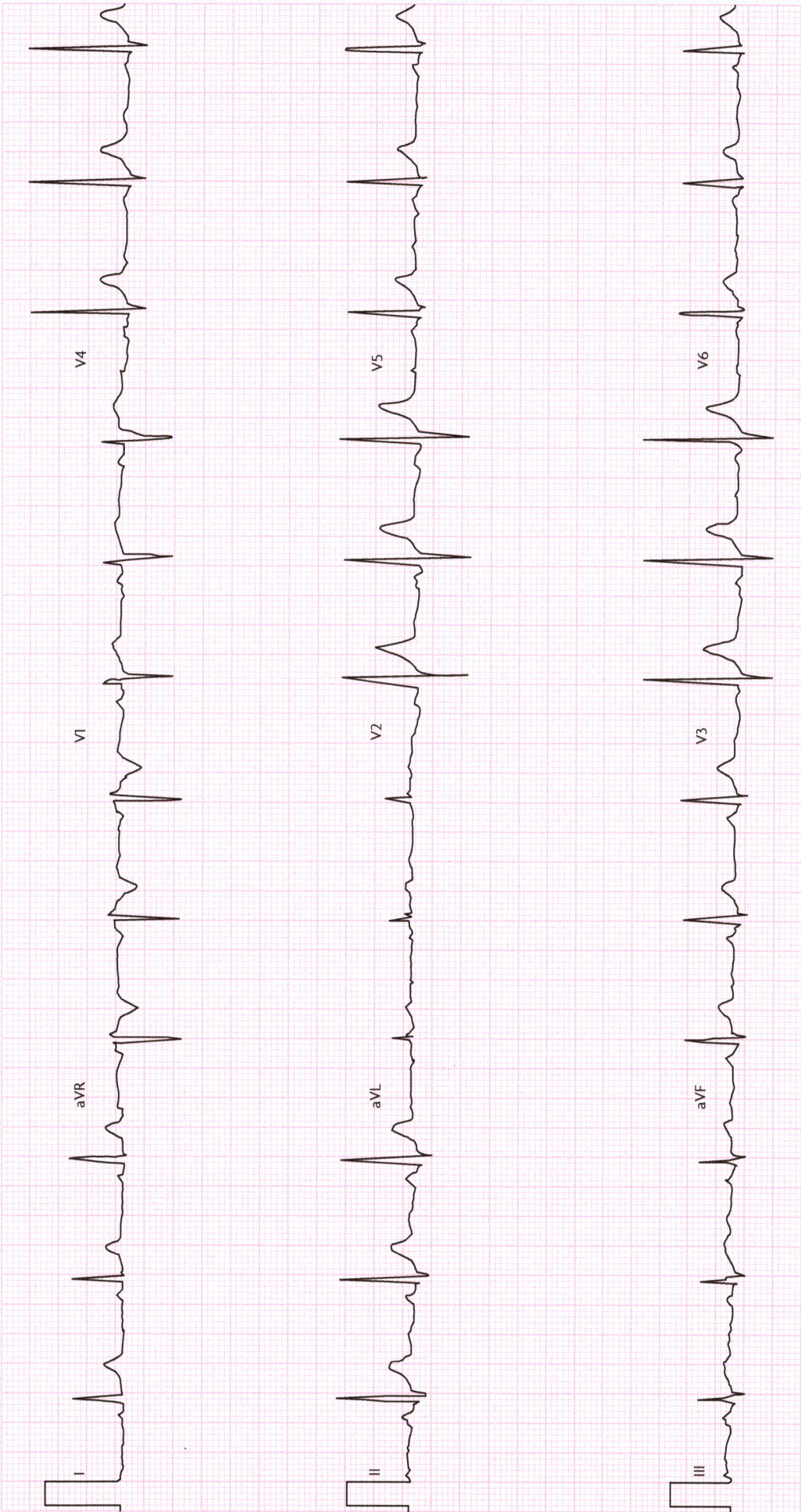

I aVR V1 V4

II aVL V2 V5

III aVF V3 V6

Case Scenario 4.2.4   27-year-old male, drug overdose

David has been under significant stress and anxiety in recent months and this all came to a head five days ago. He tells you that this caused him to go on a 'bender'; for three days in a row he drank alcohol and energy drinks to excess, used cocaine and hardly slept. This 'bender' ended yesterday; he has still hardly slept and feels terrible, both mentally and physically. He tells you that during the bender and since, he has been taking double doses of his anti-depressants, hoping that it would make him feel better. It has not. For the last four hours he has been experiencing palpitations, fatigue and shortness of breath. He says he thought it was an anxiety attack but when it didn't get better as it usually does he became more concerned.

Past medical history: *Anxiety, depression.*

Medication: *Amitriptyline.*

Allergies: *None*

Social history: *Lives alone, worked as an estate agent but was recently made redundant, binge drinks alcohol, smokes when drinking, uses cocaine several times a year.*

Family history: *He thinks mother and father are both well.*

Review of systems: *No chest pain or discomfort, no difficulty breathing.*

Examination: *Rapid and irregular radial pulse.*

Clinical Observations

SpO$_2$	%	EtCO$_2$	kPa	NIBP	mmHg
			5.4		139
	97	RR	20	(104)	87

T°	Blood Glucose	GCS
36.8°C	4.3 mmol/l	15 (E4 / S5 / M6)

Questions

a) Use the 9-step ECG interpretation tool to assess David's ECG.
b) What rhythm is the ECG?
c) What is your working diagnosis?

ECG Steps   Remember to look at every ECG lead view, not just lead II

1	What is the rate and rhythm?
2	Are there any P waves and what is their relationship with the QRS complex?
3	What is the duration and morphology of the QRS complex?
4	Is the ST segment isoelectric, depressed or elevated?
5	Are the QT intervals and T waves normal?

Clinical Steps

6	Is the heart generating a palpable pulse of appropriate rate and providing adequate perfusion?
7	Is the rhythm unstable and at risk of deterioration?
8	Does the presenting rhythm support or change your working diagnosis?
9	Are any clinical interventions required?

Case Scenario ECG 4.2.4

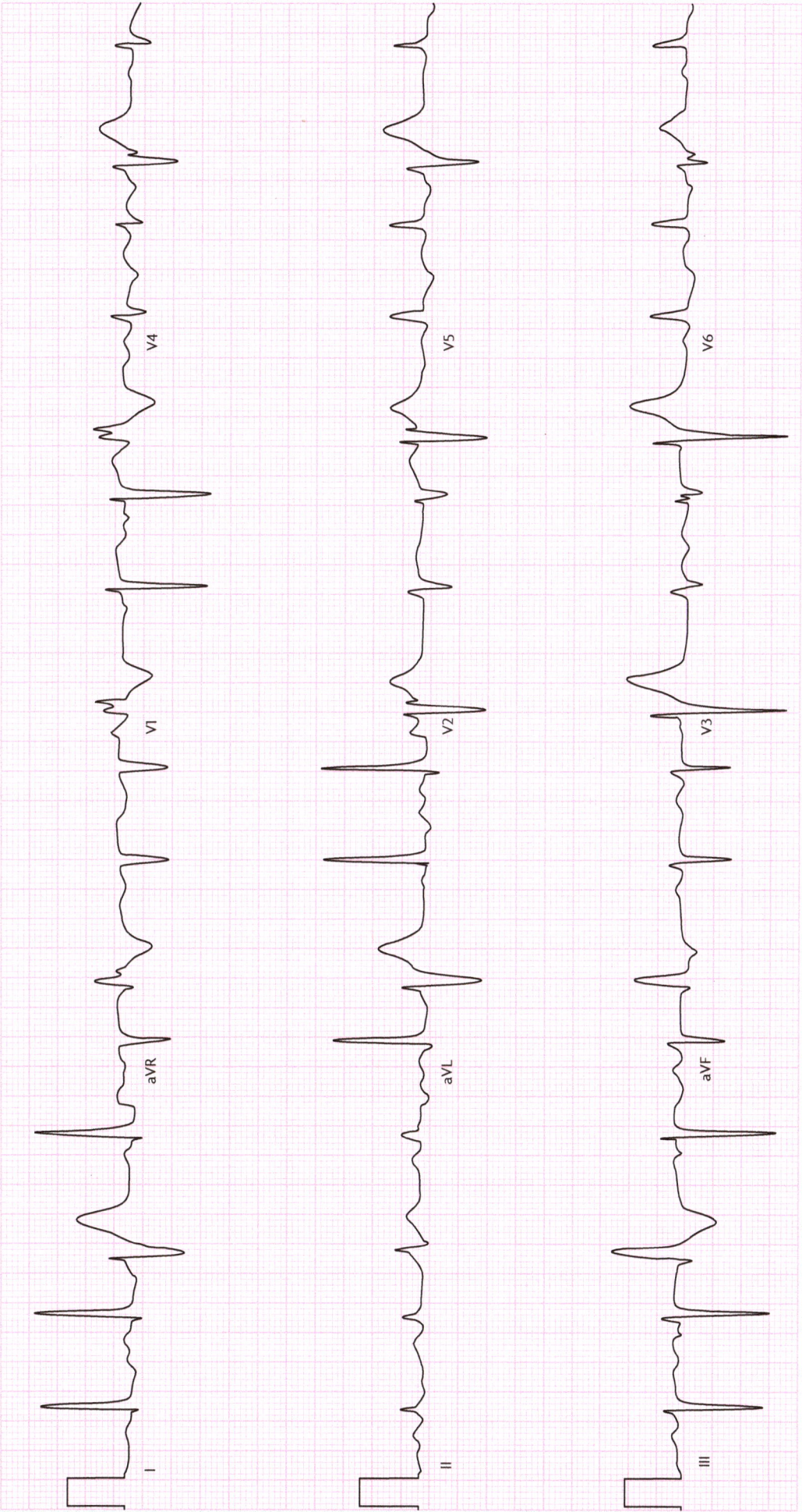

I

II

III

aVR

aVL

aVF

V1

V2

V3

V4

V5

V6

Case Scenario 4.2.5	32-year-old male with chest pain

Ali has experienced a sudden onset of chest pain whilst driving about 30 minutes ago. He has pulled into a lay-by and called for help. He describes his pain as a tight pressure across his chest. He scores it as 8/10 and says that it does not radiate anywhere. He also feels short of breath and anxious.

Past medical history: *None.*

Medication: *None.*

Allergies: *None.*

Social history: *Lives with his parents and younger siblings, does not drink alcohol, smoke or use illicit drugs.*

Family history: *Father has survived two MIs at age 36 and 45. Ali's older brother had an MI at age 40.*

Review of systems: *No palpitations, no abdominal pain, no back pain, no difficulty breathing.*

Examination: *Regular radial pulse. Pale and clammy.*

Clinical Observations

SpO$_2$	%	EtCO$_2$	kPa	NIBP	mmHg	T°	Blood Glucose	GCS
	97	RR	5.3 / 18	(99)	143 / 77	36.3°C	8.2 mmol/l	15 (E4 / S5 / M6)

Questions

a) What are your differential diagnoses for Ali?
b) Use the 9-step ECG interpretation tool to assess Ali's ECG.
c) What rhythm is the ECG?
d) What is your working diagnosis?

ECG Steps
Remember to look at every ECG lead view, not just lead II

1. What is the rate and rhythm?
2. Are there any P waves and what is their relationship with the QRS complex?
3. What is the duration and morphology of the QRS complex?
4. Is the ST segment isoelectric, depressed or elevated?
5. Are the QT intervals and T waves normal?

Clinical Steps

6. Is the heart generating a palpable pulse of appropriate rate and providing adequate perfusion?
7. Is the rhythm unstable and at risk of deterioration?
8. Does the presenting rhythm support or change your working diagnosis?
9. Are any clinical interventions required?

Case Scenario ECG 4.2.5

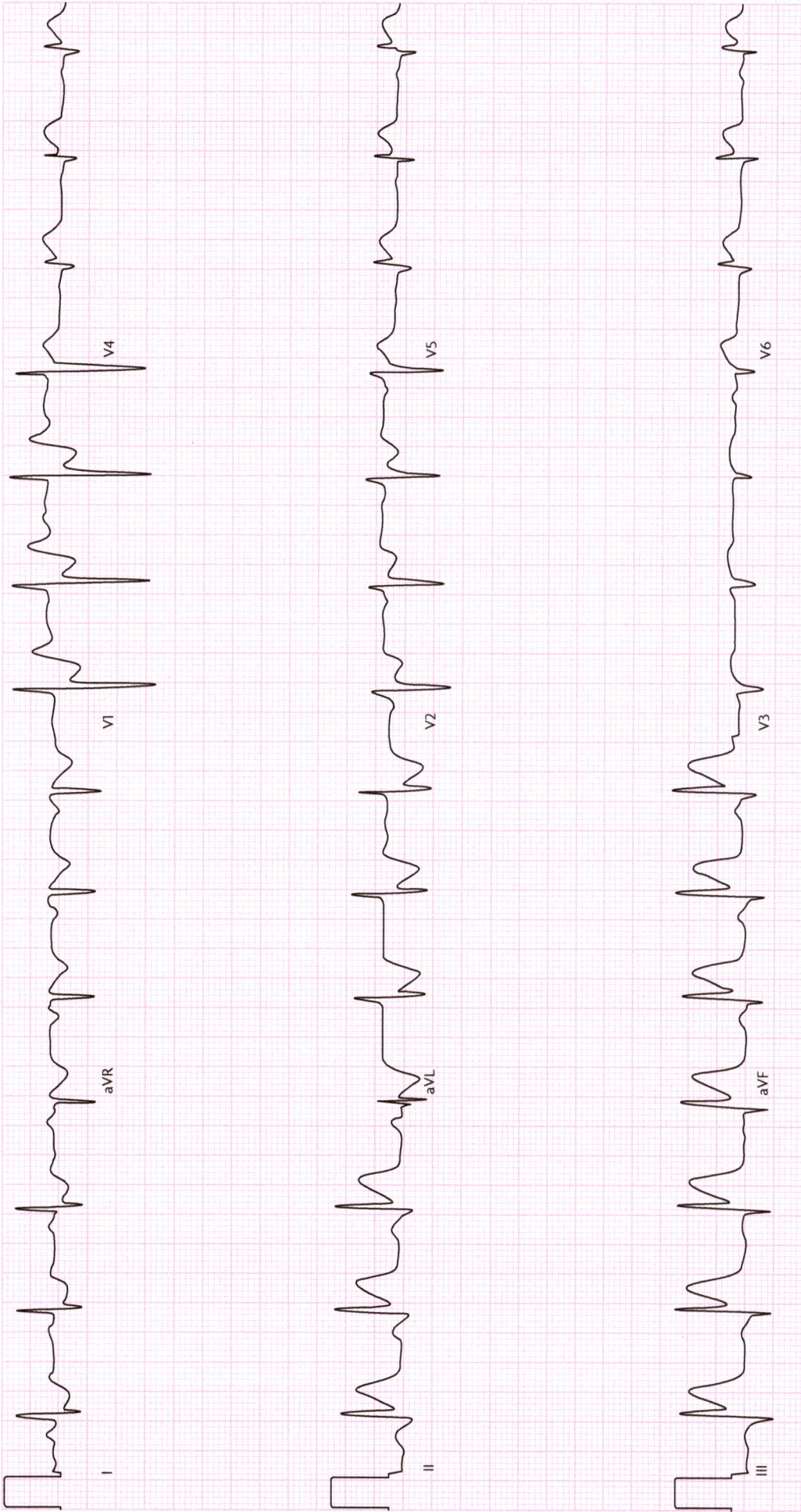

Case Scenarios Set 3

Case Scenario 4.3.1	89-year-old female with fatigue

Phyllis has been unwell for the last nine days. She is waiting for an appointment with her GP in two weeks' time. She has been feeling increasingly short of breath on exertion and struggling to climb the stairs to bed. For the last six nights she has slept sitting up in her chair downstairs; she says this feels more comfortable at the moment anyway. She has had a productive cough, with white/yellow sputum. She has also been feeling increasingly fatigued, spending a lot more time resting during the day.

Past medical history: *Osteoarthritis, stress incontinence, diverticular disease, age-related macular degeneration.*

Medication: *Ibuprofen, duloxetine.*

Allergies: *None.*

Social history: *Lives alone and is independent. Daughter lives nearby, visits regularly and helps with the weekly shop. Does not drink, smoke or use illicit drugs.*

Family history: *Parents died in old age; she cannot remember details.*

Review of systems: *No chest pain or discomfort, no palpitations, no back pain, no difficulty breathing, no current abdominal pain though did have upper epigastric pain 10 days ago lasting a few hours.*

Examination: *Regular radial pulse. Pale. Auscultation of lungs reveals bibasal crepitations.*

Clinical Observations

SpO$_2$	%	EtCO$_2$	kPa	NIBP	mmHg
			4.9		141
	94	RR	22	(106)	89

T°	Blood Glucose	GCS
36.6°C	6.5 mmol/l	15 (E4 / S5 / M6)

Questions

a) What are your differential diagnoses for Phyllis?
b) Use the 9-step ECG interpretation tool to assess Phyllis's ECG.
c) What rhythm is the ECG?
d) What is your working diagnosis?

ECG Steps	Remember to look at every ECG lead view, not just lead II
1	What is the rate and rhythm?
2	Are there any P waves and what is their relationship with the QRS complex?
3	What is the duration and morphology of the QRS complex?
4	Is the ST segment isoelectric, depressed or elevated?
5	Are the QT intervals and T waves normal?

Clinical Steps	
6	Is the heart generating a palpable pulse of appropriate rate and providing adequate perfusion?
7	Is the rhythm unstable and at risk of deterioration?
8	Does the presenting rhythm support or change your working diagnosis?
9	Are any clinical interventions required?

Case Scenario ECG 4.3.1

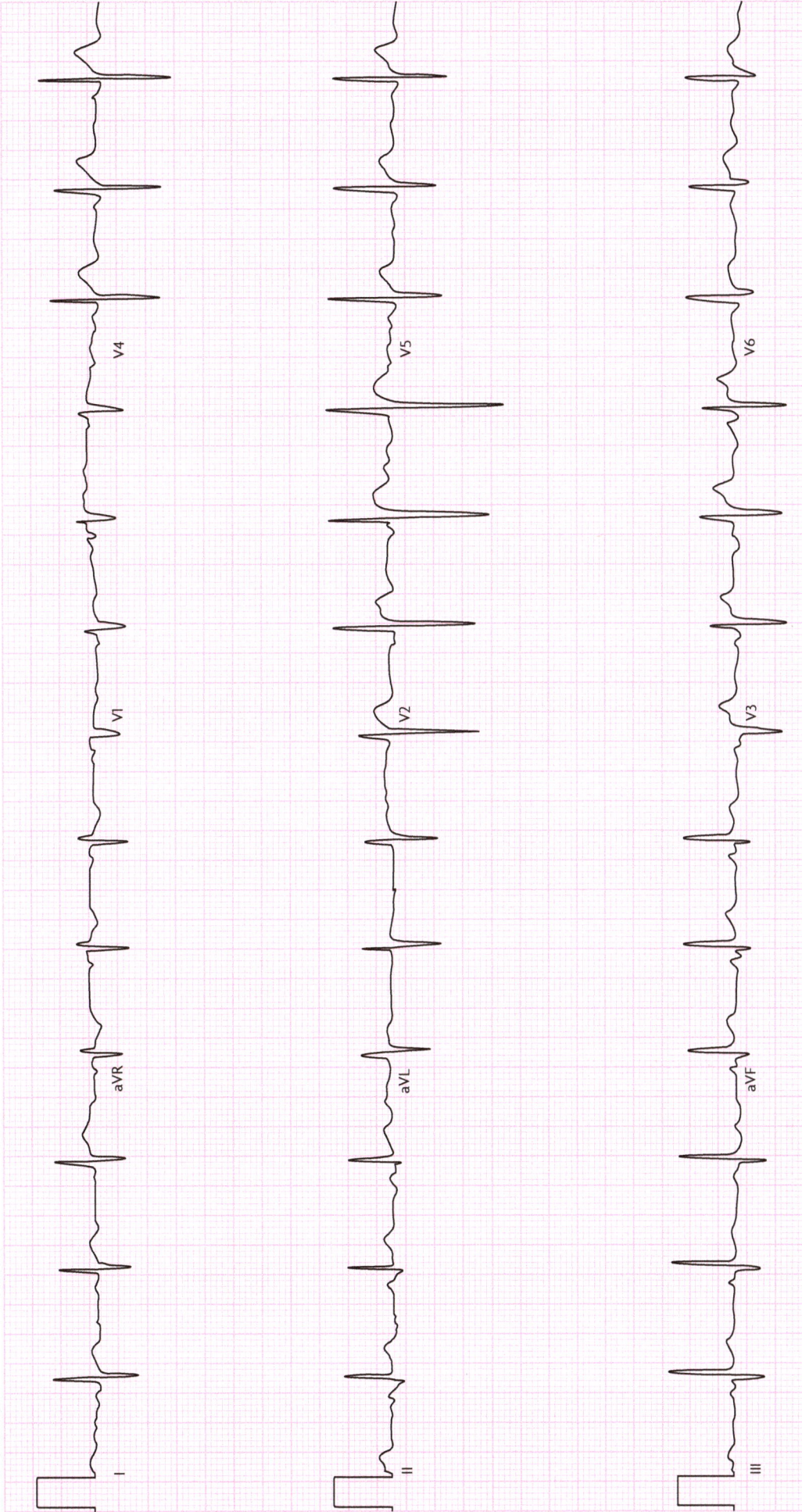

Case Scenario 4.3.2   21-year-old male with abdominal pain

Zachary has been unwell for five days. He has had lower right-sided sharp abdominal pain. It has become suddenly worse in the last three hours and he scores it as 5/10. He has also been suffering from diarrhoea for two days.

Past medical history: *Cardiac surgery at birth and at three years old.*

Medication: *None.*

Allergies: *None.*

Social history: *Lives with friends. Drinks several alcoholic drinks each weekend, does not smoke or use illicit drugs.*

Family history: *Mother and father both well.*

Review of systems: *No chest pain or discomfort, no back pain, no difficulty breathing. No vomiting.*

Examination: *Regular and rapid radial pulse. Flushed. Lungs clear on auscultation. Abdomen tender on palpation.*

Clinical Observations

SpO$_2$	%	EtCO$_2$	kPa	NIBP	mmHg
			5.0		112
	96	RR	22	(85)	71

T°	Blood Glucose	GCS
38.6°C	7.1 mmol/l	15 (E4 / S5 / M6)

Questions

a) What are your differential diagnoses for Zachary?
b) Use the 9-step ECG interpretation tool to assess Zachary's ECG.
c) What rhythm is the ECG?
d) What is your working diagnosis?

ECG Steps   Remember to look at every ECG lead view, not just lead II

1	What is the rate and rhythm?
2	Are there any P waves and what is their relationship with the QRS complex?
3	What is the duration and morphology of the QRS complex?
4	Is the ST segment isoelectric, depressed or elevated?
5	Are the QT intervals and T waves normal?

Clinical Steps

6	Is the heart generating a palpable pulse of appropriate rate and providing adequate perfusion?
7	Is the rhythm unstable and at risk of deterioration?
8	Does the presenting rhythm support or change your working diagnosis?
9	Are any clinical interventions required?

Case Scenario ECG 4.3.2

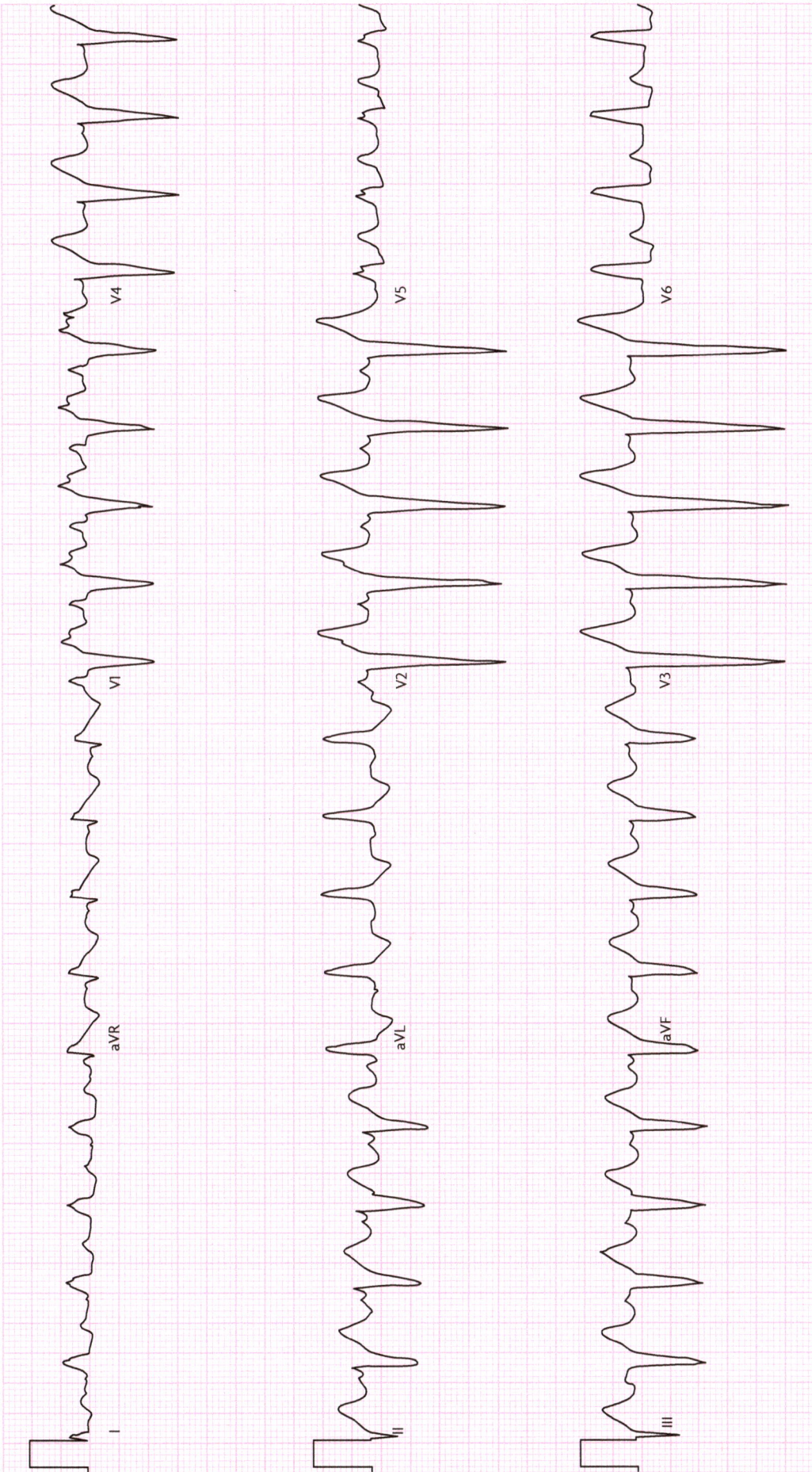

Case Scenario 4.3.3   72-year-old male, collapsed

Eric has been found collapsed in his hallway by a neighbour. She has not been able to wake him. It is unclear how long Eric has been on the floor; it is lunchtime and he is wearing different clothes from yesterday, so his neighbour believes he must have collapsed since he got up today, not last night.

Past medical history: *COPD, hypertension.*

Medication: *Spiriva inhaler, felodipine, perindopril.*

Allergies: *None.*

Social history: *Lives alone. Drinks a couple of alcoholic drinks most days, smokes 15/day.*

Family history: *Unknown.*

Review of systems: *Unable.*

Examination: *Extremely slow, regular central pulse. Radial pulses absent. Extremely pale.*

Clinical Observations

SpO$_2$	%	EtCO$_2$	kPa	NIBP	mmHg
			6.2		63
	89	RR	12	(42)	32

T°	Blood Glucose	GCS
35.8°C	4.5 mmol/l	6 (E1 / S2 / M3)

Questions

a) What are your differential diagnoses for Eric?
b) Use the 9-step ECG interpretation tool to assess Eric's ECG.
c) What rhythm is the ECG?
d) What is your working diagnosis?

ECG Steps   Remember to look at every ECG lead view, not just lead II

1	What is the rate and rhythm?
2	Are there any P waves and what is their relationship with the QRS complex?
3	What is the duration and morphology of the QRS complex?
4	Is the ST segment isoelectric, depressed or elevated?
5	Are the QT intervals and T waves normal?

Clinical Steps

6	Is the heart generating a palpable pulse of appropriate rate and providing adequate perfusion?
7	Is the rhythm unstable and at risk of deterioration?
8	Does the presenting rhythm support or change your working diagnosis?
9	Are any clinical interventions required?

Case Scenario ECG 4.3.3

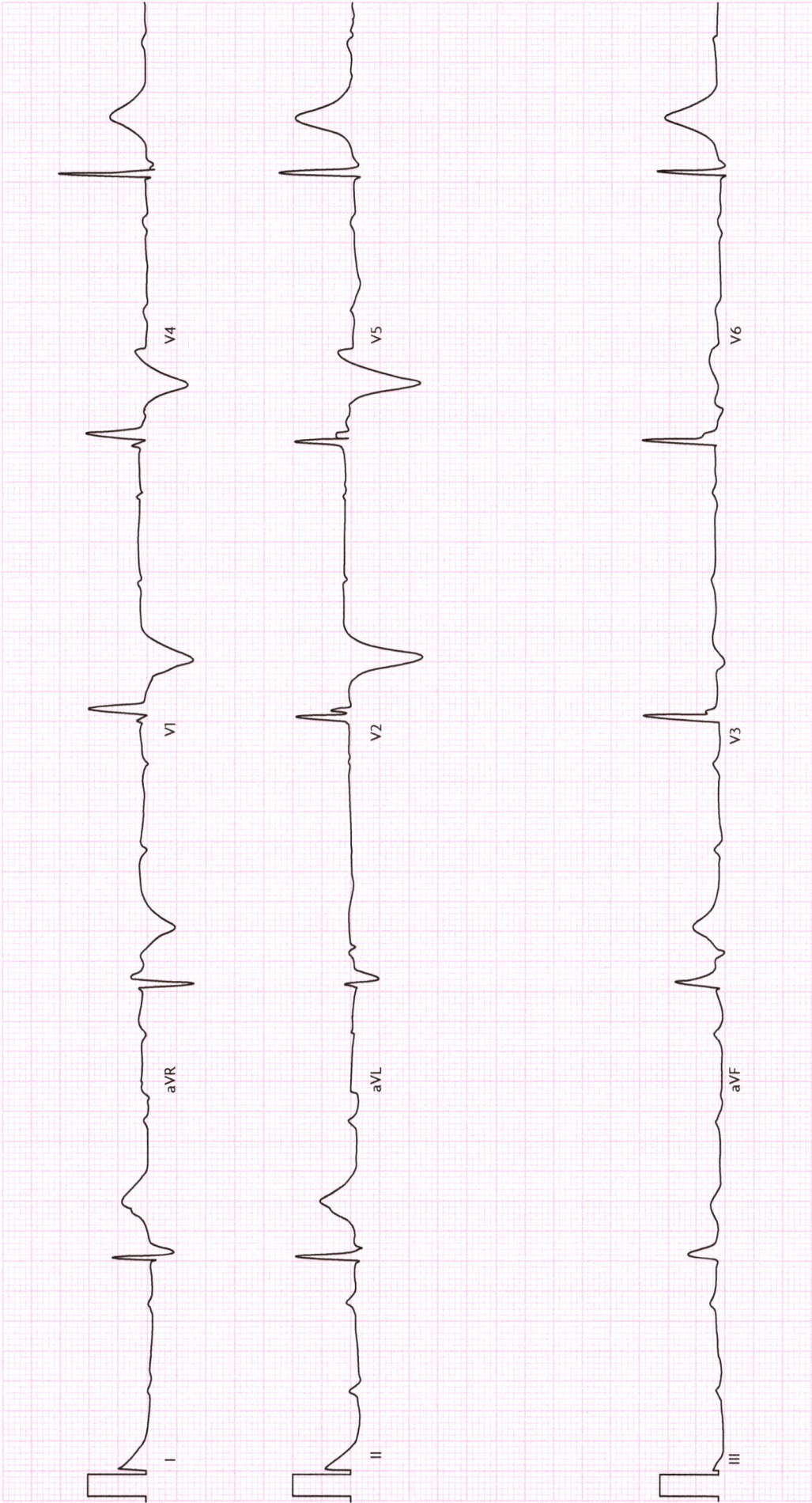

Case Scenario 4.3.4   79-year-old female feeling lethargic

Geraldine has been feeling fatigued and lethargic for the last three days. She has spent most of her time sleeping, which is unusual for her as she normally likes to spend time tending her garden. She describes the feeling as though her whole body is heavy, and as though she just wants to fall asleep, even if she has just had a nap.

Past medical history: *AF, Gilbert's syndrome, varicose veins.*

Medication: *Atenolol, rivaroxaban.*

Allergies: *None.*

Social history: *Lives alone, no carers, has meals delivered and family live nearby and visit regularly.*

Family history: *Mother and father died in old age, no siblings.*

Review of systems: *No chest pain or discomfort, no palpitations, no abdominal pain, no back pain, no difficulty breathing. No recent illness.*

Examination: *Regular radial pulse. Lungs clear on auscultation. Heart sounds S1+S2+0.*

Clinical Observations

SpO_2	%	$EtCO_2$	kPa	NIBP	mmHg	T°	Blood Glucose	GCS
			5.2		98			15
	97	RR	16	(68)	53	36.7°C	7.2 mmol/l	(E4 / S5 / M6)

Questions

a) **What are your differential diagnoses for Geraldine?**
b) **Use the 9-step ECG interpretation tool to assess Geraldine's ECG.**
c) **What rhythm is the ECG?**
d) **What is your working diagnosis?**

ECG Steps   Remember to look at every ECG lead view, not just lead II

1	**What is the rate and rhythm?**
2	**Are there any P waves and what is their relationship with the QRS complex?**
3	**What is the duration and morphology of the QRS complex?**
4	**Is the ST segment isoelectric, depressed or elevated?**
5	**Are the QT intervals and T waves normal?**

Clinical Steps

6	**Is the heart generating a palpable pulse of appropriate rate and providing adequate perfusion?**
7	**Is the rhythm unstable and at risk of deterioration?**
8	**Does the presenting rhythm support or change your working diagnosis?**
9	**Are any clinical interventions required?**

Case Scenario ECG 4.3.4

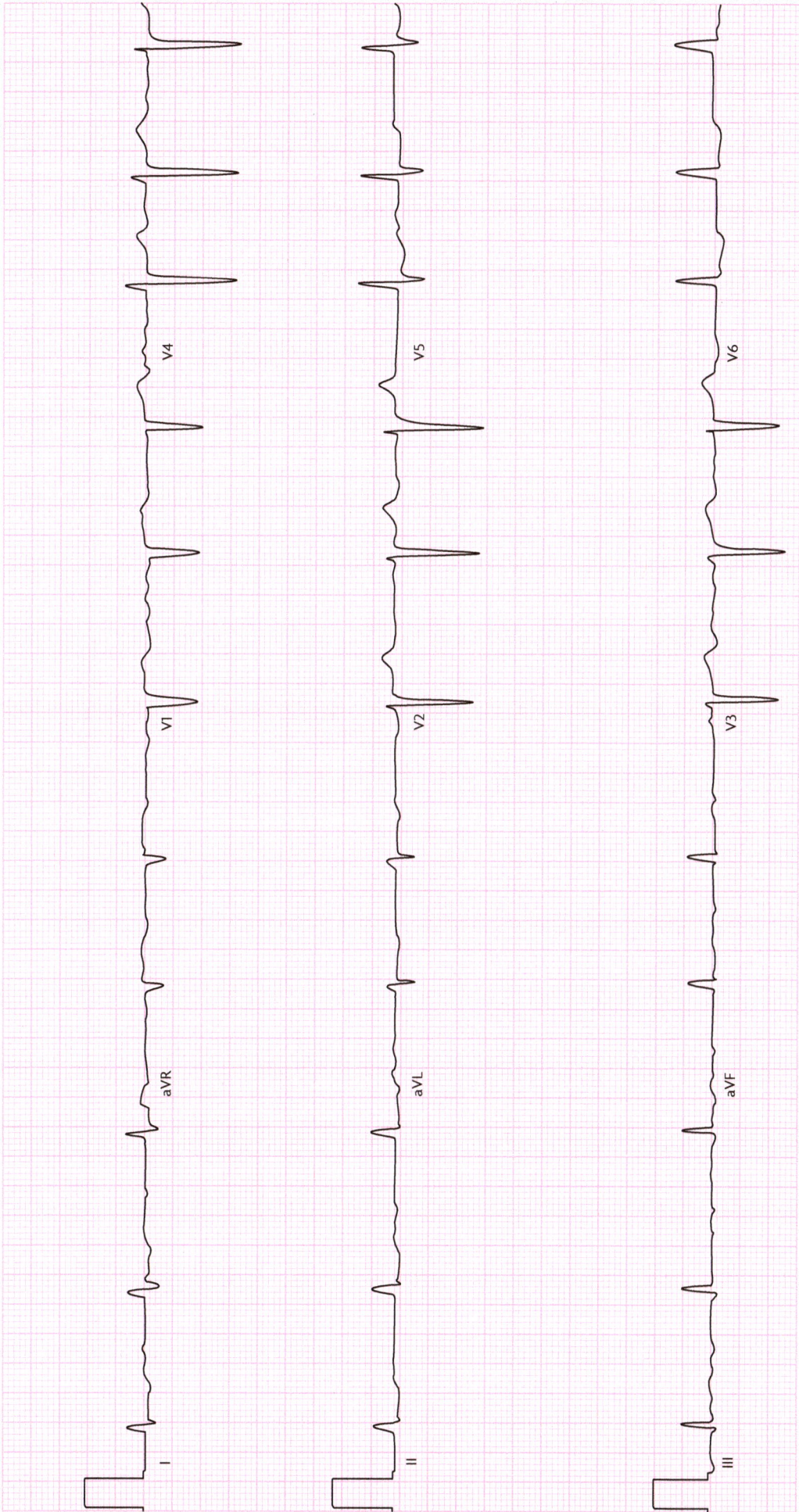

I

II

III

aVR

aVL

aVF

V1

V2

V3

V4

V5

V6

Case Scenario 4.3.5   67-year-old female, with vomiting

Marion has just returned home from Sunday lunch at a pub with her daughter, son-in-law and their children. As they were sitting in the lounge, she suddenly became pale, clammy and vomited. She has continued to vomit repeatedly and is still vomiting when you arrive. She had the same meal as the rest of the family; they all feel fine. Marion is agitated and not speaking coherently. She keeps moving her hand to her upper abdomen.

Past medical history: *Type 2 Diabetes.*

Medication: *Metformin.*

Allergies: *None.*

Social history: *Lives alone, retired. Drinks an occasional glass of wine (none today), does not smoke or use illicit drugs.*

Family history: *Unknown.*

Review of systems: *Unable. No recent illness.*

Examination: *Regular and rapid radial pulse. Pale, cold and clammy. No blood visible in the vomit.*

Clinical Observations

SpO$_2$	%	EtCO$_2$	kPa	NIBP	mmHg
			5.3		146
	93	RR	26	(113)	97

T°	Blood Glucose	GCS
36.2°C	8.9 mmol/l	15 (E4 / S3 / M6)

Questions

a) What are your differential diagnoses for Marion?
b) Use the 9-step ECG interpretation tool to assess Marion's ECG.
c) What rhythm is the ECG?
d) What is your working diagnosis?

ECG Steps   Remember to look at every ECG lead view, not just lead II

1	What is the rate and rhythm?
2	Are there any P waves and what is their relationship with the QRS complex?
3	What is the duration and morphology of the QRS complex?
4	Is the ST segment isoelectric, depressed or elevated?
5	Are the QT intervals and T waves normal?

Clinical Steps

6	Is the heart generating a palpable pulse of appropriate rate and providing adequate perfusion?
7	Is the rhythm unstable and at risk of deterioration?
8	Does the presenting rhythm support or change your working diagnosis?
9	Are any clinical interventions required?

Case Scenario ECG 4.3.5

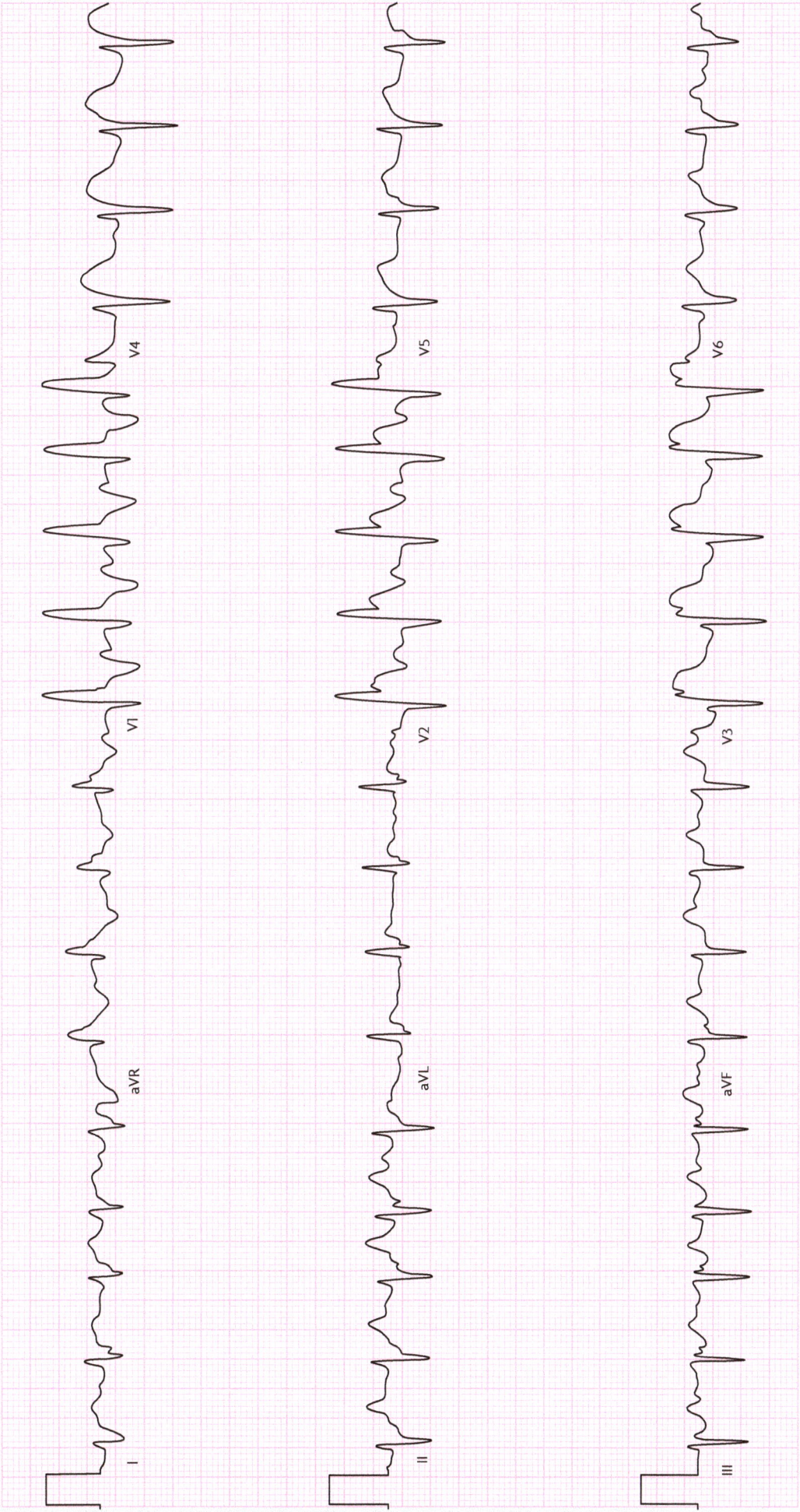

I

II

III

aVR

aVL

aVF

V1

V2

V3

V4

V5

V6

Case Scenarios Set 1 Answers

Case Scenario 4.1.1   Answers

a) **What are your differential diagnoses for Vincent?** *Differentials should include: myocardial infarction, stroke, subarachnoid haemorrhage, internal haemorrhage.*

b) **Use the 9-step ECG interpretation tool to assess Vincent's ECG.**

c) **What rhythm is the ECG?** *STEMI inferior and bradycardia.*

d) **What is your working diagnosis?** *STEMI.*

Discussion: *Vincent has clear signs of STEMI on his ECG. His clinical presentation also suggests that a sudden coronary artery occlusion has occurred and caused bradycardia and reduced cardiac output, leading to his collapse. Clinical management of Vincent is a fine balance of interventions. We can assume with relative certainty that the cause of his hypotension is cardiogenic. We can also assume that his reduced level of consciousness, his pallor and clamminess are due to this hypotension. His MAP is below 60 mmHg and his reduced GCS suggests that his brain and other organs are not adequately perfused. Atropine therapy is indicated for this symptomatic bradycardia, though technically, fluid therapy is also indicated as we have signs of impaired tissue perfusion. We also know that fluid therapy in cardiogenic shock has the serious potential to cause fluid overload and subsequent heart failure, worsening the status of an already failing heart. We must also balance the need to maintain perfusion to essential organs; his presentation suggests that his organs are not adequately perfused. Further discussion of the risks and relative benefits of fluid therapy in cardiogenic shock can be found on page 38. It is a safe decision in this situation to obtain IV access and begin atropine therapy first; if Vincent's heart responds to this therapy with increased heart rate and cardiac output, it may avoid the need for fluid therapy.*

ECG Steps

1	**What is the rate and rhythm?**	*The rate is around 55 beats/minute and the rhythm is regular.*
2	**Are there any P waves and what is their relationship with the QRS complex?**	*There is a P wave before every QRS complex and a QRS complex after every P wave.*
3	**What is the duration and morphology of the QRS complex?**	*The QRS complex is of normal morphology and the duration is less than 0.12 seconds (3 small squares).*
4	**Is the ST segment isoelectric, depressed or elevated?**	*The ST segment is displaying elevation in leads II, III and aVF, as well as leads V2–V6.*
5	**Are the QT intervals and T waves normal?**	*The T wave shape is peaked in leads with ST segment changes and the QT interval is normal.*

Clinical Steps

6	**Is the heart generating a palpable pulse of appropriate rate and providing adequate perfusion?**	*The heart is generating a palpable pulse at a bradycardic rate. The presence of weak radial pulses suggests perfusion is currently present though on the cusp of inadequacy.*
7	**Is the rhythm unstable and at risk of deterioration?**	*Yes. This ECG shows active STEMI and is at risk of further cardiac muscle damage or cardiac arrest. Bradycardia is further indication of instability and risk of deterioration.*
8	**Does the presenting rhythm support or change your working diagnosis?**	*Supports MI.*
9	**Are any clinical interventions required?**	*High flow oxygen, IV access and atropine IV are indicated for this patient. Potentially fluid therapy and ACS drugs (see discussion). Rapid transport with pre-alert call to activate local STEMI pathway and cath lab.*

Case Scenario 4.1.2 Answers

a) **What are your differential diagnoses for Prisha?** *Differentials should include: Re-entrant tachycardia, atrial flutter, atrial fibrillation, pulmonary embolism, hyperventilation syndrome.*

b) **Use the 9-step ECG interpretation tool to assess Prisha's ECG.**

c) **What rhythm is the ECG?** *Atrial fibrillation.*

d) **What is your working diagnosis?** *Atrial fibrillation.*

Discussion: *It would be easy (and wrong) for some clinicians to jump to the conclusion that Prisha was experiencing hyperventilation syndrome (anxiety attack) today. She has a history of anxiety and her presentation could be seen to fit this diagnosis. But, we know that it is wrong to jump to conclusions when formulating a diagnosis and we also know that hyperventilation syndrome is a diagnosis that can only be made by excluding other potential conditions. In this instance, Prisha's ECG immediately excludes hyperventilation syndrome as the primary diagnosis. She is likely to be experiencing some anxiety, but secondary to her cardiac arrhythmia. Her ECG shows atrial fibrillation with rapid ventricular response; this finding fits with her symptoms and thus gives us our working diagnosis.*

ECG Steps

1	**What is the rate and rhythm?**	*The rate is around 180 beats/minute and the rhythm is irregularly irregular.*
2	**Are there any P waves and what is their relationship with the QRS complex?**	*There are no visible P waves.*
3	**What is the duration and morphology of the QRS complex?**	*The QRS complex is of narrow complex morphology and the duration is less than 0.12 seconds (3 small squares).*
4	**Is the ST segment isoelectric, depressed or elevated?**	*The ST segment is displaying depression in leads I, II, aVL and V1–V3. There is also ST segment elevation in lead III.*
5	**Are the QT intervals and T waves normal?**	*The T wave is of normal shape and the QT interval is appropriate for the rate.*

Clinical Steps

6	**Is the heart generating a palpable pulse of appropriate rate and providing adequate perfusion?**	*The heart is generating a palpable pulse at a tachycardic rate. The presence of radial pulses suggests adequate perfusion is currently present.*
7	**Is the rhythm unstable and at risk of deterioration?**	*No. The rhythm is stable.*
8	**Does the presenting rhythm support or change your working diagnosis?**	*Supports diagnosis of atrial fibrillation with rapid ventricular response.*
9	**Are any clinical interventions required?**	*No interventions are required based on this ECG. The patient requires transport to hospital.*

Case Scenario 4.1.3   Answers

a) Use the 9-step ECG interpretation tool to assess Pedro's ECG
b) What rhythm is the ECG? *Sinus tachycardia.*

Discussion: *Pedro has a sinus tachycardia, but this fits with his situation. Not only has he just been exercising (and pushing himself), but he is also in severe pain having experienced a stressful accident. It is not surprising that his heart rate is high!*

Please note that it would not usually be appropriate to carry out a 12-lead ECG on a trauma patient during the initial assessment without good reason. The 12-lead ECG is given here for educational purposes.

ECG Steps

1	**What is the rate and rhythm?**	*The rate is about 120 beats/minute and the rhythm is regular.*
2	**Are there any P waves and what is their relationship with the QRS complex?**	*There is a P wave before every QRS complex and a QRS complex after every P wave.*
3	**What is the duration and morphology of the QRS complex?**	*The QRS complex is of normal shape and the duration is under 0.12 seconds (3 small squares).*
4	**Is the ST segment isoelectric, depressed or elevated?**	*The ST segment is normal.*
5	**Are the QT intervals and T waves normal?**	*The T wave is of normal shape and the QT interval is appropriate for the rate.*

Clinical Steps

6	**Is the heart generating a palpable pulse of appropriate rate and providing adequate perfusion?**	*The heart is generating a palpable pulse at an appropriate rate. The presence of radial pulses suggests adequate perfusion is currently present.*
7	**Is the rhythm unstable and at risk of deterioration?**	*No. The rhythm is stable.*
8	**Does the presenting rhythm support or change your working diagnosis?**	*Does not impact the working diagnosis for this patient.*
9	**Are any clinical interventions required?**	*No interventions are required based on this ECG. However, the patient requires analgesia and transport to further care.*

Case Scenario 4.1.4   Answers

a) **What are your differential diagnoses for Karen?** *Differentials should include: raised ICP (stroke, subarachnoid haemorrhage), drug overdose, massive pulmonary embolism.*

b) **Use the 9-step ECG interpretation tool to assess Karen's ECG.**

c) **What rhythm is the ECG?** *Sinus arrhythmia with neurological changes.*

d) **What is your working diagnosis?** *Neurological cause – stroke, subarachnoid haemorrhage.*

Discussion: *With little history to go on, it is difficult to confirm a diagnosis for Karen, although this is not necessary. We know that Karen is presenting with a significantly reduced GCS, irregular pulse and irregular respirations. This is enough to suggest that a neurological event has potentially occurred. The deep, wide and inverted T waves on her ECG, known as 'neurological T waves', further suggest that a neurological cause is an appropriate working diagnosis. What we know for sure is that Karen is acutely unwell and requires rapid transport to definitive care; we should not delay unnecessarily on scene.*

ECG Steps

1	**What is the rate and rhythm?**	*The rate is around 90 beats/minute and the rhythm is irregular.*
2	**Are there any P waves and what is their relationship with the QRS complex?**	*There is a P wave before every QRS complex and a QRS complex after every P wave.*
3	**What is the duration and morphology of the QRS complex?**	*The QRS complex is of normal morphology and the duration is less than 0.12 seconds (3 small squares).*
4	**Is the ST segment isoelectric, depressed or elevated?**	*The ST segment is isoelectric.*
5	**Are the QT intervals and T waves normal?**	*There is widespread deep and wide T wave inversion. The QT interval is normal.*

Clinical Steps

6	**Is the heart generating a palpable pulse of appropriate rate and providing adequate perfusion?**	*The heart is generating a palpable pulse at an appropriate rate.*
7	**Is the rhythm unstable and at risk of deterioration?**	*The presentation and rhythm suggest a neurological aetiology which could be unstable, though due to the neurological events, not the ECG rhythm.*
8	**Does the presenting rhythm support or change your working diagnosis?**	*Supports potential neurological cause.*
9	**Are any clinical interventions required?**	*No interventions are required based on this ECG. However, the patient requires rapid transport with pre-alert call to an appropriate receiving hospital.*

Case Scenario 4.1.5   Answers

a) **What are your differential diagnoses for Marta?** *Differentials should include: re-entrant tachycardia, long QT syndrome, neurological event.*

b) **Use the 9-step ECG interpretation tool to assess Marta's ECG.**

c) **What rhythm is the ECG?** *Polymorphic VT.*

d) **What is your working diagnosis?** *Self-limiting polymorphic VT.*

Discussion: *Marta is fortunate to have had this episode of symptomatic polymorphic VT whilst having her ECG taken. Capturing the event on ECG will make further care and treatment more swift. She requires ECG monitoring during transport to hospital as she is at risk of further episodes occurring.*

ECG Steps

1	**What is the rate and rhythm?**	*The rate is around 100 beats/minute (taken from the final two beats) and there is not enough rhythm to assess regularity.*
2	**Are there any P waves and what is their relationship with the QRS complex?**	*Assessing the final two beats: There is a P wave before every QRS complex and a QRS complex after every P wave.*
3	**What is the duration and morphology of the QRS complex?**	*Assessing the final two beats: The QRS complex is of narrow complex morphology and the duration is less than 0.12 seconds (3 small squares).*
4	**Is the ST segment isoelectric, depressed or elevated?**	*The ST segment is displaying elevation associated with LBBB. It does not meet Sgarbossa criteria.*
5	**Are the QT intervals and T waves normal?**	*The T waves and QT intervals are variable.*

Clinical Steps

6	**Is the heart generating a palpable pulse of appropriate rate and providing adequate perfusion?**	*It is unclear if a palpable pulse was present during the several seconds of polymorphic VT.*
7	**Is the rhythm unstable and at risk of deterioration?**	*Yes. The rhythm is at risk of recurrent polymorphic VT which could remain and not self-limit.*
8	**Does the presenting rhythm support or change your working diagnosis?**	*Confirms diagnosis of polymorphic VT.*
9	**Are any clinical interventions required?**	*No interventions are required based on this ECG. The patient does require ECG monitoring and transport to hospital.*

Case Scenarios Set 2 Answers

Case Scenario 4.2.1   Answers

a) **What are your differential diagnoses for Alisha?** *Differentials should include: re-entrant tachycardia, long QT syndrome, pulmonary embolism.*

b) **Use the 9-step ECG interpretation tool to assess Alisha's ECG.**

c) **What rhythm is the ECG?** *Narrow complex tachycardia, likely re-entrant tachycardia.*

d) **What is your working diagnosis?** *Re-entrant tachycardia.*

Discussion: *Alisha's presentation fits that of re-entrant tachycardia. There is no specific reason for her to be extremely tachycardic; she has not been exercising, she is not experiencing pain or particular distress. The symptoms started suddenly and without warning. This is in keeping with a re-entrant tachycardia. The rate of 180 beats/minute is at the top end of her physiological range for sinus tachycardia; to be sinus tachycardia at this rate she would need to be in an extreme state such as severe sepsis, major trauma or prolonged high intensity exercise. It is not possible to completely confirm the diagnosis, but based on the information available, the working diagnosis firmly sits as re-entrant tachycardia.*

ECG Steps

1	**What is the rate and rhythm?**	*The rate is around 180 beats/minute and the rhythm is regular.*
2	**Are there any P waves and what is their relationship with the QRS complex?**	*There are no visible P waves.*
3	**What is the duration and morphology of the QRS complex?**	*The QRS complex is of narrow complex morphology and the duration is less than 0.12 seconds (3 small squares).*
4	**Is the ST segment isoelectric, depressed or elevated?**	*The ST segment is displaying ST segment depression in leads V3–V6 and lead II. Likely due to rate.*
5	**Are the QT intervals and T waves normal?**	*The T wave is of normal shape and the QT interval is appropriate for the rate.*

Clinical Steps

6	**Is the heart generating a palpable pulse of appropriate rate and providing adequate perfusion?**	*There is a palpable pulse but the rate is inappropriately fast. The presence of the radial pulse suggests there is currently adequate perfusion.*
7	**Is the rhythm unstable and at risk of deterioration?**	*No. Re-entrant tachycardia may spontaneously revert or persist. But no specific risk of deterioration.*
8	**Does the presenting rhythm support or change your working diagnosis?**	*Supports diagnosis of re-entrant tachycardia.*
9	**Are any clinical interventions required?**	*Vagal manoeuvres could be attempted based on local protocols. However, the patient requires ECG monitoring and transport to hospital.*

Case Scenario 4.2.2   Answers

a) **What are your differential diagnoses for Harry?** *Differentials should include: acute coronary syndrome, pulmonary embolism, pericarditis, respiratory infection.*

b) **Use the 9-step ECG interpretation tool to assess Harry's ECG.**

c) **What rhythm is the ECG?** *Sinus rhythm with widespread ST segment elevation.*

d) **What is your working diagnosis?** *Pericarditis.*

Discussion: *Harry's presentation is a textbook example of pericarditis. He has recently recovered from a viral illness and has sharp chest pain that worsens when lying flat. He is also displaying signs of infection with pyrexia and a borderline tachycardia. His ECG shows widespread ST segment elevation and ST segment depression in lead aVR. These changes could indeed be due to STEMI, but his clinical presentation is much more suggestive of pericarditis. Because we are unable to completely rule out ACS, and because the pericarditis requires treatment, Harry requires transport to hospital – if possible, one with cath lab capabilities in case the emergency department discover he is having a STEMI.*

ECG Steps

1	**What is the rate and rhythm?**	*The rate is around 100 beats/minute and the rhythm is regular.*
2	**Are there any P waves and what is their relationship with the QRS complex?**	*There is a P wave before every QRS complex and a QRS complex after every P wave.*
3	**What is the duration and morphology of the QRS complex?**	*The QRS complex is of narrow complex morphology and the duration is less than 0.12 seconds (3 small squares).*
4	**Is the ST segment isoelectric, depressed or elevated?**	*The ST segment is displaying ST segment elevation in leads I, II, aVL and V2–V6. With ST segment depression in lead aVR.*
5	**Are the QT intervals and T waves normal?**	*The T wave is peaked and the QT interval is appropriate for the rate.*

Clinical Steps

6	**Is the heart generating a palpable pulse of appropriate rate and providing adequate perfusion?**	*The heart is generating a palpable pulse at an appropriate rate. The presence of a radial pulse suggests perfusion is currently present.*
7	**Is the rhythm unstable and at risk of deterioration?**	*No. The ST segment elevation is likely due to pericarditis so does not hold the same risks of sudden cardiac arrest as ST segment elevation in ACS.*
8	**Does the presenting rhythm support or change your working diagnosis?**	*Supports diagnosis of pericarditis.*
9	**Are any clinical interventions required?**	*No interventions are required based on this ECG. The patient does require analgesia and transport to hospital.*

	Case Scenario 4.2.3 Answers

a) **What are your differential diagnoses for Melissa?** *Differentials should include: hyperventilation syndrome, pulmonary embolism, re-entrant tachycardia.*
b) **Use the 9-step ECG interpretation tool to assess Melissa's ECG.**
c) **What rhythm is the ECG?** *Sinus rhythm.*
d) **What is your working diagnosis?** *Hyperventilation syndrome.*

Discussion: *Melissa has experienced the classic signs and symptoms of hyperventilation syndrome (anxiety attack). However, to confirm this diagnosis we need to exclude other, potentially sinister, causes. The swift resolution of her symptoms is reassuring, alongside her stable baseline observations. Heart and lung sounds may further reassure us, to some extent, though normal heart or lung sounds do not rule out a heart or lung problem, so we must not overly rely on those findings. Her ECG shows sinus rhythm; again this does not mean that there is not, or was not, a problem with her heart. Based on all of our findings, we can reasonably exclude any serious or sinister pathologies, and reach the diagnosis of hyperventilation syndrome. However, we must be diligent and provide detailed and appropriate safety netting advice to Melissa.*

ECG Steps

1	What is the rate and rhythm?	*The rate is around 70 beats/minute and the rhythm is regular.*
2	Are there any P waves and what is their relationship with the QRS complex?	*There is a P wave before every QRS complex and a QRS complex after every P wave.*
3	What is the duration and morphology of the QRS complex?	*The QRS complex is of narrow complex morphology and the duration is less than 0.12 seconds (3 small squares).*
4	Is the ST segment isoelectric, depressed or elevated?	*The ST segment is isoelectric.*
5	Are the QT intervals and T waves normal?	*The T wave is of normal shape and the QT interval is appropriate for the rate.*

Clinical Steps

6	Is the heart generating a palpable pulse of appropriate rate and providing adequate perfusion?	*Yes.*
7	Is the rhythm unstable and at risk of deterioration?	*No.*
8	Does the presenting rhythm support or change your working diagnosis?	*Supports a non-cardiac cause.*
9	Are any clinical interventions required?	*No interventions are required based on this ECG.*

Case Scenario 4.2.4   Answers

a) **Use the 9-step ECG interpretation tool to assess David's ECG.**
b) **What rhythm is the ECG?** *Trigeminy.*
c) **What is your working diagnosis?** *Trigeminy.*

Discussion: *David has multiple factors that could explain the trigeminy on his ECG. His binge drinking, lack of sleep and high levels of stress, combined with cocaine use and increased doses of his tricyclic anti-depressant, are all likely to have contributed to his current state.*

ECG Steps

1	**What is the rate and rhythm?**	*The rate is around 100 beats/minute and the rhythm is regularly irregular.*
2	**Are there any P waves and what is their relationship with the QRS complex?**	*There is a P wave before every QRS complex that is not a PVC and a QRS complex after every P wave.*
3	**What is the duration and morphology of the QRS complex?**	*The sinus QRS complex is of narrow complex morphology and the duration is less than 0.12 seconds (3 small squares).*
4	**Is the ST segment isoelectric, depressed or elevated?**	*The ST segment is isoelectric.*
5	**Are the QT intervals and T waves normal?**	*There is widespread T wave inversion. The QT interval is normal.*

Clinical Steps

6	**Is the heart generating a palpable pulse of appropriate rate and providing adequate perfusion?**	*The heart is generating a palpable pulse at an appropriate rate. The presence of a radial pulse suggests perfusion is currently present.*
7	**Is the rhythm unstable and at risk of deterioration?**	*No.*
8	**Does the presenting rhythm support or change your working diagnosis?**	*Confirms diagnosis of trigeminy.*
9	**Are any clinical interventions required?**	*No interventions are required based on this ECG. However, the patient requires ECG monitoring and transport to hospital.*

Case Scenario 4.2.5   Answers

a) **What are your differential diagnoses for Ali?** *Differentials should include: acute coronary syndrome, pulmonary embolism.*

b) **Use the 9-step ECG interpretation tool to assess Ali's ECG.**

c) **What rhythm is the ECG?** *STEMI inferior, lateral and signs of right sided / posterior.*

d) **What is your working diagnosis?** *STEMI.*

Discussion: *Ali is presenting with classic signs and symptoms of ACS. His ECG shows widespread ST segment elevation and meets STEMI criteria. The ST segment depression in leads V1 and V2 is suggestive of posterior MI and the ST segment elevation being greater in lead III than lead II also suggests potential for right ventricular involvement. A right-sided ECG and posterior ECG should be obtained. Ali is comparatively young to be having an MI, though his family history indicates that he is at increased risk of MI at a young age. It is important to remember that MI can occur at any age, and we should not rule it out simply because a patient is younger than we expect.*

ECG Steps

1	**What is the rate and rhythm?**	*The rate is around 90 beats/minute and the rhythm is regular.*
2	**Are there any P waves and what is their relationship with the QRS complex?**	*There is a P wave before every QRS complex and a QRS complex after every P wave.*
3	**What is the duration and morphology of the QRS complex?**	*The QRS complex is of narrow complex morphology and the duration is less than 0.12 seconds (3 small squares).*
4	**Is the ST segment isoelectric, depressed or elevated?**	*The ST segment is displaying elevation in leads II, III, aVF and V4–V6. There is ST segment depression in leads I, aVL, V1 and V2.*
5	**Are the QT intervals and T waves normal?**	*The T waves are inverted in lead aVL. The QT interval is normal.*

Clinical Steps

6	**Is the heart generating a palpable pulse of appropriate rate and providing adequate perfusion?**	*The heart is generating a palpable pulse at an appropriate rate. The presence of a radial pulse suggests perfusion is currently present.*
7	**Is the rhythm unstable and at risk of deterioration?**	*Yes. This ECG shows active STEMI a risk of further cardiac muscle damage or cardiac arrest.*
8	**Does the presenting rhythm support or change your working diagnosis?**	*Supports MI.*
9	**Are any clinical interventions required?**	*High-flow oxygen, IV access and ACS drugs are indicated for this patient. Right-sided and posterior ECGs should be obtained to assess for further ST segment elevation and potential for right ventricular involvement. Rapid transport with pre-alert call to activate local STEMI pathway and cath lab.*

Case Scenarios Set 3 Answers

Case Scenario 4.3.1   Answers

a) What are your differential diagnoses for Phyllis? *Differentials should include: acute coronary syndrome, pulmonary embolism, heart failure, chest infection.*

b) Use the 9-step ECG interpretation tool to assess Phyllis' ECG

c) What rhythm is the ECG? *Sinus rhythm with LVH and pathological Q waves.*

d) What is your working diagnosis? *Heart failure secondary to MI.*

Discussion: *Phyllis is displaying multiple signs and symptoms suggestive of worsening heart failure. Her recent deterioration and fatigue, combined with her productive cough, bibasal crepitations, low oxygen saturations and shortness of breath on exertion, point towards heart failure and pulmonary oedema. Another subtle clue is that she has a new preference for sleeping while sitting up in her chair, further suggesting the presence of pulmonary oedema. The absence of a high temperature helps us move away from chest infection as a working diagnosis, though she is at increased risk of respiratory infection due to the pulmonary oedema. A significant clue is that she experienced upper epigastric pain 10 days ago, prior to the development of all the other symptoms. This may have been an atypically presenting MI, which has caused cardiac damage and led to heart failure. This is further supported by the signs on her ECG, LVH and pathological Q waves, which suggest previous cardiac muscle damage.*

ECG Steps		
1	**What is the rate and rhythm?**	*The rate is around 90 beats/minute and the rhythm is regular.*
2	**Are there any P waves and what is their relationship with the QRS complex?**	*There is a P wave before every QRS complex and a QRS complex after every P wave.*
3	**What is the duration and morphology of the QRS complex?**	*The QRS complex is of narrow complex morphology and the duration is less than 0.12 seconds (3 small squares). There are deep, pathological Q waves in lead III. There are also signs of left ventricular hypertrophy.*
4	**Is the ST segment isoelectric, depressed or elevated?**	*The ST segment is mostly isoelectric, though there is some slight and subtle ST segment elevation in lead II.*
5	**Are the QT intervals and T waves normal?**	*The T wave is of normal shape and the QT interval is appropriate for the rate.*
Clinical Steps		
6	**Is the heart generating a palpable pulse of appropriate rate and providing adequate perfusion?**	*Yes.*
7	**Is the rhythm unstable and at risk of deterioration?**	*No.*
8	**Does the presenting rhythm support or change your working diagnosis?**	*Supports previous cardiac injury.*
9	**Are any clinical interventions required?**	*No interventions are required based on this ECG.*

Case Scenario 4.3.2   Answers

a) **What are your differential diagnoses for Zachary?** *Differentials should include: appendicitis, gastroenteritis.*

b) **Use the 9-step ECG interpretation tool to assess Zachary's ECG.**

c) **What rhythm is the ECG?** *Sinus tachycardia with aberrant conduction (LBBB).*

d) **What is your working diagnosis?** *Appendicitis.*

Discussion: *Zachary's history of heart surgery in childhood could explain the presence of LBBB on his ECG. His clinical presentation suggests he has appendicitis. This would explain his increased heart rate due to infection and pain. Sinus tachycardia combined with aberrant conduction can be confused with VT. But when we look more closely we can see that there are isoelectric gaps between each complex. We can also consider the rate of 120 beats/minute and the patient's presentation. The rate is on the slow side for VT and the clinical presentation gives a reasonable reason for sinus tachycardia to be present.*

ECG Steps

1	**What is the rate and rhythm?**	*The rate is around 120 beats/minute and the rhythm is regular.*
2	**Are there any P waves and what is their relationship with the QRS complex?**	*There is a P wave before every QRS complex and a QRS complex after every P wave.*
3	**What is the duration and morphology of the QRS complex?**	*The QRS complex is of LBBB morphology and the duration is greater than 0.12 seconds (3 small squares).*
4	**Is the ST segment isoelectric, depressed or elevated?**	*The ST segment is isoelectric.*
5	**Are the QT intervals and T waves normal?**	*The T wave is of appropriate shape and the QT interval is appropriate for the rate.*

Clinical Steps

6	**Is the heart generating a palpable pulse of appropriate rate and providing adequate perfusion?**	*Yes.*
7	**Is the rhythm unstable and at risk of deterioration?**	*No.*
8	**Does the presenting rhythm support or change your working diagnosis?**	*Supports a non-cardiac cause.*
9	**Are any clinical interventions required?**	*No interventions are required based on this ECG.*

Case Scenario 4.3.3   Answers

a) **What are your differential diagnoses for Eric?** *Differentials should include: acute coronary syndrome, internal haemorrhage, stroke, pulmonary embolism.*

b) **Use the 9-step ECG interpretation tool to assess Eric's ECG.**

c) **What rhythm is the ECG?** *Bradycardic 2nd degree type 2 AV block and RBBB.*

d) **What is your working diagnosis?** *Symptomatic bradycardia, cardiogenic shock.*

Discussion: *Eric is primary survey positive and in a peri-arrest state. His extremely bradycardic heart rate is due to the 2nd degree type 2 AV block. It has a 3:1 ratio, meaning that the physical heart rate is only one third of what the SA node is intending. Eric's MAP is below 60 mmHg and combined with his reduced GCS it is likely his brain and other organs are not receiving adequate perfusion. Atropine therapy is indicated for this symptomatic bradycardia, and fluid therapy is indicated as we have signs of impaired tissue perfusion and hypotension. We also know that fluid therapy in cardiogenic shock has a serious potential to cause fluid overload and subsequent heart failure, worsening the status of an already sick heart. In this case, with such extreme hypotension it is reasonable to gain IV access and initiate atropine and fluid therapy whilst being cognisant of the risks of fluid overload, and only administering the minimum amount necessary to maintain perfusion. It is to be hoped that the atropine therapy will increase heart rate and cardiac output, at which point it may be appropriate to cease fluid therapy. Further discussion of the risks and relative benefits of fluid therapy in cardiogenic shock can be found on page 38.*

ECG Steps

1	What is the rate and rhythm?	*The rate is around 30 beats/minute and the rhythm is regular.*
2	Are there any P waves and what is their relationship with the QRS complex?	*There are three P waves before every QRS complex. The first of the three P waves is hidden within the preceding T wave.*
3	What is the duration and morphology of the QRS complex?	*The QRS complex is of RBBB morphology and the duration is less than 0.12 seconds (3 small squares).*
4	Is the ST segment isoelectric, depressed or elevated?	*The ST segment is isoelectric.*
5	Are the QT intervals and T waves normal?	*The T wave is of normal shape and inverted in leads V1–V3. The QT interval is appropriate for the rate.*

Clinical Steps

6	Is the heart generating a palpable pulse of appropriate rate and providing adequate perfusion?	*No. Radial pulses are absent and the rate is absolute bradycardia.*
7	Is the rhythm unstable and at risk of deterioration?	*Yes. There is significant risk of further slowing of the rate or cardiac arrest.*
8	Does the presenting rhythm support or change your working diagnosis?	*Supports cardiogenic shock due to bradycardia.*
9	Are any clinical interventions required?	*High-flow oxygen, IV access and atropine IV are indicated for this patient along with fluid therapy. Rapid transport with pre-alert call to nearest appropriate emergency department.*

Case Scenario 4.3.4   Answers

a) **What are your differential diagnoses for Geraldine?** *Differentials should include: infection, sepsis, heart failure, acute coronary syndrome.*
b) **Use the 9-step ECG interpretation tool to assess Geraldine's ECG.**
c) **What rhythm is the ECG?** *Junctional rhythm with atrial fibrillation.*
d) **What is your working diagnosis?** *Junctional rhythm, potential cardiac cause.*

Discussion: *Geraldine has already been diagnosed with AF, but we can also identify a junctional rhythm on the ECG. This is a tricky diagnosis which might easily have been missed (I have discussed this scenario with over 200 paramedic students and only a handful have been able to determine the correct diagnosis in class). The main clue here is that the QRS complexes are (mostly) regular, which we know should not be the case in AF, where we would expect an irregularly irregular rhythm. This tells us that the rhythm for the QRS complexes originates from somewhere other than the fibrillating atria. The QRS complexes are narrow, meaning the only possible location for the rhythm to originate from is the AV node or bundle of His. This leads us to a junctional rhythm. What we do not know is what has caused this junctional rhythm. The ST segment depression and T wave inversion in the lateral leads could suggest to us that cardiac damage has occurred and might be to blame. The absence of cardiac symptoms does not rule this out as Geraldine is at increased risk of having an atypically presenting MI.*

ECG Steps

1	**What is the rate and rhythm?**	*The rate is around 65 beats/minute and the rhythm is regular.*
2	**Are there any P waves and what is their relationship with the QRS complex?**	*There are no P waves visible.*
3	**What is the duration and morphology of the QRS complex?**	*The QRS complex is of narrow complex morphology and the duration is less than 0.12 seconds (3 small squares).*
4	**Is the ST segment isoelectric, depressed or elevated?**	*The ST segment has some slight depression in lateral leads I and V5–V6.*
5	**Are the QT intervals and T waves normal?**	*There is T wave inversion in lateral leads V5–V6. The QT interval is appropriate for the rate.*

Clinical Steps

6	**Is the heart generating a palpable pulse of appropriate rate and providing adequate perfusion?**	*The presence of radial pulses suggests there is adequate perfusion and the rate is appropriate.*
7	**Is the rhythm unstable and at risk of deterioration?**	*Potentially. We do not know the cause of the junctional rhythm; as such, we are unable to assess the risk of further deterioration.*
8	**Does the presenting rhythm support or change your working diagnosis?**	*Supports a cardiac cause.*
9	**Are any clinical interventions required?**	*No interventions are required based on this ECG.*

Case Scenario 4.3.5   Answers

a) **What are your differential diagnoses for Marion?** *Differentials should include: gastroenteritis, acute coronary syndrome, pulmonary embolism, internal haemorrhage, stroke.*
b) **Use the 9-step ECG interpretation tool to assess Marion's ECG.**
c) **What rhythm is the ECG?** *Sinus tachycardia with anterior STEMI and RBBB.*
d) **What is your working diagnosis?** *STEMI.*

Discussion: *Marion is presenting with an atypical MI. Her symptoms do not fit with the 'classic' set of symptoms, but she is having an MI nonetheless. We can see significant ST segment elevation in the anterior leads. Cases like this emphasise the importance of having a low threshold for obtaining a 12-lead ECG in patients with undifferentiated presentations, as there is a danger that her symptoms might be diagnosed incorrectly as gastroenteritis due to the vomiting and her recent meal. Missing the diagnosis of STEMI would be likely to have fatal consequences.*

ECG Steps

1	**What is the rate and rhythm?**	*The rate is around 120 beats/minute and the rhythm is regular.*
2	**Are there any P waves and what is their relationship with the QRS complex?**	*There is a P wave before every QRS complex and a QRS complex after every P wave.*
3	**What is the duration and morphology of the QRS complex?**	*The QRS complex is of RBBB morphology and the duration is greater than 0.12 seconds (3 small squares).*
4	**Is the ST segment isoelectric, depressed or elevated?**	*There is ST segment elevation in leads V2–V5, with ST segment depression in leads I, II, aVF and V6.*
5	**Are the QT intervals and T waves normal?**	*The T wave is inverted in leads V1–V2. The QT interval is appropriate for the rate.*

Clinical Steps

6	**Is the heart generating a palpable pulse of appropriate rate and providing adequate perfusion?**	*The rate is appropriate, and the presence of radial pulses suggests adequate perfusion is present. Though Marion's clinical presentation is suggestive of cardiogenic shock.*
7	**Is the rhythm unstable and at risk of deterioration?**	*Yes. This ECG shows active STEMI and is at risk of further cardiac muscle damage or cardiac arrest.*
8	**Does the presenting rhythm support or change your working diagnosis?**	*Supports MI.*
9	**Are any clinical interventions required?**	*Oxygen, IV access and ACS and anti-emetic drugs are indicated for this patient. Rapid transport with pre-alert call to activate local STEMI pathway and cath lab.*

Appendix 1 Obtaining a 12-Lead ECG[1,2]

As with all procedures, when obtaining an ECG it is essential that the process is clearly explained and carried out with the patient's consent. To improve electrical conduction, the skin at the sites of electrode placement must be prepared; this could include drying the skin if wet, shaving hairs, using alcohol wipes on oily skin and exfoliation by gently scraping or abrading to remove any dead skin cells from the skin surface.

Once the electrodes have been applied, connect them to the monitor and follow the specific process given for the model of monitor you are using. Request that the patient stay still and not speak while the monitor is capturing the ECG, as this will create artefact. It may be necessary or appropriate, depending on the clinical situation, to obtain several ECGs. It may also be necessary to leave the electrodes in place so that multiple ECGs can be obtained during the patient care episode and during journey to hospital.

Application of ECG Electrodes for a Standard 12-Lead ECG

Limb electrodes: Apply the four limb electrodes. These can be applied anywhere on each limb, though application closer to the torso (proximal placement) can reduce artefact.

- The right upper limb lead is usually red.
- The left upper limb lead is usually yellow.
- The right lower limb lead is usually black.
- The left lower limb lead is usually green.

Chest leads: The six chest electrodes, V1–V6, are applied in specific locations across the patient's chest (Figure 5.1). All attempts should be made, with both male and female patients, to place the electrodes in the anatomically correct positions.

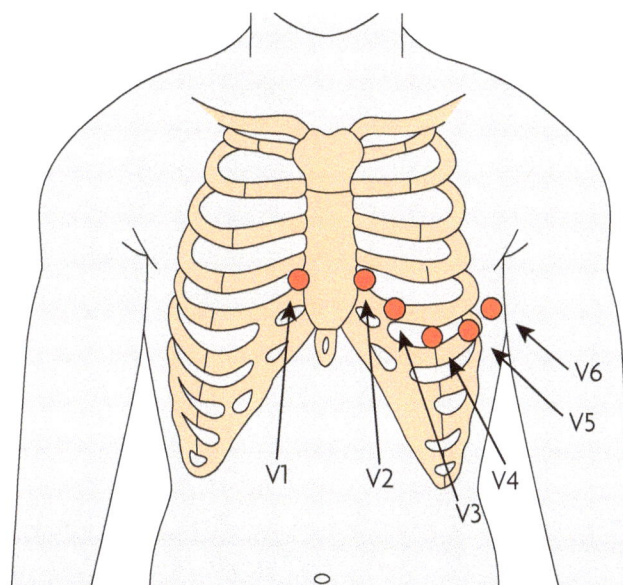

Figures 5.1 Standard 12-lead electrode placement.

■ Place the four limb leads onto the patient's four limbs, using the colour coding detailed above. This can differ by manufacturer.

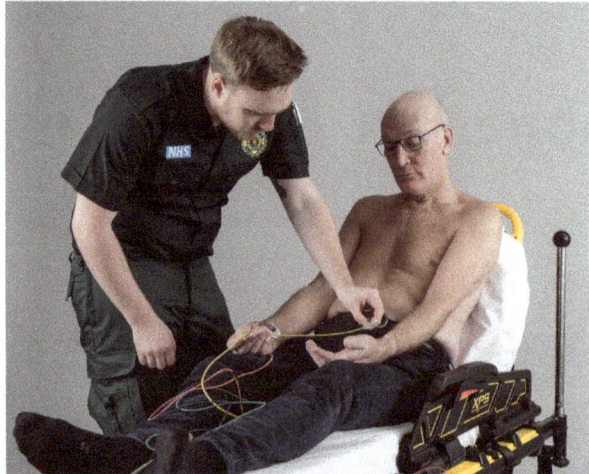

■ V1: Identify the 4th intercostal space by palpating down from the top of the manubrium until you feel a horizontal ridge (angle of Louis) which is the joint between the bottom of the manubrium and the top of the sternum. Palpate down and to the patient's right of the angle of Louis to identify the right 2nd intercostal space. Palpate down two more intercostal spaces to the 4th intercostal space. Electrode V1 is placed in the right 4th intercostal space, next to the sternum.

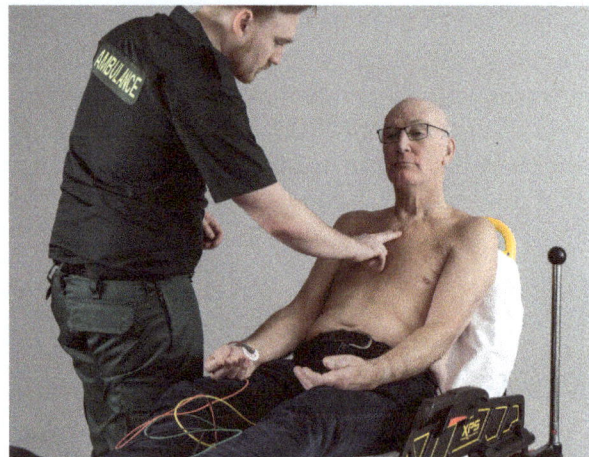

■ V2: From electrode V1, palpate to the patient's left, across the sternum, to identify the left 4th intercostal space. Electrode V2 is placed here next to the sternum, in a mirrored position of electrode V1.

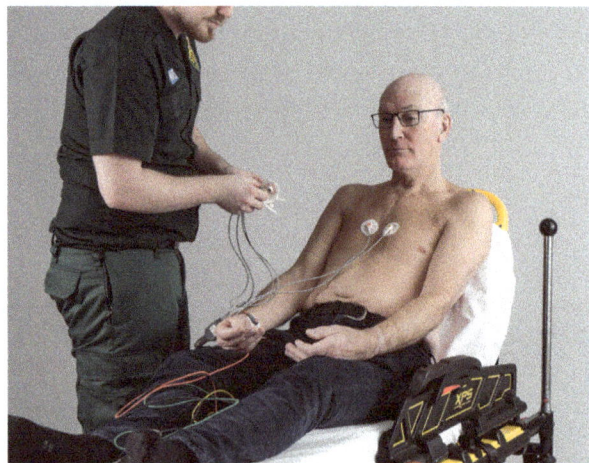

- V4: Palpate down from the 4th intercostal space to identify the 5th intercostal space on the left side of the chest. Place electrode V4 in the 5th intercostal space, in the mid-clavicular line.

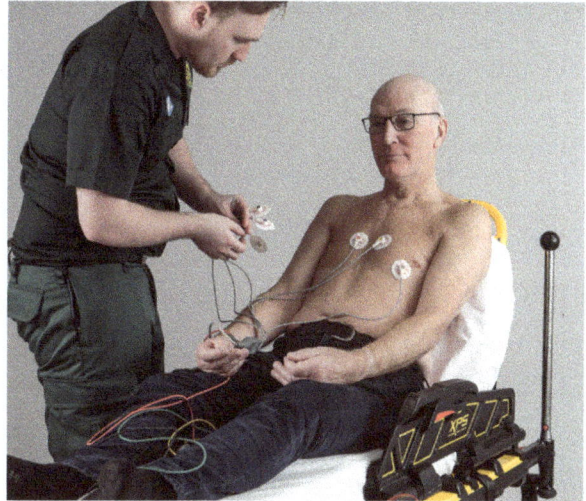

- V3: Electrode V3 is now placed midway between electrodes V2 and V4.

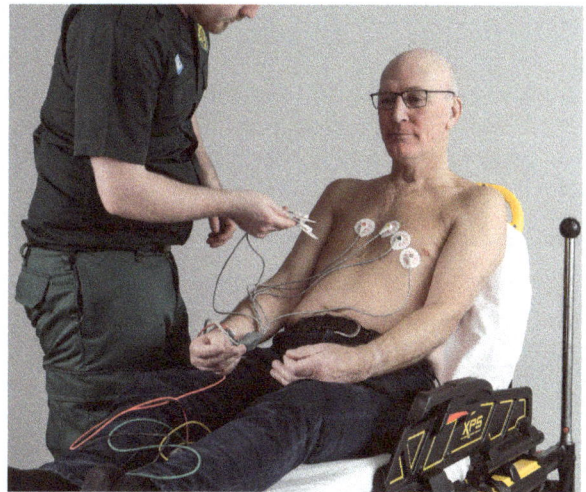

- V6: Palpate laterally from electrode V4 in the 5th intercostal space and place electrode V6 in the mid-axillary line, 5th intercostal space.

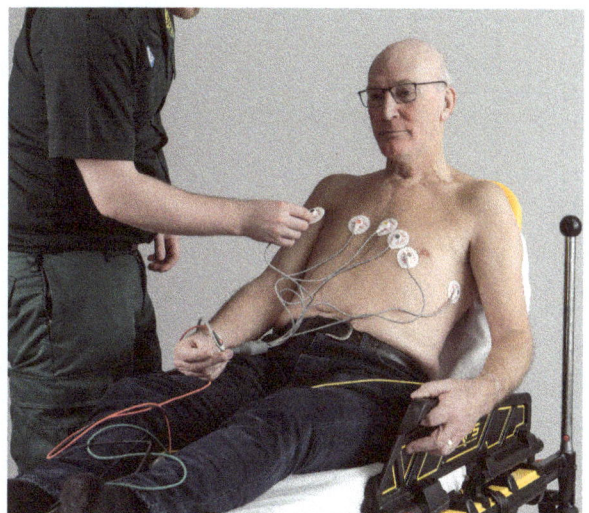

- V5: Electrode V5 is placed between electrodes V4 and V6, in the 5th intercostal space, anterior axillary line.

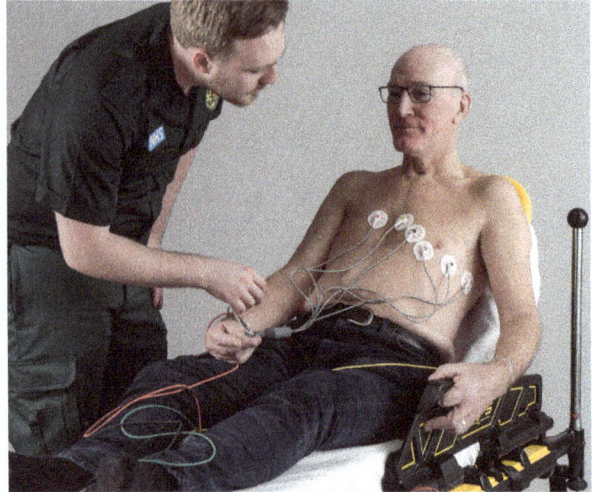

Additional ECG Lead Views Electrode Placement

To obtain additional ECG lead views, some of the electrodes need to be repositioned on the patient's chest. When obtaining additional lead views, new electrode stickers should be used, with the original electrodes remaining in the standard 12-lead ECG positions.

Right-sided ECG

A right-sided ECG is obtained by swapping the precordial electrodes to the opposite side of the chest from their standard positions (Figure 5.2). The lead views they produce now have 'R' added to their

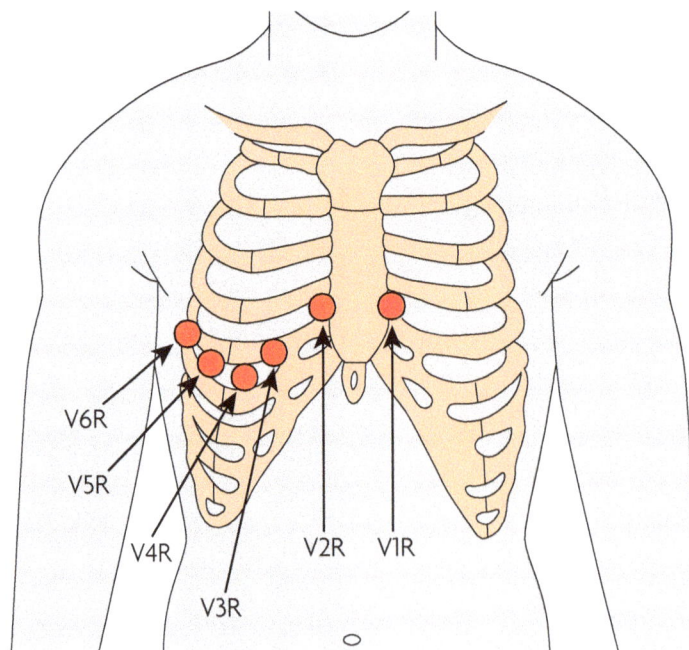

Figure 5.2 Right-sided electrode placement.

title; for example, V4R. A right-sided ECG can consist of all six precordial leads, leads V4R–V6R, or just lead V4R. For the purposes of identifying STEMI in the out-of-hospital environment, it is common to obtain just V4R or V4R, V5R and V6R. The location for electrode V4R is in the 5th intercostal space, mid-clavicular line, on the right side of the patient's chest. V6R is located in the 5th intercostal space, mid-axillary line, also on the right side of the chest. The electrode for V5R should be placed on the right side of the chest, between electrodes V4R and V6R, in the 5th intercostal space, anterior axillary line.

Posterior ECG

A posterior ECG is obtained by repositioning the electrodes of leads V4, V5 and V6 on to the left side of the patient's back, where they become V7 (previously V4), V8 (previously V5) and V9 (previously V6) (Figure 5.3). All three electrodes are placed in the same horizontal plane as electrode V4. The location for electrode V7 is at the posterior axillary line. V8 is placed at the mid-scapular line, and V9 is placed at the spinal border.

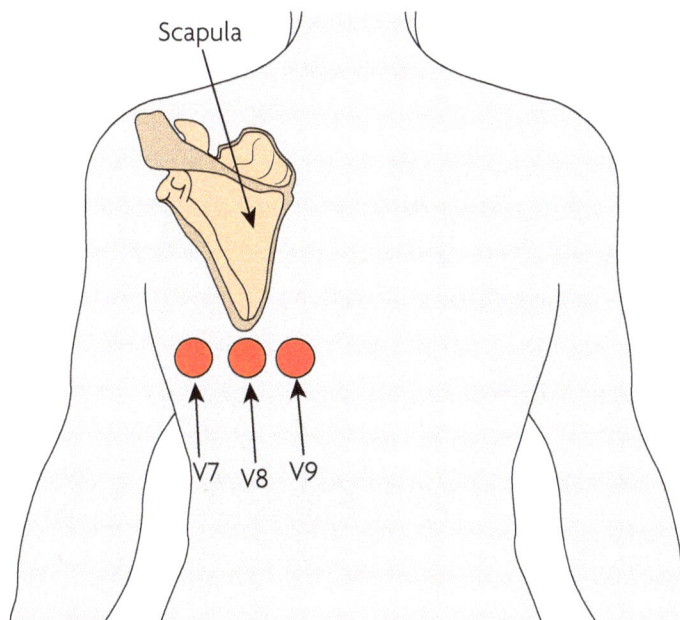

Figure 5.3 Posterior electrode placement.

Two main factors need to be considered when including an ECG as part of the out-of-hospital assessment of a paediatric patient: the age of the patient and the reason for obtaining the ECG. We must consider our reasons for obtaining an ECG in a paediatric patient. The main consideration is if the ECG will have any meaningful influence on the outcome of the patient care episode. Is it going to alter the treatment or transport plan for this child? Often the answer is no. It is likely we will not be equipped with the specialist paediatric knowledge or equipment to safely diagnose and discharge the patient with cardiac symptoms and a normal ECG.

With younger children and infants, the usual reason for obtaining a lead II ECG is either to monitor an accurate electrical heart rate or to assess for life-threatening arrhythmias in unconscious or peri-arrest patients. A significant finding is bradycardia, which in the case of children is mostly likely to be secondary to hypoxia.[3] Bradycardia can also be a sign of physiological decompensation and a warning of potential, imminent, further rapid deterioration, due to either hypoxia or another cause. With older children, the ECG becomes more of a diagnostic aid, in the same way as it functions with adult patients.

Common presentations of paediatric patients that might prompt the obtaining of an ECG include chest pain, syncope, palpitations or shortness of breath. The ECG findings for these patients are often insignificant as the majority are not due to a cardiac cause.[4] We should still seek to obtain an ECG for these presentations when possible, particularly if symptoms such as palpitations are still present, as we may capture a tracing of a transient arrhythmia.

It is also important that we remember children can and do present with illnesses and cardiac problems that are normally associated with adults. For example, although it is comparatively rare, children can present with myocardial infarction. Up to 1% of children who present to the emergency department with chest pain are found to have a cardiac problem and around 15% are found to have an abnormal ECG.[4]

Obtaining a 12-lead ECG in an acutely unwell child could potentially cause delay in critical treatment and transport of the patient. For example, around 11% of ECGs obtained from paediatric patients who have had a seizure are considered to be abnormal,[5] but this would not normally be a relevant finding when managing an acutely unwell child who has had a seizure while in the out-of-hospital environment. While lead II monitoring is most often appropriate to monitor for a tachyarrhythmia or bradyarrhythmia, we need to carefully consider if it is appropriate to potentially delay transport for the time needed to obtain a 12-lead ECG in this situation. The priority in this time-critical situation would be to monitor and manage the patient's ABCs, ensure oxygenation, control further seizures where required and provide rapid transport to an appropriate hospital.[3]

Clinical Conditions and ECG Abnormalities That May Present in Paediatric Patients[6, 7, 8]

- Wolff-Parkinson-White syndrome.
- Long QT syndrome.
- Pericarditis.
- Hyperkalaemia.
- Atrial fibrillation.
- Complete heart block.
- Right bundle branch block.

Findings on a Paediatric ECG That May Be Normal[6, 7, 8]

- Heart rate above 100 beats per minute.
- Sinus arrhythmia (variable p-p interval).
- 1st degree or 2nd degree type 1 AV block.
- Short sinus pauses (under 1.8 seconds).
- Ectopic beats.
- Shortened P wave and PR interval.
- Q waves in inferior and lateral leads II, III, aVF and V5–V6.
- Dominant R waves in leads V1–V3.
- Shortened QRS duration.
- Shortened QT interval.
- T wave inversion in leads V1–V3.

Appendix 6 Human Factors in ECG Interpretation

Gary Rutherford and Charles L. Till

Recording and interpreting an ECG can be considered an example of a technical skill. However, the College of Paramedics highlights how non-technical skills are also required in order to facilitate 'safe, effective and efficient task performance'.[9] Therefore, well-applied non-technical skills will optimise the interpretation of the ECG.

Shippey and Rutherford (2020), state that non-technical skills are an aspect of 'human factors' related to cognitive functions and individual behaviours which are of relevance to paramedic practice.[10] They suggest that non-technical skills such as situation awareness, decision making, teamwork, leadership and communication may be highly applicable as practised by paramedics in the field. Situation awareness and aspects of decision making are of particular relevance to ECG interpretation.

Situation awareness is described as 'the process by which we perceive stimuli (for example visual images), make meaning from those inputs, and then project forward to generate an expectation of what will happen next'.[10] Therefore, if we do not optimally perceive or understand the visual image of the ECG, we may not be able to make the best decision on what to do next. Our situation awareness can be affected by many factors such as tunnel vision, distraction, stress, fatigue, workload, experience and training.[11] The designed layout of the ECG on the screen or paper may also influence our ability to perceive the required information, for example if the lead views are presented in a different layout to the one previously encountered.

Once we have perceived and understood the ECG, we then need to project what is likely to happen next and make a decision on what to do. There are many theories and models of decision making, although the popular belief that we mostly make rational, carefully calculated decisions is likely to be inaccurate. In fact, humans are much more likely to attempt to make a fast, intuitive decision without slowing their thinking down to consider options.[12] This type of rapid decision making is susceptible to error and bias. A bias is a type of subconscious error where judgement has been unduly influenced by other factors.[13] It may be possible, yet difficult, to recognise situations where we should try actively to slow our thinking down, in order to maximise situation awareness and optimal decision making, and minimise the influence of these biases.

Examples of Biases That May Influence Decision Making[10, 13, 14]

Confirmation bias occurs when someone only looks for information (or clinical findings) that supports their initial hypothesis (or potential diagnosis) and dismisses information (or clinical findings) that does not support it. In other words, *keep an open mind* in regard to ECG interpretation and be willing to revise your initial ECG diagnosis should new or unexpected findings arise. Confirmation bias is similar to **anchoring bias**, which occurs when an individual depends too heavily on an initial piece of information to make a judgement or decision and cannot adjust that decision in the light of further information.

Availability bias occurs when recent experiences or memories of making a decision unduly influence the current decision that needs to be made. **Saliency bias** occurs when the decision is overly influenced by a memory of a recent success (such as a correct ECG diagnosis). These two biases may often occur together.

Multiple alternatives bias occurs when decision making becomes more difficult with an availability of multiple choices. People may revert to more simple or basic decisions between two options and disregard others. In ECG interpretation there are always multiple alternatives. Multiple alternative bias can be protected against by adopting a conscious decision to retain an open mind towards ECG interpretation.

Task Focused

When performing a stressful or challenging task, or a task that demands the majority of your attention, you can become so focused that you lose situation awareness and may miss or overlook things that are happening around you. This can occur when studying a 12-lead ECG in clinical practice. While it is important to try to keep one eye on the wider situation and the patient's condition while interpreting the ECG, this will be challenging in practice. A strategy could be to verbalise the risk and ask that a crewmate monitor the patient and alert you to changes because you may become very task focused while interpreting the ECG.

References

1. B. Campbell et al., 'Clinical guidelines by consensus: recording a standard 12-lead electrocardiogram. An approved method by the Society for Cardiological Science and Technology (SCST)', *The Journal of the Society for Cardiological Science and Technology*, vol. 7, no. 8, 2017, 1–25.

2. R. Pilbery and K. Lethbridge, *Ambulance Care Practice*. Bridgwater: Class Publishing, 2019.

3. Joint Royal College Ambulance Liaison Committee and Association of Ambulance Chief Executives, *JRCALC Clinical Guidelines 2019*. Bridgwater: Class Professional Publishing, 2019.

4. S. Gandhi et al., 'Predictors of abnormal electrocardiograms in the pediatric emergency department', *Annals of Pediatric Cardiology*, vol. 11, no. 3, 2018, pp. 255–260.

5. A. G. Pompa et al., 'Utility of ECGs in the pediatric emergency department for patients presenting with a seizure', *American Journal of Emergency Medicine*, vol. 38, no. 7, 2020, pp. 1362–1366.

6. J. S. Jheeta, O. Narayan and T. Krasemann, 'Accuracy in interpreting the paediatric ECG: a UK-wide study and the need for improvement', *Archives of Disease in Childhood*, vol. 99, no. 7, 2014, pp. 646–648.

7. D. F. Dickinson, 'The normal ECG in childhood and adolescence', *Heart*, vol. 91, 2005, pp. 1626–1630.

8. S. Goodacre and K. McLeod, 'Paediatric electrocardiography', *BMJ*, vol. 324, 2002, pp. 1382–1385.

9. The College of Paramedics, *Paramedics Curriculum Guidance*, 4th edn. Bridgwater: College of Paramedics, 2017.

10. B. Shippey and G. Rutherford, 'Situation awareness and decision making', in G. Rutherford, ed., *Human Factors in Paramedic Practice*. Bridgwater, Class Professional Publishing, 2020.

11. M. R. Endsley, 'Towards a theory of situation awareness in dynamic systems', *Human Factors*, vol. 37, no. 1, 1995, pp. 32–64.

12. D. Kahneman, *Thinking, Fast and Slow*, London: Penguin Books, 2012.

13. P. Crosskerry, G. Singahl and S. Mamede, 'Cognitive debiasing 1: origins of bias and theory of debiasing', *BMJ Quality and Safety*, vol. 22, 2013, pp. 58–64.

14. M. Cristofaro, 'Reducing biases of decision-making processes in complex organizations', *Management Research Review*, vol. 40, no. 3, 2017, pp. 270–290.

Index

References to illustrations are in **bold.**

www.ingramcontent.com/pod-product-compliance
Lightning Source LLC
Chambersburg PA
CBHW041153220326
41598CB00045B/7422